ADHD: Non-Pharmacologic Interventions

Editors

STEPHEN V. FARAONE
KEVIN M. ANTSHEL

CHILD AND ADOLESCENT PSYCHIATRIC CLINICS OF NORTH AMERICA

www.childpsych.theclinics.com

Consulting Editor
HARSH K. TRIVEDI

October 2014 • Volume 23 • Number 4

ELSEVIER

1600 John F. Kennedy Boulevard • Suite 1800 • Philadelphia, Pennsylvania, 19103-2899

http://www.theclinics.com

CHILD AND ADOLESCENT PSYCHIATRIC CLINICS OF NORTH AMERICA Volume 23, Number 4
October 2014 ISSN 1056–4993, ISBN-13: 978-0-323-32601-8

Editor: Joanne Husovski
Developmental Editor: Stephanie Carter

Child and Adolescent Psychiatric Clinics of North America (ISSN 1056-4993) is published quarterly by Elsevier Inc., 360 Park Avenue South, New York, NY 10010-1710. Months of issue are January, April, July, and October. Business and Editorial Offices: 1600 John F. Kennedy Boulevard, Suite 1800, Philadelphia, PA 19103-2899. Periodicals postage paid at New York, NY and additional mailing offices. Subscription prices are $310.00 per year (US individuals), $491.00 per year (US institutions), $155.00 per year (US students), $360.00 per year (Canadian individuals), $598.00 per year (Canadian institutions), $200.00 per year (Canadian students), $430.00 per year (international individuals), $598.00 per year (international institutions), and $200.00 per year (international students). International air speed delivery is included in all *Clinics* subscription prices. All prices are subject to change without notice. **POSTMASTER:** Send address changes to *Child and Adolescent Psychiatric Clinics of North America*, Elsevier Health Sciences Division, Subscription Customer Service, 3251 Riverport Lane, Maryland Heights, MO 63043. **Customer Service: 1-800-654-2452 (U.S. and Canada); 314-447-8871 (outside U.S. and Canada). Fax: 314-447-8029. E-mail: JournalsCustomer Service-usa@elsevier.com (for print support) or journalsonlinesupport-usa@elsevier.com (for online support).**

Reprints. For copies of 100 or more of articles in this publication, please contact the Commercial Reprints Department, Elsevier Inc., 360 Park Avenue South, New York, New York 10010-1710 Tel.: 212-633-3874; Fax: 212-633-3820, E-mail: reprints@elsevier.com.

Child and Adolescent Psychiatric Clinics of North America is covered in *MEDLINE/PubMed (Index Medicus), ISI, SSCI, Research Alert, Social Search, Current Contents,* and *EMBASE/Excerpta Medica.*

Contributors

CONSULTING EDITOR

HARSH K. TRIVEDI, MD
Executive Director and Chief Medical Officer, Behavioral Health Vice Chair for Clinical
Affairs; Associate Professor of Psychiatry, Vanderbilt University School of Medicine,
Nashville, Tennessee

CONSULTING EDITOR EMERITUS

ANDRÉS MARTIN, MD, MPH

FOUNDING CONSULTING EDITOR

MELVIN LEWIS, MBBS, FRCPSYCH, DCH

EDITORS

STEPHEN V. FARAONE, PhD
Distinguished Professor of Psychiatry, Departments of Psychiatry and of Neuroscience
and Physiology, SUNY Upstate Medical University, Syracuse, New York

KEVIN M. ANTSHEL, PhD
Director of Clinical Psychology Program; Associate Professor of Psychology, Department
of Psychology, Syracuse University, Syracuse, New York

AUTHORS

KEVIN M. ANTSHEL, PhD
Director of Clinical Psychology Program; Associate Professor of Psychology, Department
of Psychology, Syracuse University, Syracuse, New York

L. EUGENE ARNOLD, MD, M.Ed
Professor Emeritus of Psychiatry, Nisonger Center, The Ohio State University Medical
Center, Columbus, Ohio

OLGA G. BERWID, PhD
Assistant Professor, Psychology Department, York College, The City University of New
York (CUNY), Jamaica, New York

MICHAEL H. BLOCH, MD, MS
Child Study Center, Department of Psychiatry, Yale University, New Haven, Connecticut

DANIEL BRANDEIS, PhD
Department of Child and Adolescent Psychiatry, University of Zürich, Zürich, Switzerland;
Department of Child and Adolescent Psychiatry and Psychotherapy, Central Institute of
Mental Health, Medical Faculty Mannheim, Heidelberg University, Mannheim, Germany

SAMUELE CORTESE, MD, PhD
Consultant Child Psychiatrist, Department of Child Psychiatry, Cambridge University Hospitals NHS Foundation Trust, Cambridge, United Kingdom; Division of Psychiatry, Institute of Mental Health, University of Nottingham, Nottingham, United Kingdom

GEORGE J. DUPAUL, PhD
Professor of School Psychology, Department of Education and Human Services, Lehigh University, Bethlehem, Pennsylvania

THERESA EGAN, MA
Department of Psychology, Center for Intervention Research in Schools, Ohio University, Athens, Ohio

STEVEN W. EVANS, PhD
Professor of Psychology, Department of Psychology, Center for Intervention Research in Schools, Ohio University, Athens, Ohio

GREGORY A. FABIANO, PhD
Department of Counseling, School, and Educational Psychology, University at Buffalo, SUNY, Buffalo, New York

STEPHEN V. FARAONE, PhD
Distinguished Professor of Psychiatry, Departments of Psychiatry and of Neuroscience and Physiology, SUNY Upstate Medical University, Syracuse, New York

MATTHEW J. GORMLEY, MEd
Doctoral Student in School Psychology, Department of Education and Human Services, Lehigh University, Bethlehem, Pennsylvania

LAUREN M. HAACK, PhD
Clinical Psychology Fellow, Department of Psychiatry, University of California, San Francisco, San Francisco, California

JEFFREY M. HALPERIN, PhD
Distinguished Professor, Psychology Department, Queens College and the Graduate Center, The City University of New York (CUNY), Flushing, New York

XINMIN HAN, MD, PhD
Department of Pediatrics of Chinese Medicine, Nanjing University of Traditional Chinese Medicine, Nanjing, China

MARTIN HOLTMANN, MD
LWL-University Hospital for Child and Adolescent Psychiatry, Ruhr University Bochum, Hamm, Germany

KATHLEEN HOLTON, PhD, MPH
Assistant Professor, School of Education, Teaching and Health, Center for Behavioral Neuroscience American University, Washington, DC

ELIZABETH A. HURT, PhD
Postdoctoral Fellow, School of Professional Psychology, Wright State University, Dayton, Ohio

MARY JIA, BSc
Department of Psychology, University of British Columbia, Vancouver, British Colombia, Canada

JOSHUA M. LANGBERG, PhD
Associate Professor of Psychology, Department of Psychology, Virginia Commonwealth University, Richmond, Virginia

SETH D. LARACY, MEd
Doctoral Student in School Psychology, Department of Education and Human Services, Lehigh University, Bethlehem, Pennsylvania

SHUANG LEI, MD, PhD
Department of Pediatrics of Chinese Medicine, Nanjing University of Traditional Chinese Medicine, Nanjing, China

AMORI YEE MIKAMI, PhD
Associate Professor, Department of Psychology, University of British Columbia, Vancouver, British Colombia, Canada

STEPHEN J. MOLITOR, BA
Department of Psychology, Virginia Commonwealth University, Richmond, Virginia

JILIAN MULQUEEN, BA
Child Study Center, Yale University, New Haven, Connecticut

JENNIFER JIWON NA, BSc
Department of Psychology, University of British Columbia, Vancouver, British Colombia, Canada

XINQIANG NI, MD, PhD
Department of Pediatrics of Chinese Medicine, Nanjing University of Traditional Chinese Medicine, Nanjing, China

JOEL T. NIGG, PhD
Professor, Departments of Psychiatry and Behavioral Neurosciencce, Oregon Health & Science University, Portland, Oregon

SARAH O'NEILL, PhD
Assistant Professor, Psychology Department, The City College, The City University of New York (CUNY), New York, New York

AMY K. OLSZEWSKI, MS
Research Associate, Department of Psychology, Syracuse University, Syracuse, New York

WILLIAM E. PELHAM Jr, PhD
Department of Psychology, Florida International University, Miami, Florida

LINDA J. PFIFFNER, PhD
Professor of Psychiatry, University of California, San Francisco; Director, Hyperactivity, Attention and Learning Problems (HALP) Clinic, San Francisco, California

ARTHUR L. ROBIN, PhD
Director of Psychology Training, Child Psychiatry and Psychology Department, Children's Hospital of Michigan; Professor of Psychiatry & Behavioral Neurosciences, Wayne State University School of Medicine, Detroit, Michigan

NICOLE K. SCHATZ, PhD
Department of Counseling, School, and Educational Psychology, University at Buffalo, SUNY, Buffalo, New York

LARRY J. SEIDMAN, PhD
Professor of Psychology, Harvard Medical School Departments of Psychiatry, Beth
Israel Deaconess Medical Center, and Massachusetts General Hospital, Boston,
Massachusetts

TERRI L. SHELTON, PhD
Vice Chancellor for Research and Economic Development; Professor of Psychology,
University of North Carolina at Greensboro, Greensboro, North Carolina

EDMUND SONUGA-BARKE, PhD
Developmental Brain-Behaviour Laboratory, Psychology, Institute for Disorders of
Impulse & Attention, University of Southampton, Southampton, United Kingdom;
Department of Experimental Clinical & Health Psychology, Ghent University, Ghent,
Belgium

JICHAO SUN, MD
Department of Pediatrics of Chinese Medicine, Nanjing University of Traditional Chinese
Medicine, Nanjing, China

AMANDA P. WILLIFORD, PhD
Research Assistant Professor, Center for Advanced Study of Teaching and Learning,
Curry School of Education, University of Virginia, Charlottesville, Virginia

YANLI ZHANG-JAMES, PhD
Department of Psychiatry, SUNY Upstate Medical University, Syracuse, New York

RONGYI ZHOU, MD
Department of Pediatrics of Chinese Medicine, Nanjing University of Traditional Chinese
Medicine, Nanjing, China

Contents

> Children with attention-deficit/hyperactivity disorder (ADHD) experience
> significant difficulties with behavior, social functioning, and academic
> performance in elementary school classrooms. Although psychotropic
> medication may enhance classroom behavior, pharmacologic treatment
> is rarely sufficient in addressing the many challenges encountered by indi-
> viduals with ADHD in school settings. This article describes 3 evidence-
> based strategies including behavioral, academic, and self-regulation
> interventions. Future directions for research on school-based interventions
> are discussed.

> The development and evaluation of psychosocial treatments for adoles-
> cents with attention-deficit/hyperactivity disorder has lagged behind the
> treatment development work conducted with children with the disorder.
> Two middle school–based and high school–based treatment programs
> have the most empirical work indicating beneficial effects. Treatment
> development research addressing many of the basic questions related
> to mediators, moderators, and sequencing of treatments is needed. Impli-
> cations for future treatment development research are reviewed, including
> the potential benefits of combining treatments of a variety of modalities to
> address the large gaps in the literature.

> This article summarizes behavior management strategies for preschool
> children who are at high risk for attention-deficit/hyperactivity disorder
> that have found to be effective in improving child behavior. Both parent
> and teacher training programs are reviewed, as these have been backed
> by substantial research evidence. In addition, multimodal treatments that
> include some combination of parent training, teacher training, and social
> skills training are also reviewed. Interventions emphasize the need for a
> strong adult–child relationship combined with proactive behavior man-
> agement strategies to improve child behavior.

Behavior management treatments are the most commonly used nonpharmacologic approaches for treating attention-deficit/hyperactivity disorder (ADHD) and associated impairments. This review focuses on behavioral parent training interventions for school-age children in the home setting and adjunctive treatments developed to extend effects across settings. Empirical support includes numerous randomized clinical trials, systematic reviews, and meta-analyses showing positive effects of these interventions on child compliance, ADHD symptoms and impairments, parent-child interactions, parenting and parenting stress. These studies support categorization of behavior management treatment as a well-established, evidence-based treatment of ADHD. Factors for consideration in clinical decision making and directions for research are provided.

Adolescents with attention deficit hyperactivity disorder (ADHD) and their parents experience a great deal of conflict and coercion because the executive function deficits of ADHD interact with the parents' characteristics, family stress, and parenting practices. This article provides a step-by-step description of the defiant teen approach to family therapy, which is designed to help adolescents with ADHD and their parents reduce conflict and coercion. The article also summarizes 2 studies supporting the effectiveness of the defiant teen approach.

Interventions with Patients

Children with attention-deficit/hyperactivity disorder (ADHD) require intensive treatments to remediate functional impairments and promote the development of adaptive skills. The summer treatment program (STP) is an exemplar of intensive treatment of ADHD. STP intervention components include a reward and response-cost point system, time-out, use of antecedent control (clear commands, establishment of rules and routines), and liberal praise and rewards for appropriate behavior. Parents also participate in parent management training programming to learn how to implement similar procedures within the home setting. There is strong evidence supporting the efficacy of the STP as an intervention for ADHD.

Children with attention-deficit/hyperactivity disorder (ADHD) have prominent social impairment, which is commonly manifested in unskilled behaviors in social situations and difficulties in being accepted and befriended by peers. This social impairment often remains after administration of medication and behavioral contingency management treatments that address the core symptoms of ADHD. This article reviews traditional social skills training (SST) approaches to remediating social impairment, and presents the evidence for their efficacy and significant limitations to their efficacy. The article introduces potential reasons why the efficacy of traditional SST may be limited, and concludes with some promising alternative SST approaches.

Considerable scientific effort has been directed at developing effective treatments for attention-deficit/hyperactivity disorder (ADHD). Among alternative treatment approaches, neurofeedback has gained some promising empirical support in recent years from controlled studies as a treatment of core ADHD symptoms. However, a recent stringent meta-analysis of 8 randomized controlled trials published in 2013 found that the effects were stronger for unblinded measures and 3 recent subsequently published well-controlled trials found no effects for the most blinded ADHD outcome. Firmer conclusions must await upcoming evidence from larger controlled studies and future meta-analyses contrasting different forms of neurofeedback and different outcome measures.

There has been an increasing interest in and the use of computer-based cognitive training as a treatment of attention-deficit/hyperactivity disorder (ADHD). The authors' review of current evidence, based partly on a stringent meta-analysis of 6 randomized controlled trials (RCTs) published in 2013, and an overview of 8 recently published RCTs highlights the inconsistency of findings between trials and across blinded and nonblinded ADHD measures within trials. Based on this, they conclude that more evidence from well-blinded studies is required before cognitive training can be supported as a frontline treatment of core ADHD symptoms.

Attention deficit/hyperactivity disorder (ADHD) often persists into adolescence and has the same functional impairments as were present during childhood. Medications lessen ADHD symptoms yet do not reliably affect functioning. Thus, there exists a great need for psychosocial treatments in adolescents with ADHD. Nonetheless, relative to the vast literature that has been reported on children with ADHD, much less data have been reported about psychosocial interventions for adolescents with ADHD. Cognitive behavioral therapy interventions that are being used with adolescents rely more on traditional behavioral principles than cognitive therapy tenets.

Stimulants are the primary treatment for ADHD. Psychotherapy may augment pharmacologic treatment. In this article, we discuss strategies psychotherapists may use in working with teenagers and adults, including individuals who reject medications or take them suboptimally. Individuals with ADHD often have other psychiatric issues, including affective or cognitive comorbidities. Having ADHD does not protect people from the difficulties of life, and psychotherapy can help to disentangle "ADHD" from other issues. A psychotherapist knowledgeable about ADHD assessment can improve diagnostic precision. Psychotherapy can integrate forms of treatment in which the central goal is increasing mastery and competence of the individual.

This review covers an introduction of traditional Chinese medicine (TCM) in treating attention-deficit/hyperactivity disorder (ADHD), focusing on the traditional theoretic basis from the perspective of TCM regarding ADHD's cause, pathogenesis, methods of syndrome differentiation, and rationale for treatment. The authors present commonly accepted and successfully practiced clinical procedures used in China for diagnosis and treatment of ADHD by TCM clinicians along with the supportive clinical evidence. The authors hope to inspire more research to better understand the mechanisms underlying the therapies and to promote appropriate incorporation of TCM therapies with Western pharmacologic treatment to better help patients with ADHD.

Diet and Lifestyle Interventions

Polyunsaturated fatty acid supplementation appears to have modest benefit for improving ADHD symptoms. Melatonin appears to be effective in treating chronic insomnia in children with ADHD but appears to have minimal effects in reducing core ADHD symptoms. Many other natural supplements are widely used in the United States despite minimal evidence of efficacy and possible side effects. This review synthesizes and evaluates the scientific evidence regarding the potential efficacy and side effects of natural supplements and herbal remedies for ADHD. We provide clinicians with recommendations regarding their potential use and role in overall ADHD treatment.

Data from animal studies provide convincing evidence that physical exercise enhances brain development and neurobehavioral functioning in areas believed to be impaired in children with attention-deficit/ hyperactivity disorder (ADHD). To a lesser but still compelling extent, results from studies in typically developing children and adults indicate beneficial effects of exercise on many of the neurocognitive functions that have been shown to be impaired in children with ADHD. Together, these data provide a strong rationale for why a program of structured physical exercise might serve as an effective intervention for children with ADHD.

Food elimination diets are defined and the history of their investigation in relation to attention-deficit/hyperactivity disorder (ADHD) is reviewed. After noting that a consensus has emerged that an elimination diet produces a small but reliable aggregate effect, the present review provides updated quantitative estimates of effect size and clinical response rates to elimination diets. It then highlights key issues that require research attention, in particular characterization of dietary responders. Finally, because some children may benefit, clinical guidelines at the present state of knowledge are summarized. It is concluded that updated trials of elimination diets are sorely needed for ADHD.

Dietary and herbal interventions for attention-deficit/hyperactivity disorder (ADHD) have been proposed by practitioners of Western medicine and traditional Chinese medicine. Children who are suspected to have nutritional deficiencies, insufficiencies, and/or food allergies should be evaluated and, if the suspicion is confirmed, treated with supplementation or specific food elimination as part of standard care. Limited research exists on the efficacy and safety of dietary intervention as an adjunct to conventional medication; thus, improvement and side effects should be closely monitored.

We have created an evidence-based guide for clinicians to the relative utility of nonpharmacologic treatments for attention-deficit/hyperactivity disorder (ADHD). This article uses the term evidence-based in the sense applied by the Oxford Center for Evidenced-Based Medicine to help readers understand the degree to which nonpharmacologic treatments are supported by the scientific literature. This article also reviews the magnitude of the treatment effect expressed as the standardized mean difference effect size (also known as Cohen D). It then describes a meta-algorithm to describe how to integrate pharmacologic and nonpharmacologic treatments for ADHD.

CHILD AND ADOLESCENT PSYCHIATRIC CLINICS

FORTHCOMING ISSUES

Top Topics in Child & Adolescent Psychiatry
Harsh K. Trivedi, *Editor*

School Mental Health
Margaret Benningfield and
Sharon Stephan, *Editors*

Global Mental Health
Paramjit Joshi, *Editor*

Family Based Treatment in Child Psychiatry
Thomas Roesler and Michelle Rickerby,
Editors

RECENT ISSUES

July 2014
Alternative and Complementary Therapies for Children with Psychiatric Disorders, Part 2
Deborah R. Simkin and Charles W. Popper,
Editors

April 2014
Disaster and Trauma
Stephen J. Cozza, Judith A. Cohen, and
Joseph G. Dougherty, *Editors*

January 2014
Acute Management of Autism Spectrum Disorders
Matthew Siegel and Bryan H. King, *Editors*

October 2013
Psychosis in Youth
Jean A. Frazier and Yael Dvir, *Editors*

RELATED INTEREST

Molecular Genetics of Attention Deficit Hyperactivity Disorder
Stephen V. Faraone and Eric Mick, *Authors*
in
Psychiatric Clinics of North America, March 2010 (Vol. 33, No. 1, Pages 159–180)
Psychiatric Genetics
James B. Potash, *Editor*

DOWNLOAD Free App!

Review Articles
THE CLINICS

NOW AVAILABLE FOR YOUR iPhone and iPad

Preface

ADHD: Non-Pharmacologic Interventions

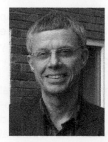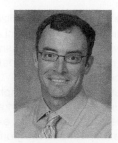

Stephen V. Faraone, PhD   Kevin M. Antshel, PhD
Editors

Welcome to the Nonpharmacologic Interventions for ADHD issue of the *Child and Adolescent Psychiatric Clinics of North America*. We hope that you find this issue to be a useful compendium on the current state-of-the-art nonpharmacologic interventions that clarify their evidence base for managing ADHD in children and adolescents.

While pharmacological interventions are an evidence-based intervention for ADHD treatment, we elected to focus on the nonpharmacologic interventions for several reasons. First and foremost, ADHD is a very public and popular topic in print, on television, and on the Internet. Opinions and various folk remedies abound about nonpharmacologic treatment of ADHD. While increased access to information is indeed positive, not all of the information that is published is accurate. In an attempt to help clinicians better guide the families with whom they treat, in this issue, we assembled the leading ADHD intervention researchers in the world to provide current information on the application of nonpharmacologic interventions.

In the past decade, new nonpharmacologic interventions have been developed, such as working memory, intensive school-based interventions for adolescents, and neurofeedback training, and much more research on older treatments (eg, dietary modifications) has been published. We aim to help the clinician to decipher the literature base in an attempt to make informed decisions and recommendations for the families that they treat.

Several of the most well-researched nonpharmacologic interventions, such as behavioral parent training (Dr Pfiffner's group) and school-based contingency management interventions (Dr DuPaul's group), will be familiar to clinicians who have treated children with ADHD. These nonpharmacologic interventions have been employed for 30+ years with children with ADHD. More preschool children are being diagnosed with ADHD than in the past; thus, we included an article on ADHD management in preschool children (Dr Shelton's group). These authors have synthesized volumes of research to provide expert clinical direction advice about the implementation of these nonpharmacologic treatments.

Child Adolesc Psychiatric Clin N Am 23 (2014) xiii–xiv
http://dx.doi.org/10.1016/j.chc.2014.06.004
1056-4993/14/$ – see front matter © 2014 Elsevier Inc. All rights reserved.

childpsych.theclinics.com

Intensive multimodal programs also represent an important evidence-based non-pharmacologic intervention for managing ADHD. Summer treatment programs (Dr Fabiano and his group) and school-based interventions for middle- and high-school students (Dr Evans and his group) have demonstrated effectiveness for managing ADHD. These are comprehensive and intensive interventions. These authors explain how to divide treatment subcomponents to target functional domains in a manner that should be quite useful for clinicians.

Traditional clinic-based interventions continue to be utilized in ADHD. Articles on psychotherapy (Dr Seidman), social skills training (Dr Mikami and her group), cognitive behavioral therapy for adolescents with ADHD (Dr Antshel), and family therapy (Dr Robin) are also included to provide readers with an updated description of the interventions and the supporting evidence base.

Readers will also benefit from several articles on nonpharmacologic, biological treatments. Articles on computer training (Dr Sonuga-Barke and his group), neurofeedback (Dr Holtmann), dietary supplements (Dr Bloch), exercise (Dr Halperin and his group), traditional Chinese medicine (Dr Han and his group), herbal and nutritional products (Dr Arnold and his group), and restriction and exclusion dietary treatments (Dr Nigg and his group) are also included. Each group has provided a thoughtful and comprehensive review that hopefully can provide valuable insights to clinicians.

We wish to commend the authors for their strong and appreciated contributions to this issue. We are grateful to our authors for not only sharing their vast knowledge base but also providing clinical insights to the readers of *Child and Adolescent Psychiatric Clinics of North America*. To help the readers of these articles, the authors adhered to a specific article structure designed to describe the nonpharmacologic intervention, both theoretically and practically, as well as to provide clinically useful information regarding who is most likely to respond and which outcomes are most likely to be affected by treatment. Likewise, authors included information on adverse effects/contraindications of the nonpharmacologic treatments and how treatments should be sequenced and/or integrated with other treatments. Our fundamental goal was to have authors translate science into clinical practice that can be easily digested and applied. The resulting issue strikes the right balance between reviewing the evidence base and providing clinically useful information.

Finally, we wish to sincerely thank Joanne Husovski at Elsevier for her patience, guidance, and assistance as we worked with authors to make this issue as accurate, up-to-date, and clinically useful as possible. Her optimistic approach, patience, and attention to detail were quite valuable to us both.

Stephen V. Faraone, PhD
Departments of Psychiatry and
Neuroscience and Physiology
SUNY Upstate Medical University
750 East Adams Street
Syracuse, NY, 13210, USA

Kevin M. Antshel, PhD
Department of Psychology
Syracuse University
802 University Avenue, Syracuse, NY 13244, USA

E-mail addresses:
sfaraone@childpsychresearch.org (S.V. Faraone)
kmantshe@syr.edu (K.M. Antshel)

School-Based Interventions for Elementary School Students with ADHD

George J. DuPaul, PhD*, Matthew J. Gormley, MEd,
Seth D. Laracy, MEd

KEYWORDS

- Attention-deficit/hyperactivity disorder • Elementary school • Behavioral intervention
- Academic intervention • Self-regulation intervention

KEY POINTS

- Children with attention-deficit/hyperactivity disorder experience significant behavioral, academic, and social difficulties in elementary school classrooms.
- Although stimulant and other medications can reduce symptoms, these are rarely sufficient in comprehensively addressing school functioning.
- Teachers and other school personnel can implement behavioral, academic, and self-regulation interventions to directly target symptoms and associated impairment.
- Empiric evidence supporting classroom interventions is relatively strong, particularly for behavioral treatment.

INTRODUCTION/BACKGROUND

Children with attention-deficit/hyperactivity disorder (ADHD) frequently experience significant difficulties in school settings. This should not be surprising given that the *Diagnostic and Statistical Manual of Mental Disorders* (Fifth Edition) (*DSM-5*) criteria for this disorder require symptoms to be associated with impairment in academic and/or social functioning.[1] There are at least 3 areas that must be targeted by

Disclosure Statement: G.J. DuPaul receives author royalties from the American Psychological Association, Brookes Publishing Company, and Guilford Press for books and videos related to attention-deficit/hyperactivity disorder. M.J. Gormley and S.D. Laracy report no actual or potential conflicts of interest.
Department of Education and Human Services, Lehigh University, 111 Research Drive, Bethlehem, PA 18015, USA
* Corresponding author.
E-mail address: gjd3@lehigh.edu

Child Adolesc Psychiatric Clin N Am 23 (2014) 687–697
http://dx.doi.org/10.1016/j.chc.2014.05.003 **childpsych.theclinics.com**

Abbreviations	
ADHD	Attention-deficit/hyperactivity disorder
CAI	Computer-assisted instruction
CWPT	Classwide peer tutoring
DRC	Daily report card
OCEBM	Oxford Centre for Evidence-Based Medicine

school-based interventions. First, the symptomatic behaviors (ie, inattention and hyperactivity/impulsivity) comprising ADHD can significantly disrupt classroom activities to a degree that deleteriously affects the learning of all children, not just those with ADHD. Thus, the reduction of disruptive, off-task behavior is an important goal for treatment. Second, symptomatic behaviors also negatively impact children's interactions with peers, teachers, and other school professionals. A common goal for school-based treatment is increased positive social interactions with concomitant reduction in verbal and physical aggression. Third, inattentive and hyperactive–impulsive behaviors frequently compromise learning and academic achievement. Thus, the success of school-based interventions is judged not only on reduction of disruptive, off-task behavior, but also with respect to improvement in the completion and accuracy of academic work.

The need for treatment of ADHD in school settings is clear from both theoretical and empiric perspectives. From a theoretical or conceptual standpoint, it would be hard to design a more problematic setting for individuals with ADHD than the typical elementary school classroom. Students are expected to sit still, listen to academic instruction, follow multistep directions, complete independent work, wait their turn, and behave appropriately with peers and teachers. In particular, they are expected to delay responding and think before acting. These requirements are exceptionally challenging for students with ADHD given underlying difficulties in delaying their response to the environment,[2] motivation,[3] and executive functioning.[4] Thus, it is not surprising that children with ADHD experience significantly lower standardized achievement scores and school grades and higher rates of grade retention and school dropout compared with their same-aged peers.[5] In fact, one of the most ubiquitous and problematic long-term outcomes associated with ADHD is educational underachievement.[6]

The purpose of this article is to describe and review the empiric evidence supporting the use of treatment strategies to address ADHD symptoms and associated impairment in elementary classroom settings. A guide to clinical decision making is provided, and the authors discuss future directions for research and practice in this area.

INTERVENTIONS

Three broad types of intervention have been used to address symptoms and impairment exhibited by elementary school students with ADHD, including behavioral, academic, and self-regulation strategies. Theoretical context, description, and empiric support are described separately for each intervention approach.

Behavioral Interventions

Theoretical overview
Behavioral interventions aim to replace socially undesirable behavior (eg, calling out) with socially appropriate behavior (eg, working quietly). From the behavioral perspective, each behavior must be understood in the context of its antecedents and

consequences.[7] More specifically, behavior is theorized to serve one of 4 main functions: (1) escape or avoidance of a nonpreferred activity or setting, (2) gain attention, (3) gain access to materials or preferred settings, or (4) sensory stimulation.[8] Proactive behavioral interventions target the antecedents of disruptive behaviors, making students less likely to engage in such behaviors (eg, reviewing classroom expectations). Conversely, reactive behavioral interventions target the consequences of a given behavior, reinforcing desirable behavior and ignoring or punishing interfering behaviors (eg, verbal reprimand for calling out). Successful interventions are those that facilitate the function (eg, attention) of the student's interfering behavior (eg, calling out) by reinforcing a socially appropriate replacement behavior (eg, raising his or her hand[5]).

Description

Proactive strategies The use of cues and prompts has been found to increase compliance with desired behavior.[9] By providing students with age-appropriate, nonequivocal rules regarding classroom expectations, teachers can improve classroom behavior.[10] There are several basic strategies that have been found to help maintain positive classroom behavior for students with ADHD:

  Remind students of classroom rules throughout the day and publically praise students for appropriate behavior
  Maintain appropriate eye contact with students
  Remind students of behavioral expectations prior to the start of a new activity
  Actively monitor students by moving throughout the classroom
  Use nonverbal cues to redirect behavior
  Maintain appropriate pacing for classroom activities
  Provide a clear schedule of activities[5]

Teacher attention

Differential teacher attention has also been found effective for students with ADHD.[11] Teachers should catch their students being good and provide positive attention for the socially desirable behavior. Praise should occur immediately following the desired behavior and should be specific in nature (eg, "James, you're doing a great job completing your worksheet!"). Additionally, teachers can extinguish minor disruptive behaviors (eg, tapping a pencil) through ignoring. It should be noted, however, that ignoring minor behaviors may sometimes lead to more intrusive behaviors (eg, calling out), because students are not gaining the attention that they desire and have not been provided a socially acceptable replacement.[8] Conversely, evidence also suggests that teacher reprimands can be effective in reducing interfering behaviors.[12] Redirections should be brief and specific and should be consistently delivered immediately following the negative behavior in a calm and quiet manner.

Token reinforcement/response–cost

Token reinforcement is a reactive strategy that provides students an immediate reinforcer (eg, a sticker) for achieving a specific behavioral expectation (eg, completing a worksheet). These initial reinforcers or tokens are exchanged for back-up reinforcers (eg, additional computer time) later in the day or at the end of the week.[8] Token reinforcement programs are particularly helpful for students with ADHD who often require immediate feedback and reward in order to change behavior. Further, token reinforcement offers valuable flexibility as the criteria to earn both immediate and back-up reinforcers can be made increasingly stringent to help elicit longer periods or higher levels of appropriate behavior.

Response–cost systems are conceptually similar to token reinforcement interventions; however, within a response–cost system, students begin with access to their reward (eg, 10 minutes of computer time) and are fined for each occurrence of undesirable classroom behavior or interval in which behavioral expectations were not met.[8] Although both token reinforcement and response–cost have been demonstrated as effective in improving classroom behavior, their combination generally leads to greater efficacy, enhanced maintenance, and higher ratings of acceptability.[13,14] In fact, in analog classroom settings, the combination of response–cost and token reinforcement has produced behavioral gains greater than those observed with stimulant medication.[15]

Daily report cards

There are many different forms of DRCs; however, they are designed to improve student behavior through frequent feedback to students regarding their behavior and regular communication between school and home.[16,17] Further, the DRC allows for both proactive (eg, review of behavioral expectation) and positive reactive (eg, earning reinforcers) strategies.[18] Specifically, DRCs consist of a list of clearly defined target behaviors (eg, leaves work area fewer than 3 times) and a mechanism to rate the target behavior (eg, frequency, percentage, and/or duration) across multiple periods of the day (eg, class periods[18]). Ideally, students provide the DRC to their parents, who then provide a predetermined reward (eg, time to play video games) if students met the behavioral requirements. This type of home reward DRC method has been shown to be effective for students with ADHD, with additional evidence suggesting programs that link school and home are more effective relative to those that are only implemented at school.[17,19] In cases in which parents may be unable or unwilling to participate in the DRC intervention, the teacher could administer the reinforcement to the student as in the case of a token reinforcement system.

Empiric support

The empiric support for classroom behavioral interventions for elementary students with ADHD has been well documented across single-subject research,[20] group research,[15] systematic literature reviews,[17] and meta-analyses.[21] Results of systematic literature reviews and meta-analyses have indicated that behavioral classroom management techniques meet the requirements for consideration as a well-established treatment. Using Oxford Centre for Evidence-Based Medicine (OCEBM) criteria, classroom behavioral interventions for elementary students with ADHD are a level 1 intervention.

Academic Interventions

Theoretical overview

In contrast to behavioral and self-regulation interventions that target ADHD symptoms, academic intervention strategies are directed at functional impairment associated with symptoms. Specifically, these interventions aim to enhance reading and math skill development as well as performance on academic tasks. Although behavioral and self-regulation interventions are effective in improving student attention and reducing disruptive behavior, changes to ADHD symptoms alone do not necessarily lead to concomitant gains in academic skill acquisition and achievement.[21] Further, based on studies available to date, treatment approaches directed at presumed underlying cognitive deficits (eg, working memory) have not been found to significantly impact academic achievement.[22] Thus, interventions must directly target the specific academic skills that are impaired for a given student with ADHD.

Description
Interventions to address academic skill acquisition and performance difficulties associated with ADHD can include explicit instruction, computer-assisted instruction, and peer tutoring. The most effective way to address academic underachievement is for teachers to use principles of explicit instruction when working with students. Explicit instruction is a direct approach to teaching that involves

Providing clear information to students about what is to be learned
Instructing skills in small steps using concrete, multiple examples
Continuously assessing student understanding
Supporting active student participation that ensures success[23]

A critical attribute of explicit teaching is the use of instructional momentum that involves lesson pacing (eg, using a predictable lesson process that includes varied instructional activities) and managing instructional transitions (eg, giving clear directions for transitions).[24] Explicit instruction is comprised of 5 major components including daily review and prerequisite skill check, teaching of new content, guided practice, independent practice, and weekly/monthly review of skill attainment.[25]

From a conceptual standpoint, computer-assisted instructional (CAI) programs have great potential to capture the attention and increase the motivation of students with ADHD.[5] Specifically, CAI programs typically include clear goals and objectives, highlight important material, simplify tasks, provide both immediate error correction and feedback regarding accuracy, and many also use an engaging, game-like format. Students with ADHD would presumably be more attentive to these types of teaching methods than to lectures or individual written assignments. Several controlled case studies suggest that these methods are helpful for at least some students with ADHD[26] and may be considered as an adjunct to other academic or behavioral interventions.

Similar to CAI, peer tutoring is an intervention strategy that directly addresses the needs of students with ADHD by providing immediate, frequent performance feedback and allows for active responding at the student's pace.[5] Peer tutoring involves students working in pairs and helping each other practice academic skills, typically reading, math, and spelling. The most prominent and widely studied peer tutoring program is class-wide peer tutoring (CWPT[27]) in which all students are paired for tutoring with a classmate. Students are first trained in the rules and procedures for tutoring their classmates in an academic area (eg, math, spelling, reading). The tutor reads a script (eg, math problems) to the student and awards points for correct responses. The tutor corrects erroneous responses, and the student can practice the correct response for an additional point. The script (problem list) is read as many times as possible for 10 minutes, and then the students switch roles. While students are engaged in tutoring, the teacher monitors the tutoring process and provides assistance if needed. Bonus points are awarded to pairs following all of the rules. At the end of the session, points are totaled, and those with the most points are declared the winners.

Empiric support
Relative to extensive empiric support for classroom behavioral interventions, more limited evidence is available with respect to academic intervention for students with ADHD. For example, the effects of explicit instruction on academic achievement have not been specifically studied with students with ADHD; however, there is ample empiric support for this approach for children with emotional and behavioral disorders.[25] Further, the principles underlying the explicit instruction approach have a long history of support in the behavior analytic research literature. As noted previously,

several controlled case studies have demonstrated behavioral and academic improvements associated with CAI for students with ADHD.[26] More extensive evidence is available for peer tutoring. Studies have found CWPT to enhance the on-task behavior and academic performance of unmedicated students with ADHD in general education classrooms.[28] A meta-analysis of 26 single-case research design studies including over 900 students from the general school population (including those with and without disabilities) found moderate-to-large effects of peer tutoring on academic achievement.[29] Peer tutoring effects were consistently strong across dosage (ie, duration, intensity, and number of sessions), grade level, and disability status. Of particular relevance for the use of this strategy with students with ADHD, the strongest effects were found for youth with emotional and behavioral disorders relative to other disability groups. Finally, a recent meta-analysis of school-based intervention for ADHD studies indicated moderate-to-large effects of academic interventions on reading and math outcomes, primarily in the context of within-subject and single-subject design studies.[21] It is noteworthy that academic interventions were also associated with moderate effects on behavioral outcomes, suggesting that treatment targeting academic impairment may also improve ADHD symptoms. Using OCEBM criteria, academic interventions for elementary students with ADHD are a level 1 intervention.

Self-Regulation Interventions

Theoretical overview
Self-regulation interventions aim to improve students' ability to exert increased self-control in environments in which they are experiencing some functional impairment. Such interventions typically include teaching students to identify and record a target response, possibly with reinforcement for improved performance or accurate recording.[30] These interventions are a good conceptual fit for treating ADHD, as they target skills that may be affected by key deficits underlying the disorder. Children with ADHD have demonstrated reduced brain activity associated with cognitive control and error detection.[31] These findings support the theory that the core deficit associated with ADHD is related to response inhibition, which in turn leads to the difficulties with self-control and executive functioning that ultimately manifest as inattention and impulsivity.[2] These core skills in cognitive control and executive functioning are directly targeted by self-regulation interventions.

Description
Self-monitoring interventions begin by teaching students to consistently identify target behaviors and to record some measure of these behaviors. Beyond this common component, research on self-regulation supports a variety of techniques depending on the needs and goals of a particular student. Choosing the most appropriate self-regulation intervention for a student requires making several decisions.

First, a target behavior must be selected. Students diagnosed with ADHD are most commonly taught to recognize and record attention to assigned tasks or some component of academic performance, such as the number of math problems completed. One study has indicated that targeting on-task behavior and academic performance leads to similar gains in attention, but that greater gains in academic performance are associated with monitoring attention.[32] Still, self-regulation interventions targeting both attention and academic performance have received empiric support.[30]

Next, a recording method must be selected. One common method is to create a paper form on which students can record data related to the target behavior. Electronic devices may also be used to facilitate recording.[33] A recording schedule (eg, every

3 minutes) and a method of providing a prompt (eg, an unobtrusive electronic device) should be selected. The recording method can be used throughout the school day or may be limited to classes in which the student is showing the most impairment.

Next, a practitioner must decide whether to evaluate the accuracy of a student's self-monitoring. Another individual, typically the teacher, may be asked to collect data in the same manner as the student, and the agreement between student and teacher is calculated. Although self-regulation interventions have demonstrated efficacy without any checks on accuracy,[30] providing students with feedback about accuracy may help to develop stronger self-monitoring skills.

Finally, a decision must be made regarding reinforcement. A range of different reinforcement structures has been supported by research.[30] First, self-regulation strategies may be implemented with no contingent reinforcement. Alternatively, reinforcement may be provided for either reaching a target level of performance or achieving a desired level of agreement with a teacher's ratings. Reinforcement is typically provided by the teacher and may be implemented as part of an ongoing system, such as a token economy. Students who are motivated and able to accurately monitor their own behavior may also be trained to provide reinforcers to themselves when performance goals are met.

Empiric support

Several studies employing single-case designs have examined the effects of self-regulation interventions on students diagnosed with ADHD. Reid and colleagues[30] reviewed 16 studies that provided self-regulation interventions to 51 students displaying symptoms associated with ADHD. Self-regulation interventions were associated with effect sizes of 0.6 or greater for 70% of dependent variables included in these studies (eg, increasing on-task behavior, decreasing disruptive behavior, and, importantly, improving academic productivity and accuracy). Similar findings of moderate effects on both behavioral and academic outcomes were found in a meta-analysis of school-based interventions for students with ADHD.[21] Despite the promising results from primarily single-case design studies, self-regulation interventions have yet to be examined using randomized controlled group designs. Using OCEBM criteria, self-regulation interventions for elementary students with ADHD are a level 1 intervention.

CLINICAL DECISION MAKING

The extant literature does not offer strong empiric evidence indicating moderators of treatments for ADHD or contraindications and adverse effects for behavioral treatments. For example, none of the investigated child or family characteristics in the Mulitmodal Treatment Algorithm Study of Children with ADHD (eg, prior medication, conduct problems, anxiety, intelligence, ADHD symptom severity, public assistance, parental depression, or maternal education) were related to response to behavioral treatment.[34] The exclusive use of single-subject research to investigate self-regulation intervention precludes strong conclusions about moderators of treatment effect for these strategies. Still, research has indicated that initially targeting academic behaviors may be most appropriate for students with ADHD and academic difficulties, as improvements in academics may also help improve behavior.[5] Behavioral interventions may be successful in reducing symptoms of ADHD and may be implemented before, after, or in combination with medication. Some evidence suggests that medication or a combination of medication and behavioral treatment may produce the greatest reduction in ADHD symptoms,[35] although behavioral treatment alone shows comparable efficacy to medication or combination treatment among children who display significant anxiety symptoms.[36] Still, given the strong empiric support for the efficacy of both medication and the behavioral, academic, and self-regulatory interventions discussed in this article, considerable weight should be given to the acceptability and feasibility of potential interventions to parents and other stakeholders.

FUTURE DIRECTIONS

Recent epidemiologic evidence indicates that parent-reported prevalence of ADHD has increased by 42% over the last 8 years, with the median age of diagnosis occurring at age 6, indicating an increasing need for service delivery in elementary school.[37] To meet this growing need, there are at least 4 areas for additional research on school-based interventions.

First, given that schools are primarily tasked with educating students, the efficacy of any intervention must be measured in relation to its ability to improve the academic outcomes of students with ADHD. School-based interventions should include specific programming to enhance academic outcomes for students with ADHD. Alternatively, researchers could report the impact of the intervention on the teacher's time spent in instruction. More specifically, the extent to which implementing the intervention procedure (eg, token economy) increases time instructing relative to typical procedures (eg, reprimands) may be a valuable metric for classroom interventions.

Second, future research should seek to identify the relative efficacy of varying dosages (eg, low, medium, high) of interventions across demographic and contextual variables (eg, socioeconomic status, ethnicity, educational placement). Such information is critical for practitioners to select not only evidence-based interventions, but also the intervention with the greatest opportunity for success for a given student in a particular context.

Third, future work needs to investigate the acceptability of, and, ultimately, how to increase the utilization of evidence-based interventions in classrooms. Researchers need to work with practitioners to modify existing interventions to increase usage. Alternatively, translational or participatory action research methodologies could be used to develop interventions to meet the academic, behavioral, and social needs of students while accounting for possible constraints (eg, limited resources) in classrooms.

Finally, given that ADHD is a chronic disorder, the needs of elementary students will likely persist across grade-level and school-level transitions. Research should investigate how best to provide continuous care to students from the time they enter kindergarten through their transition into middle school. Thus, clinicians must work with teachers and other school personnel (eg, counselors) to implement behavioral, academic, and self-regulation interventions.

SUMMARY

Although pharmacologic treatment (primarily stimulant medication) is effective in reducing ADHD symptoms, effects are rarely sufficient in addressing the many academic and social difficulties experienced by children with ADHD.[15,34] Thus, psychosocial and educational interventions should be used not only to improve symptomatic behaviors (ie, inattention and hyperactivity/impulsivity) but also directly address associated impairment in social and/or academic functioning (**Box 1**). Clinicians should work with teachers and school personnel (eg, counselors) to implement behavioral, academic, and/or self-regulation interventions throughout and across school years. Behavioral interventions will include some combination of proactive strategies (ie, manipulation of antecedent events), teacher attention contingent on appropriate

---

Box 1
Interventions for elementary school students with ADHD

Recommendations for clinicians

1. Classroom interventions should target both symptomatic behaviors and associated impairment in social and/or academic functioning.

2. Clinicians should consult with teachers and other school personnel (eg, counselors) to support implementation of evidence-based treatment strategies.

3. Behavioral interventions have the strongest research support and include proactive strategies (eg, systematic teaching of classroom rules), teacher attention contingent on appropriate behavior, token reinforcement and response cost systems, and DRCs.

4. Interventions that directly target academic skill acquisition and performance should be used, including explicit instruction, CAI, and peer tutoring.

5. Self-regulation strategies can supplement and extend behavioral interventions by training children to monitor, evaluate, and/or reinforce their own behavior.

---

behavior, token reinforcement and response–cost systems, and DRCs. Evidence supporting the use of behavioral interventions in elementary school classrooms is strong (OCEBM level 1), owing to multiple single-subject design and randomized controlled trial studies as well as several systematic reviews and meta-analyses.[17,21] Academic interventions directly target achievement difficulties and involve strategies such as explicit instruction, CAI, and peer tutoring. The level of evidence for academic interventions is not as strong as for behavioral treatment; however, it is still at OCEBM level 1 given multiple single-subject design, at least 1 randomized controlled trial,[38] and 2 meta-analyses.[21] Finally, self-regulation interventions are designed to change symptoms and associated impairment by assisting children in monitoring, evaluating, and/or reinforcing their own behavior. These interventions may be particularly helpful in weaning children off of externally controlled reinforcement systems and enhancing the probability that behavior gains will generalize across settings and time. Again, the level of evidence, while not as strong as for behavioral interventions, is at OCEBM level 1 given multiple single-subject design studies as well as at least 1 systematic[30] and meta-analytic[21] review. Randomized controlled trials of these and other classroom interventions are necessary to further explicate strategies that can be used within and across academic years to comprehensively address the many chronic and debilitating challenges students with ADHD face in school settings.

REFERENCES

1. American Psychiatric Association. Diagnostic and statistical manual of mental disorders. 5th edition. Washington, DC: American Psychiatric Press; 2013.
2. Barkley RA. ADHD and the nature of self-control. New York: Guilford Press; 2006.
3. Haenlein M, Caul W. Attention deficit disorder with hyperactivity: a specific hypothesis of reward dysfunction. J Am Acad Child Adolesc Psychiatry 1987;26:356–62.
4. Brown TL. A new understanding of ADHD in children and adults: executive function impairments. New York: Routledge; 2013.
5. DuPaul GJ, Stoner G. ADHD in the schools: assessment and intervention strategies. 3rd edition. New York: Guilford; 2014.
6. Barkley RA. Attention-deficit/hyperactivity disorder: a handbook for diagnosis and treatment. 4th edition. New York: Guilford Press; 2014.

7. O'Neill R, Horner RH, Albin RW, et al. Functional assessment for problem behaviors: a practical handbook. 2nd edition. Pacific Grove (CA): Brooks/Cole; 1997.

8. Cooper JO, Heron TE, Heward WL. Applied behavior analysis. 2nd edition. Upper Saddle River (NJ): Pearson; 2007.

9. Sulzer-Azaroff B, Mayer GR. Behavior analysis for lasting change. Fort Worth (TX): Holt, Rinehart & Winston; 1991.

10. Johnson TC, Stoner G, Green SK. Demonstrating the experimenting society model with classwide behavior management interventions. School Psych Rev 1996;25:198–213.

11. Pelham WE, Fabiano GA, Gnagy EM, et al. The role of summer treatment programs in the context of comprehensive treatment for attention-deficit/hyperactivity disorder. In: Hibbs ED, Jensen PS, editors. Psychosocial treatments for child and adolescent disorders: empirically based strategies for clinical practice. 2nd edition. Washington, DC: American Psychological Association; 2005. p. 377–410.

12. Pfiffner LJ, O'Leary SG. School-based psychological treatments. In: Matson JL, editor. Handbook of hyperactivity in children. Boston: Allyn & Bacon; 1993. p. 234–55.

13. Curtis DF, Pisecco S, Hamilton RJ, et al. Teacher perceptions of classroom interventions for children with ADHD: a cross-cultural comparison of teachers in the United States and New Zealand. Sch Psychol Q 2006;21:191–6.

14. Jurbergs N, Palcic J, Kelley ML. School–home notes with and without response cost: increasing attention and academic performance in low-income children with attention-deficit/hyperactivity disorder. Sch Psychol Q 2007;22:358–79.

15. Fabiano GA, Pelham WE, Gnagy E, et al. The single and combined effects of multiple intensities of behavior modification and methylphenidate for children with attention deficit hyperactivity disorder in a classroom setting. School Psych Rev 2007;36:195–216.

16. Kelley ML. School–home notes: promising children's classroom success. New York: Guilford; 1990.

17. Evans SW, Owens JS, Bunford N. Evidence-based psychosocial treatments for children and adolescents with attention-deficit/hyperactivity disorder. J Clin Child Adolesc Psychol 2013. [Epub ahead of print].

18. Volpe RJ, Fabiano GA. Daily behavior report cards: an evidence-based system of assessment and intervention. New York: Guilford; 2013.

19. Vannest KJ, Davis JL, Davis CR, et al. Effective intervention for behavior with a daily behavior report card: a meta-analysis. School Psych Rev 2010;39:654–72.

20. Gormley MJ, DuPaul GJ. Teacher to teacher consultation: facilitating consistent and effective intervention across grade levels for students with ADHD. Psychol Sch, in press.

21. DuPaul GJ, Eckert TL, Vilardo B. The effects of school-based interventions for attention deficit hyperactivity disorder: a meta-analysis 1996-2010. School Psych Rev 2012;41:387–412.

22. Rapport MD, Orban SA, Kofler MJ, et al. Do programs designed to train working memory, other executive functions, and attention benefit children with ADHD? A meta-analytic review of cognitive, academic, and behavioral outcomes. Clin Psychol Rev 2013;33:1237–52.

23. Nelson JR, Benner GJ, Mooney P. Instructional practices for students with behavioral disorders: strategies for reading, writing, and math. New York: Guilford; 2008.

24. Rosenshine B, Stevens R. Teaching functions. In: Wittrock MC, editor. Handbook of research on teaching. 3rd edition. New York: Macmillan; 1986. p. 376–91.

25. Nelson JR, Benner GJ, Bohaty J. Addressing the academic problems and challenges of students with emotional and behavioral disorders. In: Walker HM, Gresham FM, editors. Handbook of evidence-based practices for emotional and behavioral disorders: applications in schools. New York: Guilford; 2014. p. 363–77.

26. Mautone JA, DuPaul GJ, Jitendra AK. The effects of computer-assisted instruction on the mathematics performance and classroom behavior of children with ADHD. J Atten Disord 2005;9:301–12.

27. Greenwood CR, Maheady L, Delquadri J. Classwide peer tutoring programs. In: Shinn MR, Walker HM, Stoner G, editors. Interventions for academic and behavior problems II: preventive and remedial approaches. Bethesda (MD): National Association of School Psychologists; 2002. p. 611–50.

28. DuPaul GJ, Ervin RA, Hook CL, et al. Peer tutoring for children with attention deficit hyperactivity disorder: effects on classroom behavior and academic performance. J Appl Behav Anal 1998;31:579–92.

29. Bowman-Perrott L, Davis H, Vannest K, et al. Academic benefits of peer tutoring: a meta-analytic review of single-case research. School Psych Rev 2013;42: 39–55.

30. Reid R, Trout AL, Schartz M. Self-regulation interventions for children with attention deficit/hyperactivity disorder. Exceptional Children 2005;71:361–77.

31. Liotti M, Pliszka SR, Perez R, et al. Abnormal brain activity related to performance monitoring and error detection in children with ADHD. Cortex 2005;41:377–88.

32. Harris KR, Friedlander BD, Saddler B, et al. Self-monitoring of attention versus self-monitoring of academic performance: effects among students with ADHD in the general education classroom. J Spec Educ 2005;39:145–56.

33. Gulchak DJ. Using a mobile handheld computer to teach a student with an emotional and behavioral disorder to self-monitor attention. Educ Treat Children 2008;31:567–81.

34. Owens EB, Hinshaw SP, Kraemer HC, et al. Which treatment for whom for ADHD? Moderators of treatment response in the MTA. J Consult Clin Psychol 2003;71: 540–52.

35. MTA Cooperative Group. A 14-month randomized clinical trial of treatment strategies for attention-deficit/hyperactivity disorder. Multimodal treatment study of children with ADHD. Arch Gen Psychiatry 1999;56:1073–86.

36. MTA Cooperative Group. Moderators and mediators of treatment response for children with attention-deficit/hyperactivity disorder: the multimodal treatment study of children with attention-deficit hyperactivity disorder. Arch Gen Psychiatry 1999;56:1088–96.

37. Visser SN, Danielson ML, Bitsko RH, et al. Trends in parent-report of health care provider-diagnosed and medicated attention-deficit/hyperactivity disorder: United States, 2003-2011. J Am Acad Child Adolesc Psychiatry 2014;53:34–46.e2.

38. DuPaul GJ, Jitendra AK, Volpe RJ, et al. Consultation-based academic interventions for children with ADHD: effects on reading and mathematics achievement. J Abnorm Child Psychol 2006;34:633–46.

Middle School–based and High School–based Interventions for Adolescents with ADHD

Steven W. Evans, PhD[a],*, Joshua M. Langberg, PhD[b],
Theresa Egan, MA[a], Stephen J. Molitor, BA[b]

KEYWORDS

- Adolescents • ADHD • Schools • Psychosocial treatment • Organization
- Academic impairment • Social impairment

KEY POINTS

- Evidence indicates that the Challenging Horizons Program and Homework, Organization, and Planning Skills program are likely to be effective treatments for many adolescents with attention-deficit/hyperactivity disorder (ADHD).
- There is inadequate evidence to make scientifically informed decisions about moderators and mediators of treatment effects as well as optimal sequencing of treatment modalities.
- Benefits of treatment seem greatest when sessions are once or twice per week and continued over many months.
- There are many access advantages for school-based services compared with clinic-based care. Services integrated within the school day seem to have advantages for keeping students engaged compared with after-school services.
- Treatment development work is needed to address many of the challenging areas of impairment shown by adolescents with ADHD, including problems with driving, substance use, delinquency, and school dropout.

BACKGROUND

When children enter middle school they are in the midst of many developmental changes and experience significant shifts in the expectations of parents and

Disclosures: None (Dr S.W. Evans, T. Egan, S.J. Molitor). The HOPS treatment manual is available commercially and Dr J.M. Langberg receives royalties based on sales.
[a] Department of Psychology, Center for Intervention Research in Schools, Ohio University, Athens, OH 45701, USA; [b] Department of Psychology, Virginia Commonwealth University, 806 West Franklin Street, PO Box 842018, Richmond, VA 23284-2018, USA
* Corresponding author.
E-mail address: evanss3@ohio.edu

Child Adolesc Psychiatric Clin N Am 23 (2014) 699–715
http://dx.doi.org/10.1016/j.chc.2014.05.004
1056-4993/14/$ see front matter © 2014 Elsevier Inc. All rights reserved.

childpsych.theclinics.com

Abbreviations	
ADHD	Attention-deficit/hyperactivity disorder
CBT	Cognitive behavior therapy
CHP	Challenging Horizons Program
HOPS	Homework, Organization, and Planning Skills program
ISG	Interpersonal skills group (a group treatment of social impairment)
MTA	Multimodal Treatment Study of Children with ADHD
OCEBM	Oxford Center for Evidence-based Medicine
SMHP	School mental health professional (school counselors, school social workers, school psychologists)

teachers.[1] The onset of puberty coupled with increased expectations for independence from parents and teachers can be challenging, and this is particularly true for children with attention-deficit/hyperactivity disorder (ADHD). Although ratings of ADHD symptoms may decline during adolescence, they remain increased compared with peers,[2] and the transition to middle school is associated with an interruption in the decline of symptoms.[3]

Impairment in the school domain is one of the most prominent difficulties faced by adolescents with ADHD. Compared with their peers, adolescents with ADHD earn significantly lower school grades; score significantly lower on standardized achievement tests; and experience higher rates of special education placements, grade retention, and school dropout.[4–6] Adolescents with ADHD are more than 8 times more likely to drop out of school than their peers without ADHD.[4] In addition, problems with delinquency and substance use begin as young as age 11 years[7] and continue throughout adolescence.[8] Consistent with the findings related to performance in secondary school, adolescents with ADHD are far less likely than their peers to receive any postsecondary education or training.[9] As a result, addressing the social, behavioral, and academic problems of adolescents with ADHD is a high priority for parents of these youth and important for promoting positive long-term outcomes.

There continues to be a great deal of treatment development work being conducted for adolescents with ADHD.[10,11] Much of this work has focused on school-based treatments because of the considerable academic and social impairment shown at school. Providing treatment within a school allows providers to observe the students in structured and unstructured settings (eg, classroom and cafeteria), speak regularly with the students' teachers, observe the direct effects of treatment, and provide services on a frequent basis over an extended period of time. These advantages of school mental health services are well suited to address the chronic and pervasive problems of adolescents with ADHD.

As a result, most of the psychosocial treatment outcome research for adolescents with ADHD has been conducted in schools, it is important to critically review this literature in order to understand future directions for the development and evaluation of services. Future development of other clinic-based and community-based services may be informed by such a review because some of the most effective approaches may be provided and coordinated across multiple settings. This article begins by providing a description of the school-based services that have been developed and evaluated for adolescents with ADHD, followed by a review of the evidence for each treatment. The implications of this work related to modalities of treatment, models of care, and future treatment development and evaluation research are also discussed.

INTERVENTIONS AND OTHER SERVICES
Accommodations

The nonpharmacologic services most frequently provided to adolescents with ADHD in schools are often referred to as accommodations, and these include adjustments to educational practices such as allowing students with ADHD extended time to complete tests and assignments, providing them with notes from class prepared by a teacher or peer, and reducing the length of assignments. Adolescents with ADHD often qualify for and receive these services through individualized education plans or Section 504 plans. The purpose of these services is notably different from psychosocial interventions because there is no expectation that the adolescent will develop new or improved skills from these services. For example, a student may be provided with additional time to complete tests for many years, but there is no expectation that being afforded extended time will eventually lead to the student being able to complete tests independently within the expected time frame. When an adolescent is only provided accommodations, the parents and educators are not focusing on improving the student's ability to independently meet age-appropriate expectations, but instead are reducing expectations to help the student get by with a deficient skill set. A recent review of these services revealed that there was no evidence that any of these services met the criteria for being an accommodation and only minimal evidence that any provide direct benefits to the students.[12] Furthermore, these services do not address social impairment or disruptive or delinquent behavior. As a result, the most frequently provided school-based services for adolescents with ADHD have little to no evidence to support their use.

Interventions

There have been individual school-based interventions evaluated for adolescents with ADHD as well as comprehensive programs. In addition, there have been multiple secondary school–based interventions evaluated with samples that likely included participants with ADHD but that did not specifically examine the effects of the interventions on adolescents with ADHD (eg, Check and Connect[13]; Family Check-Up[14]). Studies were only included in this review if they specifically evaluated the impact of a school-based psychosocial intervention on the functioning of adolescents with ADHD. Although research and development of school-based treatments for elementary school–aged children goes back a few decades (see Ref.[15]), adolescents rarely participated in these studies throughout the 1990s.[16] Research in this area increased at the start of the new century and the first review of school-based interventions specifically for adolescents with ADHD was published in 2008.[17] The treatment development work completed to date has focused on 2 specific interventions as well as 2 comprehensive programs.

Note taking

Two common struggles for adolescents with ADHD in the school setting are attending to tasks and organizing information. Both of these problems can reduce learning and academic performance. One academic intervention that addresses both of these issues is note-taking training.[18] In the only study of note-taking training for adolescents with ADHD completed to date, instruction and practice in taking notes was integrated into teacher instruction in an analog classroom for a 2-week period. After 2 weeks, the effects of taking notes and having notes provided on on-task behavior, daily assignment accuracy scores (ie, classwork), and on quiz scores (ie, brief tests on the lecture material) were examined in a within-subject 2-by-2 design study. Evans and colleagues[18] found that having students actively take notes improved time on-task and taking and having notes improved scores on daily out-of-class assignments. The within-subject effect size for on-task behavior across conditions was approximately 0.81 for taking notes. The effect sizes for improved scores on daily assignments ranged between 0.38 and 0.96 for the difference between not taking or having notes and all 3 combinations of taking notes or having notes provided. However, adolescents' performance on quizzes was not improved by this intervention, suggesting that the benefits of note-taking interventions may need to be paired with study skills interventions to improve quiz/test performance. This study also showed that middle-school adolescents could learn to take notes with 2 weeks of instruction embedded into classroom instruction on American History (7 of 9 indices of quality of notes improved; $P<.05$). Thus the evidence from this study suggests that note-taking training is an intervention that is likely to be feasible to implement in a secondary school classroom, but, because of the lack of additional research, according to the Oxford Centre for Evidence-Based Medicine[19] the level of evidence for this intervention is level 3.

Self-management
When adolescents enter middle school, they are often expected to manage their own classwork and homework completion behaviors with minimal external supports (eg, from teachers). Therefore, teaching adolescents to self-manage these responsibilities becomes important for academic success. There is a large literature evaluating the effects of self-management training;[20] however, only 2 studies have evaluated its effects in secondary school settings with students with ADHD.[21,22] In these 2 studies, students were taught to monitor and track behaviors related to preparing for class and homework completion through frequent brief meetings with a school psychologist. In these meetings, self-management goals were established (eg, bring paper and pencil to class) and adjusted, problems meeting goals were addressed, and progress was encouraged. Gureasko-Moore and colleagues[21,22] found that the self-management intervention successfully improved classroom preparation and homework completion behaviors and that these behaviors were maintained as the intervention was faded over time. Further, students and teachers rated the intervention as acceptable for improving the students' classroom behaviors.

Although these findings are promising, across both samples there were only 9 total participants (all male) with no comorbidities, and therefore the validity of generalizing these findings may be limited. Analyses conducted included visual analyses of means and raw data points within conditions and percentage of nonoverlapping data between conditions. Based on the results of these 2 studies, self-management for adolescents with ADHD is classified as level 4 using the Oxford Center for Evidence-based Medicine (OCEBM) levels of evidence.[19]

Challenging Horizons Program
The Challenging Horizons Program (CHP) is a comprehensive school-based treatment program for middle-school and high-school students with ADHD. It includes interventions targeting social, academic, and family impairment and was first developed and evaluated in 1999. Two versions of the CHP have been evaluated, including an after-school model and mentoring model, and a third version is currently under development and evaluation.

After-school model The after-school model of the CHP has been provided between 2 and 3 days per week for 2.5 hours per session over the course of an academic year. Interventions include interpersonal skills group (ISG), academic skills training, sports skills, mentoring, and parent meetings. The CHP after-school interventions have been provided by undergraduate students in the role of counselors with graduate students or faculty serving as supervisors. The ISG is conducted in a group format and targets social impairment in a manner substantially different than traditional social skills training. The techniques in ISG: address the developmental goal of defining a personal identity, teach adolescents to understand the cause-and-effect relationships between their behavior and this identity, and help them learn to engage in a constant monitoring and revising process pertaining to their interpersonal behavior so that it aligns with their goals for their identity. The academic skills training involves training in organization of academic materials and tracking of assignments, training in note taking (discussed earlier), and creating flashcards and using both notes and flashcards for studying. Sports skills training is included to provide an opportunity to practice interpersonal skills learned in ISG and to develop skills and knowledge in common sports to allow adolescents to participate in these recreational and social activities in the community and at school. Brief mentoring meetings with CHP counselors occur at every CHP session and provide adolescents with opportunities to share their concerns of the day, initiate special interventions to augment program services, and receive coaching and encouragement on treatment goals. In addition, there are monthly parent meetings that involve providing parents with information about ADHD and adolescence and helping them learn effective parenting practices. In order to monitor progress, identify areas of concern, and assess implementation of skills, CHP counselors communicate with parents and teachers regularly and observe students in structured and unstructured school settings.

Mentoring model The mentoring model of the CHP was an attempt to provide a subset of the CHP interventions provided in the after-school model, during the school day. In the mentoring model, school mental health professionals (SMHPs; ie, counselors, social workers, school psychologists), teachers, and other staff meet weekly with the students to provide the organization and homework tracking interventions. These specific interventions were prioritized for the mentoring model because of their effect on skills important to classroom functioning such as completing assignments and preparing for tests. CHP staff consult with mentors on a regular basis to monitor their implementation of the CHP organization interventions and help them address problems that arise. CHP mentors are also encouraged to teach a problem-solving model to students and use this model throughout the academic year to address issues related to the CHP interventions or other problems that arise for the students. A similar version of the mentoring model was also tried in high schools, but services were provided by school-based research staff instead of school-employed staff, as has been done in the middle schools. The mentoring model of the CHP was the first attempt to integrate CHP interventions into the school day in a model that is likely to be more feasible than the after-school program.

Evidence supporting the efficacy of the CHP To date, there have been 9 empirical articles published focusing on the efficacy of the CHP, reporting results from 3 randomized trials, 1 trial using a quasiexperimental design, and other small studies from the treatment development process. Three studies of CHP have included random assignment to CHP or to a control group[23–25] and 1 included random assignment of schools, but not participants.[26] Sample sizes in these 4 studies ranged from 20 to 79 and 3 were conducted at the middle-school level and 1 in high schools.

Combining results across all studies there is evidence for meaningful gains in social, academic, and family functioning. Some of the findings are compared with the results of the Multimodal Treatment Study of Children with ADHD (MTA) in order to examine the efficacy of these studies with adolescents in relation to best practices with children. In the high-school CHP study[24] the percentage of respondents achieving reliable change (RC)[27] on parent ratings of functioning on the Impairment Rating Scale[28] were calculated. The percentage of participants ranged from 17.3% to 47.3% with estimates based on those receiving the optimal dosage of CHP in the 40% to 60% range. Although the MTA investigators did not report percentage of respondents meeting RC criteria in any of the articles we could find, the percentage achieving RC on parent ratings for participants in any of the 3 active treatment groups can be calculated from analyses of MTA data reported by Karpenko and colleagues.[29] Based on their report of parent ratings of participants in the medication-only, behavior therapy–only, and combined groups (active treatment groups), at the 14-month evaluation 36% of participants met RC on the Columbia Impairment Scale, 48% on the Home Situation Questionnaire, 54% on the Homework Problems Checklist, and 60% on the Social Skills Rating Scale. These percentages are based on results from well-established treatments for children between the ages of 7 and 9 years. In the only study that we found of treatment of adolescents with ADHD that reported RC, Barkley and colleagues[30] reported that between 0% and 24% of participants showed reliable improvement on parent ratings of a variety of functioning domains at home related to parent/child interactions. Thus, the CHP evaluated in high schools resulted in percentages that were lower, but with overlapping percentages, than those that resulted from the combination of all 3 active treatment conditions in the MTA (behavioral, medication, and combined), but participants receiving the optimal dosage of the CHP produced equivalent percentages.

An examination of between-group effect sizes after 14 months of the CHP mentoring condition[26] and the MTA behavior treatment condition after 14 months provides an additional point of comparison.[31] Both studies reported data from similar parent rating scales of symptoms and the same parent rating scale of social functioning (Social Skills Rating Scale).[32] Effect sizes based on between-group differences between treatment (behavioral treatment in MTA) and control revealed that the effect sizes in the CHP study were more than twice as large on parent ratings of symptoms (CHP, 0.45 Hyperactivity/Impulsivity (HI) and 0.31 Inattention; MTA, 0.15 HI and 0.13 Inattention) and also larger on parent ratings of gains in social skills (CHP, 0.39; MTA, 0). Thus, based on these effect size data and percentage of the sample achieving RC, the effects of the CHP mentoring intervention are equivalent, with some advantages and disadvantages, compared with the evidence-based psychosocial treatments for children. As a result, the CHP meets criteria for level 2 using the OCEBM levels of evidence.[19]

Homework, organization, and planning skills intervention

The Homework, Organization, and Planning Skills (HOPS) intervention is an offshoot of the CHP intervention. Given the importance of organization, time-management, and planning skills for the academic functioning of adolescents with ADHD,[33] the HOPS intervention focuses entirely on teaching these skills (ie, classroom/school behavior and interpersonal skills are not targeted). Similar to the CHP intervention, the HOPS intervention manual clearly operationalizes what it means for an adolescent to show effective organization, time-management, and planning skills. Consistent with a behavioral therapeutic approach, these definitions allow realistic and achievable goals to be established and progress with skills implementation to be consistently monitored and rewarded. The HOPS intervention includes the use of a structured materials organization system in which adolescents learn to self-manage a specific system of binder, book-bag, and locker/desk organization. An organizational skills checklist containing the operationalized organization criteria (eg, no loose papers are in the book bag) is used by an SMHP to evaluate adolescents' adherence to the system.

The HOPS intervention is delivered by an SMHP through 16 sessions that take place during the school day (ie, pullout services). Skills are taught in an established and specific order and sessions take no longer than 25 minutes to implement (mean session length, 20 minutes). Approximately halfway through the intervention, sessions with the SMHP change from 2 times per week to once per week, and the intervention is completed in 1 semester. Although similar to the CHP mentoring condition, the HOPS is more structured and regimented because skills are always taught in a specific, session-by-session order, and in a time-limited fashion. Further, HOPS is always delivered by SMHPs and no outside consultation is provided.

The HOPS intervention also includes two 1-hour family meetings that adolescents and their parents/guardians attend with the SMHP. All adolescents who participate in HOPS have a rewards system in place starting at session 1 and the points and rewards systems used are consistent across all adolescents receiving the intervention. The primary purpose of these meetings is to promote generalization of the HOPS skills and to transfer the monitoring and rewarding duties to the parent. During these meetings the SMHP works with the parents and adolescents to establish an effective and feasible home-based point system whereby the adolescents are sufficiently motivated to implement, self-monitor, and continually improve their organization and time-management skills. Small, daily rewards that do not cost money (eg, privileges such as 15 minutes' additional video-game time) are emphasized and consequences are not used.

The HOPS intervention also includes a heavy focus on time-management and planning skills. Students are taught to use their school planners or electronic planners to break projects and studying for tests down into small pieces and to schedule times to complete each task. Adolescents are taught to create evening schedules that list all of the activities to be completed after school each day (eg, sports practice, dinner, and bedtime) and to input all of their planned homework and studying tasks into the schedule. A time-management checklist that provides operationalized definitions of the HOPS time-management and planning skills (eg, the adolescent recorded an upcoming test in the planner at least 1 day in advance) is completed by the SMHP every session, and the adolescent earns points depending on the complexity of planning skills shown.

Evidence supporting the efficacy of the HOPS intervention To date, there have been 4 empirical articles published focusing on the HOPS intervention, reporting results from 3 distinct intervention trials. Two studies of HOPS have included random assignment to HOPS or to a control group,[34,35] 1 of the studies was a small open trial,[36] and the fourth study focused on evaluating predictors of response and mechanisms of change.[37] The sample sizes associated with these studies have been modest, with the largest trial containing 47 middle school–aged adolescents with ADHD.[35]

To date, treatment outcome findings have been consistent across the various studies of HOPS. Adolescents with ADHD have made large gains (Cohen d effect size of >0.8) in parent-rated organization and time-management/planning skills and large improvements in the severity of parent-rated homework problems.[35] These gains have been found to persist out to 3 months after completion of the intervention, which is the longest follow-up conducted to date.[35] Adolescents in the studies have also shown moderate improvements in ADHD symptoms of inattention, likely because multiple Diagnostic and Statistical Manual of Mental Disorders inattentive items focus on forgetfulness, organization, and procrastination. In contrast, teacher ratings suggest that adolescents with ADHD make small (eg, $d = 0.28$)[34] and statistically nonsignificant improvements in organization and time-management/planning skills. However, multiple studies with HOPS suggest that adolescents who receive the intervention do make small to moderate effect size improvements in their grades.[34] In summary, the HOPS intervention has been evaluated in 2 moderate-size, randomized trials with well-defined samples (middle school–aged adolescents with ADHD) that have included short-term (8-week and 3-month) follow-up assessments. The HOPS intervention accordingly meets the OCEBM criteria for a level 2 treatment.[19]

WHAT HAS BEEN LEARNED ABOUT TREATING ADOLESCENTS WITH ADHD?
Treatment Development

At present, many of the treatments reviewed in this article are not widely available in community or school settings. This unavailability is not a problem unique to treatments for adolescents with ADHD because interventions are frequently developed and tested under controlled conditions with minimal consideration given to the feasibility of implementation under real-world conditions.[38] If psychosocial treatments for adolescents with ADHD are to be widely disseminated, they must be feasible for providers to implement using existing infrastructure. Weisz and colleagues[39] proposed the Deployment Focused Model (DFM) as a method of developing treatments that can ultimately be widely disseminated. This model stipulates that interventions should be developed in collaboration with stakeholders with a focus on ensuring that the intervention being developed is feasible to implement if efficacy testing shows that it is a viable treatment option. The treatments reviewed in this article have been evaluated in schools and many of them were implemented by SMHPs. Furthermore, many effective treatments that are feasible to implement in schools often spend considerable time evolving at the earliest levels of the DFM. For example, the CHP started as a collaborative development project between administrators and educators at a middle school and the first author. The goal of the collaboration was to develop a set of school-based interventions that could feasibly be provided at a middle school and effectively improve the social, behavioral, and academic impairment of students with ADHD. Interventions were added to the CHP based on the empirical literature and teacher experience. During the first few years of the program, many interventions were tried, omitted, modified, and replaced based on clinical experience with the students and analyses from small samples. Organization interventions and ISG evolved out of this iterative process. The CHP began as an after-school program to accommodate the need to make frequent modifications to the program as we developed and examined many versions of the interventions.

The iterative process continues through later stages of development. For example, 2 main findings from the CHP studies that inform future treatment development include evidence that dosage matters and that attrition differs between models. First, larger dosages within a fixed amount of time[24,40] or larger dosages over an extended period of time (ie, cumulative benefit over 2.5 years)[26] lead to greater improvements in parent ratings of academic and social functioning. A second primary finding is that there are many important benefits to integrating the program within the school activities.[40] One such advantage has to do with attrition. In a large recently completed trial approximately 80% of the participants in the after-school model of the CHP remained in treatment for the entire academic year. Although this is a substantial majority, more than 95% of those in the mentoring version of the model remained in care. Based on these findings, current CHP development work is focused on a model that will provide a large dosage within the school day in order to maximize benefits and minimize attrition.

Modalities of Treatment

One unique aspect of the treatments described earlier is that most of them do not involve manipulating the contingencies in the environments in which outcomes are being measured. Best practices for children with ADHD involve changing the contingencies involving rewards and punishment in classrooms and homes by training parents and teachers how to effectively manage behavior.[10] The primary mechanism of action for the interventions reviewed earlier involves training adolescents to show behavior in other settings. For example, in these school-based treatments, adolescents are trained to follow a system of organizing materials, interact effectively with peers, plan their time at home, and follow classroom rules. When rewards are provided, they are usually provided during times other than those when they are expected to show the new behaviors. In the latest review of evidence-based treatments for children and adolescents with ADHD for the Society of Clinical Child and Adolescent Psychology,[10] this distinction between traditional behavior management treatments and training interventions is described. Training interventions, like those described in this article, have many advantages for adolescents. They are supportive of adolescents' attempts to gain independence and self-reliance[41] and are feasible in that they do not rely on the need to manage all of the various environments in which adolescents exist. Teenagers have many teachers at school, move through school independently, and spend an increasing amount of time outside their parents' direct supervision when not at school. These reasons, along with others, have led those developing school-based treatments for adolescents with ADHD to focus primarily on training interventions instead of the behavior management techniques that are best practices for younger children.

CLINICAL DECISION MAKING
Who Can Benefit?

The CHP and HOPS intervention studies reviewed earlier included adolescents with commonly occurring comorbidities, such as learning disorders, oppositional defiant disorder, and mood disorders. To date, there has not been any association found between the presence of these comorbid conditions and before-to-after improvements in functioning[37]; however, future research is needed to confirm this finding. One limitation related to who can benefit is that the adolescent must be attending school. Given the higher rate of dropout for adolescents with ADHD compared with other students, this requirement may exclude some of the most impaired adolescents. In contrast, adolescents who are attending middle or high school do not have to attend clinics to receive these services. School-based services therefore provide a large access advantage for adolescents, because attending clinics usually requires substantial support from parents In terms of time and financial resources. We have observed that many of the most impaired adolescents enrolled in our treatment outcome studies have not received services at clinics because the teenagers are reluctant to go and their parents either cannot or will not support them receiving clinic-based services. In a recent review[10] it was noted that many clinic-based treatment studies include children with higher scores on cognitive ability tests and families with higher income than children in school-based treatment studies. In summary, there do not seem to be comorbid conditions that alter response to these treatments or contraindicate the treatments, and access advantages and limitations exist.

Predictors of Response to Intervention

As with many psychosocial interventions, the working alliance between the student and the service provider may be an important factor in predicting response to intervention for adolescents with ADHD. The term working alliance, broadly defined, refers not only to the bond between a therapist and client but also to the therapist's and client's ability to work together collaboratively and to agree on treatment goals.[42] In each of the interventions described in this article, setting realistic and achievable goals for skills implementation, motivating the adolescent to work toward those goals, and establishing realistic and achievable goals for the adolescent's own self-management are considered critical intervention components. If these components do not occur, it is unlikely that the intervention will succeed. In at least one study of the HOPS intervention, adolescents' ratings of the therapeutic working alliance were strong predictors of improvement in parent-rated organization and planning skills.[37] After examining many different demographic variables and possible mechanisms of change, the only factor that predicted improvement more strongly than the working alliance was how well the adolescent adopted and adhered to the binder materials organization system. In summary, whether or not the adolescent agrees with the goals of the intervention and is motivated to work with the clinician to achieve the goals is an important predictor of outcomes.

The impact of psychotropic medication use has also been evaluated as a predictor of response to the CHP and HOPS interventions. Stimulant medications are an effective treatment of adolescents with ADHD[11]; however, there is minimal evidence that the short-term gains in academic productivity associated with medication use translate into long-term improvements in academic outcomes such as grades.[43] Across studies of CHP and HOPS, approximately 50% to 70% of participants were taking ADHD medications while receiving the psychosocial interventions (eg, 67%[23]; 69%[35]), with a smaller proportion of participants taking medications for comorbid mood disorders (eg, 27%[23]). None of the studies completed to date have found medication use to be significantly associated with outcomes. For example, in the study by Evans and colleagues,[23] there was a significant main effect for medication, whereby adolescents taking ADHD medication were rated as more severe/impaired compared with participants not taking ADHD medications; however, there were no significant interactions between condition, time, and medication status. Langberg and colleagues[37] similarly evaluated whether ADHD medication status was associated with the before-to-after gains of adolescents who received the HOPS intervention and found no effect on any of the homework problems or organizational skills outcomes. However, medication use was not controlled or purposefully manipulated in these studies (ie, they were naturalistic studies in terms of medication). A wide range of factors determine whether or not families pursue and are adherent with ADHD medication[44] and, as such, it is not yet possible to draw conclusions about the importance of medication in the context of a psychosocial treatment studies.

Sequencing Treatments

Parents face choices when they decide to pursue services to help their adolescents with ADHD. These choices may include medication, accommodations, and the treatments described in this article. However, research findings often do not inform the decisions regarding the sequencing of these services. There is a model of care called the Life Course Model[45] based on the principle that treatments should be sequenced according to their likelihood for helping the patient independently meet age-appropriate expectations. In this model, services are organized into 4 layers with the first involving treatments designed to stabilize environments that may be significantly exacerbating problems such as a chaotic home or classroom. The second layer involves psychosocial services and may include treatments provided at schools, clinics, or other locations in the community. The third layer includes medication and the fourth is accommodations. The model includes principles of care and encourages a data-based decision-making process within each layer across multiple treatments as well as when making decisions to move to the next layer. Children may receive treatments across multiple layers concurrently, but the sequence is recommended based on the guiding principle of prioritizing treatments that help patients independently meet age-appropriate expectations (ie, without continuous treatment). The rationale for the model, thorough descriptions, and additional details are provided in other publications.[45,46] In this model of care, the school-based treatments described in this article are frontline services for adolescents with ADHD.

FUTURE DIRECTIONS

Some of the most pressing research questions pertaining to both CHP and HOPS are currently being addressed in 3 large federally funded randomized trials. Results will allow the identification of characteristics of adolescents, families, and schools that may moderate treatment effects as well as aspects of the treatments that may mediate outcomes. These studies are being conducted at middle schools and high schools to allow a determination of the extent to which the age of the adolescents and differences between middle and high schools may affect access to care, engagement, and outcomes. Other important questions will not be addressed in these studies, such as sequencing of treatments and possible interactive effects of combining treatments. It may be that optimal care for some adolescents involves a combination of treatments such as medications, clinic-based or home-based care, along with school-based services.

Although much more research and development work has been conducted with school-based treatments than clinic-based services for adolescents with ADHD, there are some promising clinic-based treatments. For example, behavioral parent training interventions have been developed to specifically address the academic and school impairments of adolescents with ADHD. One such intervention, the Supporting Teens' Academic Needs Daily intervention is a parent-teen collaborative treatment model that has been evaluated with middle school–aged[47] and high school–aged[48] adolescents with ADHD, with participants making improvements in parent-rated academic functioning and ADHD symptoms. In addition, Fabiano and colleagues[49] completed a pilot study of a clinic-based family treatment of adolescents with ADHD that led to improvements in the adolescents' driving behavior. The Summer Treatment Program was modified to address the needs of adolescents with ADHD[50] and has shown promise for improving behavioral functioning and academic skills.[51] Continued development work with these interventions may lead to clinicians being able to prescribe services individually based on characteristics of the adolescent; presenting problems; and school, community, and family resources.

These studies have also provided information on directions for treatment development work that may not be as viable as the work described earlier. For example, although cognitive behavior therapy (CBT) is effective for adolescents with anxiety and depression and had some intuitive appeal for children with ADHD,[52] results indicated that it was not effective for children with ADHD[53] and there is little to suggest that the conclusion will be any different with adolescents. The efficacy of CBT for ADHD is reviewed by Antshel elsewhere in this issue. Although there have been reports of CBT being effective for adults with ADHD, there are concerns that the participants in those studies may be different in important ways from people being studied as children and adolescents with ADHD.[54] However, this characterization of CBT as unlikely to be effective is based on the traditional definition of cognitive therapy involving cognitive restructuring, changing automatic thoughts, and addressing irrational beliefs. This approach was originally included in cognitive approaches to children with ADHD related to trying to have them change their thinking to be more

---

Box 1
Summary and recommendations for clinicians treating adolescents with ADHD

- Deficits in organizational skills are common in adolescents with ADHD and are unlikely to be normalized with medication treatment.[55] For this reason, the 4 school-based interventions that have been developed for adolescents with ADHD to date (note taking, self-management, CHP, and HOPS) all target aspects of organizational skills as they apply to social, behavioral, or academic impairment.[56]

- Deficits in organizational skills are pervasive across domains of functioning and include problems with:

  o Organization of time (eg, planning ahead and time estimation)

  o Organization of materials (eg, filing and transferring school materials to and from home)

  o Organization of writing (eg, structure of writing and use of main ideas and supporting details)

  o Organization of speech and social cues (eg, turn taking, staying on topic, and concise speech)

- Deficits in organizational skills manifest clinically as:

  o Lost and misplaced homework assignments

  o Procrastination, often resulting in parent-adolescent conflict and inadequate preparation for tests

  o Lack of structure and coherent themes in writing

  o Difficulty maintaining structured and reciprocal social conversations

- Organizational skills should be assessed and monitored during treatment using standardized ratings and/or with collection of data directly from teachers. Tools for measuring organizational skills include:

  o Daily report cards (DRCs),[57] including teacher report of homework assignment completion (eg, number of assignments turned in and number of assignments due)

  o DRCs that contain operationalized definitions of binder and book-bag organization, such as that there are no loose papers in the book bag or that all homework to be taken home is in the homework folder

  o Classroom performance survey:[58] a teacher-completed rating scale that includes items related to organization and class preparation

  o Homework problems checklist:[59] a parent-completed rating scale that assesses homework materials organization and homework completion behaviors

  o Children's Organizational Skills Scale:[60] includes parent, teacher, and self-report versions that assess organization, planning, and time-management skills

  o Behavior Rating Inventory of Executive Function:[61] includes parent and teacher versions that assess organizational skills as an important aspect of executive functioning

Note: many of these resources are available at http://www.oucirs.org/resources/educator&mhprofessional.

reflective before acting.[52] A broad definition of cognitive approaches could include problem-solving techniques, and these may show more promise as part of a comprehensive treatment of adolescents with ADHD. Furthermore, CBT may be appropriate for treating comorbid depression or anxiety in adolescents with ADHD.

Note that some of the interventions reviewed in this article only addressed academic impairment (note taking and HOPS). Disruptive behavior, social impairment, and problematic family relations may be the most difficult areas of impairment to treat effectively. Self-management and ISG have shown some promise in these areas, but other treatments such as clinic-based family therapy have yielded disappointing results.[30] In addition, many related problems such as substance use, driving problems, delinquency, and transitioning to independence and adulthood require considerable attention. Adolescents with ADHD who experience these problems have no evidence-based options for treating the disorder along with the related problems.

SUMMARY

Treatment development and evaluation research on school-based treatments for adolescents with ADHD has led the way in the development of psychosocial treatments for adolescents with ADHD. The 2 treatment programs reviewed in this article (CHP and HOPS) have evidence suggesting that they are effective at improving multiple areas of impairment, but many questions remain. Given the findings related to dosage, the degree of impairment, and the chronic nature of the disorder, it is unlikely that 10 to 20 sessions of any treatment is going to be adequate to address the needs of adolescents with ADHD. Combining treatments and providing them for extended periods of time may be the best answer for many adolescents. However, the research is inadequate to inform school-based or clinic-based practitioners or parents how to proceed. Because professionals thought for many years that children grow out of ADHD when they reach puberty, the development of treatment of adolescents with the disorder has been significantly delayed and is only now gaining momentum (Box 1).

REFERENCES

1. Eccles JS, Roeser RW. School and community influences on human development. In: Bornstein MH, Lamb ME, editors. Developmental science: an advanced textbook. 6th edition. New York: Psychology Press; 2011. p. 571–643.
2. Sibley MH, Pelham WE, Molina BS, et al. Diagnosing ADHD in adolescence. J Consult Clin Psychol 2012;80:139–50.
3. Langberg JM, Epstein JN, Altaye M, et al. The transition to middle school is associated with changes in the developmental trajectory of ADHD symptomatology in young adolescents with ADHD. J Clin Child Adolesc Psychol 2008; 37:651–63.
4. Kent KM, Pelham WE, Molina BS, et al. The academic experience of male high school students with ADHD. J Abnorm Child Psychol 2011;39:451–62.
5. Molina BS, Hinshaw SP, Swanson JM, et al. The MTA at 8 years: prospective follow-up of children treated for combined-type ADHD in a multisite study. J Am Acad Child Adolesc Psychiatry 2009;48:484–500.
6. Langberg JM, Molina BS, Arnold LE, et al. Patterns and predictors of adolescent academic achievement and performance in a sample of children with attention-deficit/hyperactivity disorder. J Clin Child Adolesc Psychol 2011;40:519–31.

7. Molina BS, Flory K, Hinshaw SP, et al. Delinquent behavior and emerging substance use in the MTA at 36 months: prevalence, course, and treatment effects. J Am Acad Child Adolesc Psychiatry 2007;46:1028–40.
8. Molina BS, Hinshaw SP, Arnold LE, et al. Adolescent substance use in the multimodal treatment study of attention-deficit/hyperactivity disorder (ADHD) (MTA) as a function of childhood ADHD, random assignment to childhood treatments, and subsequent medication. J Am Acad Child Adolesc Psychiatry 2013;52: 250–63.
9. Kuriyan AB, Pelham WE, Molina BS, et al. Young adult educational and vocational outcomes of children diagnosed with ADHD. J Abnorm Child Psychol 2013;41:27–41.
10. Evans SW, Owens JS, Bunford N. Evidence-based psychosocial treatments for children and adolescents with attention-deficit/hyperactivity disorder. J Clin Child Adolesc Psychol 2013. [Epub ahead of print].
11. Sibley MH, Kuriyan AB, Evans SW, et al. Pharmacological and psychosocial treatments for adolescents with ADHD: an updated systematic review of the literature. Clin Psychol Rev 2014;34:218–32.
12. Harrison J, Bunford N, Evans SW, et al. Educational accommodations for students with behavioral challenges: a systematic review of the literature. Rev Educ Res 2013;83:551–97.
13. Anderson A, Christenson S, Sinclair M, et al. Check and connect: the importance of relationships for promoting engagement with school. J Sch Psychol 2004;42:95–113.
14. Stormshak EA, Fosco GM, Dishion TJ, et al. Implementing interventions with families in schools to increase youth school engagement: the family check-up model. School Ment Health 2010;2:82–92.
15. DuPaul GJ. Attention deficit-hyperactivity disorder: classroom intervention strategies. Sch Psychol Int 1991;12:85–94.
16. DuPaul GJ, Eckert TL. The effects of school-based interventions for attention deficit hyperactivity disorder: a meta-analysis. Sch Psychol Rev 1997;26:5–27.
17. DuPaul GJ, Evans SW. School-based interventions for adolescents with attention-deficit/hyperactivity disorder. Adolesc Med State Art Rev 2008;19: 300–12.
18. Evans SW, Pelham W, Grudberg MV. The efficacy of notetaking to improve behavior and comprehension with ADHD adolescents. Exceptionality 1995;5: 1–17.
19. OCEBM Levels of Evidence Working Group. The Oxford 2011 levels of evidence. Oxford centre for evidence-based medicine. Available at: http://www. cebm.net/index.aspx?o=5653. Accessed June 24, 2014.
20. Briesch AM, Chafouleas SM. Review and analysis of literature on self-management interventions to promote appropriate classroom behaviors (1988-2008). Sch Psychol Q 2009;24:106–18.
21. Gureasko-Moore S, DuPaul GJ, White GP. The effects of self-management in general education classrooms on the organizational skills of adolescents. Behav Modif 2006;30:159–83.
22. Gureasko-Moore S, DuPaul GJ, White GP. Self-management of classroom preparedness and homework: effects on school functioning of adolescents with attention deficit hyperactivity disorder. Sch Psychol Rev 2007;36:647–64.
23. Evans SW, Schultz BK, DeMars CE, et al. Effectiveness of the challenging horizons after-school program for young adolescents with ADHD. Behav Ther 2011; 42:462–74.

24. Evans SW, Schultz BK, DeMars CE. High school based treatment for adolescents with ADHD: results from a pilot study examining outcomes and dosage. Sch Psychol Rev 2014;43(2):185–202.

25. Molina BS, Flory K, Bukstein OG, et al. Feasibility and preliminary efficacy of an after school program for middle schoolers with ADHD: a randomized trial in a large public middle school. J Atten Disord 2008;12:207–17.

26. Evans SW, Serpell ZN, Schultz B, et al. Cumulative benefits of secondary school-based treatment of students with ADHD. Sch Psychol Rev 2007;36: 256–73.

27. Jacobson NS, Truax P. Clinical significance: a statistical approach to defining meaningful change in psychotherapy research. J Consult Clin Psychol 1991; 51:12–9.

28. Fabiano GA, Pelham WE, Waschbusch DA, et al. A practical measure of impairment: psychometric properties of the impairment rating scale in samples of children with attention deficit hyperactivity disorder and two school-based samples. J Clin Child Adolesc Psychol 2006;35:369–85.

29. Karpenko V, Owens JS, Evangelista NM, et al. Clinically significant symptom change in children with attention-deficit/hyperactivity disorder: does it correspond with reliable improvement in functioning? J Clin Psychol 2009;65:76–93.

30. Barkley RA, Edwards G, Laneri M, et al. The efficacy of problem-solving communication training alone, behavior management training alone, and their combination for parent-adolescent conflict in teenagers with ADHD and ODD. J Consult Clin Psychol 2001;69:926–41.

31. The MTA Cooperative Group. A 14-month randomized clinical trial of treatment strategies for attention-deficit/hyperactivity disorder. Arch Gen Psychiatry 1999; 56:1073–86.

32. Gresham FM, Elliot SN. Social skills rating system. Circle Pines (MN): American Guidance Service; 1990.

33. Langberg JM, Dvorsky MR, Evans SW. What specific facets of executive function are associated with academic functioning in youth with attention-deficit/hyperactivity disorder? J Abnorm Child Psychol 2013;41:1145–59.

34. Langberg JM, Epstein JN, Urbanowicz CM, et al. Efficacy of an organization skills intervention to improve the academic functioning of students with attention-deficit/hyperactivity disorder. Sch Psychol Q 2008;23:407–17.

35. Langberg JM, Epstein JN, Becker SP, et al. Evaluation of the homework, organization, and planning skills (HOPS) intervention for middle school students with attention deficit hyperactivity disorder as implemented by school mental health providers. Sch Psychol Rev 2012;41:342–64.

36. Langberg JM, Vaughn AJ, Williamson P, et al. Refinement of an organizational skills intervention for adolescents with ADHD for implementation by school mental health providers. School Ment Health 2011;3:143–55.

37. Langberg JM, Becker SP, Epstein JN, et al. Predictors of response and mechanisms of change in an organizational skills intervention for students with ADHD. J Child Fam Stud 2013;22:1000–12.

38. Hoagwood K, Burns BJ, Weisz JR. A profitable conjunction: from science to service in children's mental health. In: Burns BJ, Hoagwood K, editors. Community treatment for youth: evidence-based interventions for severe emotional and behavioral disorders. New York: Oxford University Press; 2002. p. 327–38.

39. Weisz JR, Jensen AL, McLeod BD. Development and dissemination of child and adolescent psychotherapies: milestones, methods, and a new deployment-focused model. In: Hibbs ED, Jensen PS, editors. Psychosocial treatments for

child and adolescent disorders: empirically based strategies for clinical practice. 2nd edition. Washington, DC: American Psychological Association; 2005. p. 9–45.
40. Schultz BK, Evans SW, Langberg J. Interventions for adolescents with ADHD: results of a clinical trial. The annual meeting of the National Association of School Psychologists (NASP). Washington, DC, February 20, 2014.
41. Cicchetti D, Rogosch FA. A developmental psychopathology perspective on adolescence. J Consult Clin Psychol 2002;70:6–20.
42. Martin DJ, Garske JP, Davis MK. Relation of the therapeutic alliance with outcome and other variables: a meta-analytic review. J Consult Clin Psychol 2000;68:438–50.
43. Langberg JM, Becker SP. Does long-term medication use improve the academic outcomes of youth with attention-deficit/hyperactivity disorder? Clin Child Fam Psychol Rev 2012;15:215–33.
44. Hack S, Chow B. Pediatric psychotropic medication compliance: a literature review and research-based suggestions for improving treatment compliance. J Child Adolesc Psychopharmacol 2001;11:59–67.
45. Evans SW, Owens JS, Mautone JA, et al. Toward a comprehensive, life course model of care for youth with ADHD. In: Weist M, Lever N, Bradshaw C, et al, editors. Handbook of school mental health. 2nd edition. New York: Springer; 2014. p. 413–26.
46. Evans SW, Rybak T, Strickland H, et al. The role of school mental health models in preventing and addressing children's emotional and behavioral problems. In: Walker HM, Gresham FM, editors. Handbook of evidence-based practices for students having emotional and behavioral disorders. New York: Guilford Press; 2014. p. 394–409.
47. Sibley MH, Pelham WE, Derefinko KJ, et al. A pilot trial of supporting teens' academic needs daily (STAND): a parent-adolescent collaborative intervention for ADHD. J Psychopathol Behav Assess 2013;35:436–49.
48. Sibley MH, Altszuler AR, Ross JM, et al. A parent-teen collaborative treatment model for academically impaired high school students with ADHD. Cogn Behav Pract 2014;21:32–42.
49. Fabiano GA, Hulme K, Linke S, et al. The Supporting a Teen's Effective Entry to the Roadway (STEER) program: feasibility and preliminary support for a psychosocial intervention for teenage drivers with ADHD. Cogn Behav Pract 2011;18: 267–80.
50. Evans SW, Pelham WE. Psychostimulant effects on academic and behavioral measures for ADHD adolescents in a lecture format classroom. J Abnorm Child Psychol 1991;19:537–52.
51. Sibley MH, Pelham WE, Evans SW, et al. An evaluation of a summer treatment program for adolescents with ADHD. Cogn Behav Pract 2011;18:530–44.
52. Braswell L, Bloomquist ML. Cognitive-behavioral therapy with ADHD children. New York: Guilford Press; 1991.
53. Abikoff HB. Cognitive training in ADHD children: less to it than meets the eye. J Learn Disabil 1991;24:205–9.
54. Knouse LE, Safren SA. Psychosocial treatments of adults with attention deficit hyperactivity disorder. In: Evans SW, Hoza B, editors. Treating attention deficit hyperactivity disorder: assessment and intervention in developmental context. Kingston (NJ): Civic Research Institute; 2011. p. 12-1–12-21.
55. Abikoff H, Nissley-Tsiopinis J, Gallagher R, et al. Effects of MPH-OROS on the organizational, time management, and planning behaviors of children with ADHD. J Am Acad Child Adolesc Psychiatry 2009;48:166–75.

56. Storer J, Evans SW, Langberg J. Organization interventions for children and adolescents with attention-deficit/hyperactivity disorder (ADHD). In: Weist M, Lever N, Bradshaw C, et al, editors. Handbook of school mental health. 2nd edition. New York: Springer; 2014. p. 385–98.

57. Volpe RJ, Fabiano GA. Daily behavior report cards: an evidence-based system of assessment and intervention. New York: Guilford Press; 2013.

58. Brady CE, Evans SW, Berlin KS, et al. Evaluating school impairment with adolescents: a psychometric evaluation of the classroom performance survey. Sch Psychol Rev 2012;14:429–46.

59. Anesko KM, Schoiock G, Ramirez R, et al. The homework problem checklist: assessing children's homework difficulties. Behav Assess 1987;9:179–85.

60. Abikoff H, Gallagher R. Children's organizational skills scales: technical manual. North Tonawanda (NY): Multi-Health Systems; 2008.

61. Gioia GA, Isquith PK, Guy SC, et al. Behavior rating inventory of executive function. Child Neuropsychol 2000;6:235–8.

Behavior Management for Preschool-Aged Children

Amanda P. Williford, PhD[a],*, Terri L. Shelton, PhD[b]

KEYWORDS

- ADHD • Preschool children • Early childhood • Behavior management
- Early intervention

KEY POINTS

- Parent training (PT) has been found to be an effective treatment to improve behavior outcomes for children at high risk for attention-deficit/hyperactivity disorder (ADHD).
- Teacher training is also effective in improving child behavior within the classroom context.
- Combination treatments are a strong approach to increasing young children's behavioral outcomes across contexts (ie, home, school, and peer network).

INTRODUCTION/BACKGROUND

Target of Treatment: ADHD Symptoms, Associated Features

Parent, teachers, and mental health professionals are concerned about young children who display significant impulsivity and hyperactivity because the display of these behaviors places these children at significant risk for future maladaptive outcomes.[1] On the other hand, impulsivity, hyperactivity, oppositionality, and aggression are words that accurately characterize almost all preschool children's behavior at some time or other. For about 10% to 20% of 3- and 4-year-old children, and for about 20% to 30% of young children who experience poverty,[2,3] these behaviors are displayed at levels at home and/or at child care/preschool that significantly impair their functioning within those settings and warrant early effective treatment.[4] However, preschool children who display significant levels of impulsivity and hyperactivity are not

This article was supported by grants awarded to the first author by the Institute of Education Sciences, US Department of Education, through Grants R324A100215 and R305A120323-13 to the University of Virginia. The opinions expressed are those of the authors and do not represent views of the US Department of Education.
[a] Center for Advanced Study of Teaching and Learning, Curry School of Education, University of Virginia, 350 Old Ivy Way, Suite 100, Charlottesville, VA 22903, USA; [b] The Office of Research and Economic Development, The University of North Carolina at Greensboro, 1601 MHRA Building, 1111 Spring Garden Street, Greensboro, NC 27412, USA
* Corresponding author.
E-mail address: williford@virginia.edu

Abbreviations	
ADHD	Attention deficit/hyperactivity disorder
CD	Conduct disorder
CSEFEL	Center for the Social Emotional Foundation of Early Learning
ECMHC	Early childhood mental health consultation
ODD	Oppositional defiant disorder
TACSEI	Technical Assistance Center on Social Emotional Interventions

likely to receive a formal diagnosis of ADHD because these behaviors are often transient for this age group of children, even for those who display these behaviors at high levels.[5] In addition, for young children, the behaviors specifically associated with ADHD often co-occur with externalizing behaviors such as noncompliance, aggression, and emotion dysregulation.[2] Therefore, this article focuses on the small percentage of preschool children who have a diagnosis of ADHD and the larger percentage of preschool children who are at risk for an eventual diagnosis of ADHD and co-occurring disruptive behavior disorders because they exhibit to a significant degree a broad range of externalizing behaviors within the home and/or school environments but do not have a formal ADHD diagnosis.

Need for Treatment

For many children, rates of externalizing problems decline significantly during early childhood, even without intervention, but approximately half of preschool children continue to display disruptive behaviors over time.[2,5] For a subset of these children, their behaviors continue to escalate, becoming developmentally deviant in terms of their seriousness, chronicity, and impairment in adaptive functioning, thus warranting a Diagnostic and Statistical Manual of Mental Disorders, Fourth Edition diagnosis of ADHD, oppositional defiant disorder, and/or conduct disorder.[1,5] Once established, disruptive behaviors become strikingly stable over time and are resistant to treatment.[6] The presence of early, severe, and pervasive hyperactivity, impulsivity, and inattention significantly increases the likelihood of negative outcomes across the family, school, and peer domains.[1] Developmental theory and prevention science indicate that early treatments for emerging problems, compared with later interventions, are more likely to interrupt the stabilization of behavioral, emotional, and social problems, thereby increasing children's likelihood of positive school success.[6–8]

Focus of Article

In this article, the authors review empirically supported behavior management treatments for preschool children who display hyperactivity, impulsivity, and/or inattention at levels extreme enough to place them at risk for an ADHD diagnosis. Empirically supported interventions are those that show evidence that they work either through well-controlled experimental studies or through repeated replication of positive outcomes through less rigorous quasi-experimental and observational studies.[9] Because most preschool children will not have an ADHD diagnosis and because of the importance of early intervention and prevention in improving outcomes for children exhibiting significant disruptive behavior, the authors summarize a broad range of treatments that have evidence of effectiveness. These include treatments that have been evaluated using samples of preschool children diagnosed with ADHD and samples of children who are at risk for ADHD and co-occurring disruptive behavior disorders because they exhibit to a significant degree a broad range of externalizing behaviors within the home and/or school environments.

INTERVENTIONS

The authors describe treatments that have an explicit focus on behavior management that has evidence of effectiveness. These include treatments that have been evaluated using samples of children diagnosed with ADHD, as well as treatments designed and evaluated for those children who are at risk for an eventual diagnosis of ADHD and co-occurring disruptive behavior disorders because they exhibit to a significant degree a broad range of externalizing behaviors within the home and/or school environments. Behaviorally based psychosocial treatments for preschool children who display behaviors indicating ADHD and other disruptive behaviors have strong empirical support for their effectiveness.[10] These interventions focus on improving children's outcomes through the use of parent- or teacher-implemented strategies that are based on operant conditioning principles (eg, positive reinforcement, negative reinforcement, punishment, extinction). Thus, parents and teachers are provided instruction on how to change their behavior, which in turn leads to improved child behavior.

Parent Training

Theoretic overview
A variety of PT programs have been implemented with parents of young children who are at risk for ADHD or other disruptive disorders. Most programs share common features, including the following:

1. Increasing positive, supportive, and sensitive parenting
2. Increasing parental consistency through the use of proactive, appropriate discipline strategies

The implementation of strategies to increase the sensitivity and warmth of the parent–child relationship that occurs at the beginning of most PT programs[11–13] is grounded in attachment theory and the premise that parental warmth and sensitivity are necessary for children to form a secure attachment with the parent and that a secure parent–child attachment is foundational for adaptive child functioning.[14] Recent research supports this inclusion of relationship-supporting strategies—early parenting interventions that place particular emphasis on increasing parental sensitivity and responsiveness in addition to promoting proactive and positive parenting strategies are associated with significant decreases in young children's disruptive behaviors.[15,16] In theory, a warm and responsive parent–child relationship sets a foundation that allows parents' ability to sustain the delivery of the more behaviorally grounded interventions described later.

In all well-established parenting programs, a significant portion of time is spent working with the parent to promote proactive behavior management strategies to reduce child noncompliance and negative parent–child interactions. Patterson's coercion theory,[17] which posits that children learn that negative behaviors allow them to escape unpleasant events (eg, picking up toys, going to the supermarket), provides a developmental framework for the importance of improving parents' ability to provide appropriate, proactive, and consistent discipline. The theory describes how each time the child successfully escapes an event by using aversive behaviors, those behaviors are negatively reinforced. In addition, the parent is positively reinforced for permitting the child to escape the requested task as it stops the child's negative behavior. This continued process creates a cycle that, over time, can lead to increased problematic behavior in the child and parental use of highly punitive parenting practices to control the child's behavior. In PT, this coercive cycle is disrupted as parents learn to use appropriate behavior-management techniques.

Description of parent training

PT is often delivered in a group format, but it can also be delivered to an individual caregiver or caregiver unit (eg, mother and father) or to the parent–child dyad.[12,13,18,19] There are a wide number of PT programs available; some programs have been designed specifically for children who have ADHD,[20] and others are designed more broadly for children who display a range of disruptive behaviors.[21] Particular programs have features that distinguish them from one another. One component that varies widely between programs is the number of sessions parents are required to attend to complete PT; some PT programs comprise as many as twenty-four 2-h sessions,[13] whereas other studies suggest that PT can be effective in as few as 8 sessions.[22]

PT programs designed specifically for children who are diagnosed with ADHD share many core components. As examples, well-known and studied programs that are specifically targeted to young children who display behaviors that put them at high risk for ADHD include

- Webster-Stratton's Incredible Years parent training program[13]
- Eyberg's Parent–Child Interaction Therapy[12]
- Sonuga-Barke's New Forest Parenting Program[20]

A mental health professional provides the training to one or multiple primary caregivers in a series of PT sessions.

The content of PT sessions for parents of preschool children is similar to that of older children (7–10 years of age) and include some form of special time focusing on repairing and strengthening the emotional climate of the parent–child relationship (nondirective play, praise), followed by traditional behavior management techniques including commands effectively and finally to additional specific behavioral strategies to deal with misbehavior, such as token economies and time out. Building a warm and supportive parent–child relationship is of special importance when providing PT to parents of very young children because preschool children use the parent–child relationship as a primary resource to explore new environments, situations, and activities, to help regulate their own behavior and as a model for other relationships.

Core component of parent training A core component of most PT programs is that parents regularly receive homework assignments whereby they are required to implement the strategies they have learned at home and report back the results in the next session. Therefore, a portion of each session is spent processing with parents how they have adapted their parenting practices based on the content delivered during the prior session and how changes in their parenting affected their child's behavior.

Although the major content does not change when providing treatment to parents of young children with ADHD, it is important to make sure that parents and the mental health professional who provides the service consider the developmental expectations of the preschool children. Mental health professionals should present and describe specific parenting strategies in a way that is developmentally appropriate for a young child. For instance, using effective commands is a universal component of PT. For very young children, it is especially important that parents separate commands into short and discrete steps and provide additional scaffolding (ie, providing increased support based on the child's ability) to promote the child's completion of requested tasks. A preschool child should not be expected to comply with multiple chain commands (such as "Put your toys away and wash your hands because it's time for dinner and you need to go into the kitchen to eat"), as they are unlikely to be completed successfully even by children with no behavioral problems. Instead, it is critical to deliver a series of short and simple commands whereby each command is followed by acknowledgment and praise. Entry into formal school (ie, transition to kindergarten) is important and often covered at the end of PT programs specific to preschool children to discuss topics of how parents can actively collaborate with teachers to increase their children's early school success. Depending on when PT is provided to parents, this topic can be covered during the last session or as a booster session that is timed in conjunction with the child's transition to kindergarten.[13,23]

Evidence

The support for the effectiveness of PT to manage the behavior for young children who display symptoms of ADHD and associated disruptive behaviors is well established at a Oxford Center for Evidence Based Medicine[9] (OCEBM) level 1 generally reporting moderate to large effect sizes on decreasing child disruptive behavior.[4,10,24–26]

Teacher Training

Theoretic overview

The preschool classroom is an important service setting for early prevention or intervention, as more than 60% of children younger than 6 years and not yet enrolled in kindergarten are enrolled in regularly scheduled center-based care.[27] In addition, data from a recent national study indicated that preschool children are being expelled three times more frequently than children in grades K–12.[28] Likewise, early childhood teachers indicate that addressing challenging behaviors is the area in which they most need additional training.[29]

Within the classroom context, children who display behaviors indicating ADHD and associated disruptive disorders exhibit less close relationships with teachers,[30] more negative interactions with their peers,[31] and lower engagement with learning tasks and activities.[32] An array of classroom-based intervention and prevention strategies are available for teachers to use with preschool children who display challenging behaviors. These strategies focus on improving children's outcomes by modifying child behavior using basic behavioral principles.[10,33] Many programs use the response to intervention (RtI) model of service delivery, which includes

- Early identification through universal screening
- Ongoing progress monitoring
- Use of evidence-based instructional strategies that match children's level of need
- Decision making and problem solving based on children's performance
- Documentation of implementation

This model has recently been applied to the early childhood setting.[34] The RtI model emphasizes that broad attention to the fundamental competencies underlying social-emotional development can reduce the need for more intensive, individualized treatments. Technical assistance centers such as the Center for the Social Emotional Foundation of Early Learning (CSEFEL; http://csefel.vanderbilt.edu/) and the Technical Assistance Center on Social Emotional Interventions (TACSEI; http://www.tacsei.org/) have created easily accessible materials with the goal of increasing early childhood educator's access to and use of evidence-based strategies to address children's challenging behaviors. These Web sites include extensive, user-friendly training materials, videos, and print resources that are available for teachers to use to promote children's social-emotional competence.[34]

Description
Teacher training is most often delivered via a mental health professional (eg, school psychologist, mental health consultant [MHC]) and can be conducted via a series of group-based trainings or individually via ongoing consultation. The content of training usually includes strategies that can be used at both the classroom and individual child levels. For instance, teachers may receive training on the use of effective proactive classroom management techniques, such as consistent classroom rules and routines, setting limits, and positive reinforcement to be applied to all children in the classroom or to individualize these same strategies for a particular child or children who are displaying disruptive behaviors in the classroom. When implementing an RtI approach such as the Pyramid Model, teachers typically receive group-based training on the provision of universal, targeted, and intensive/individualized strategies.

Assessment For children evidencing the highest levels of ADHD and associated disruptive behaviors, there is a strong focus on comprehensive child assessment that guides decision making about where, how, and when to intervene with a child in the school context.[34] Functional behavior assessment is considered the gold standard for the purpose whereby antecedents, behaviors, and consequences are identified along with environmental contexts in which both negative and appropriate child behaviors are observed.[24,35]

Intervention After assessment, a combination of intervention strategies is implemented by the preschool teacher for a single child in consultation with the mental health professional. In these situations, the frequency of consultation varies widely, from a single session to multiple sessions per week. Strategies used may include some or all of the following: providing choice in activities whenever possible, establishing clear and consistent classroom rules that are positively stated (eg, "walk inside the classroom" rather than "no running in the classroom"), creating quick and smooth transitions between activities, ignoring mildly inappropriate behaviors, giving positive attention to and providing specific praise for appropriate behavior, and implementing token economies.

Teacher training programs One well-researched teacher training model is Webster-Stratton's Incredible Years program, which is a group-based teacher training program that focuses on providing teachers with effective proactive classroom management techniques, including the use of classroom rules and routines, limit setting, positive reinforcement, using incentives, using natural consequences for unwanted behavior, and helping children self-monitor their own behavior. In addition, in this program, teachers are provided training on strategies to promote children's emotional literacy and self-regulation, such as problem-solving coaching. Finally, teachers are encouraged to increase parental involvement in children's schooling through strategies such as sending regular parent letters and invitations to visit the classroom. The program consists of 28 to 32 hours (4 workshop days) of group-based training usually delivered to teachers on a monthly basis.

Example The following is an example of one of the techniques taught to teachers to help children better manage their own behavior. Teachers are encouraged to use the give me five signal to help children give the teacher their full attention. In this technique, each finger on the hand represents a specific behavior in which the child needs to engage. After children are taught, using a picture, what give me five means, the teacher can simply raise her open hand to get children's attention. This technique helps children to remember which behaviors to exhibit (eg, looking at the teacher with hands in lap) and which behaviors to inhibit (eg, looking at and manipulating a toy).

There has been a focus on providing teachers training on how to improve children's behavior in the classroom using early childhood mental health consultation (ECMHC).[36] In ECMHC, a health care professional forms a collaborative partnership with early childhood care providers, such as preschool/child care teachers, teaching assistants, and program directors. The consultation is often child focused, with interventions directed to address the concerns of a particular child, but it can also be program or classroom focused, with services directed toward improving the classroom quality for all children. In this service delivery model, consultation is provided to child care/preschool staff within the context of a collaborative relationship to change teachers' skills and behaviors and promote improved classroom quality, behavior management techniques, and individual teacher-child interactions, which in turn affects children's outcomes.

Empirical support

These classroom-based, teacher-initiated behavioral intervention strategies have been found effective in decreasing children's challenging behavior, as well as in improving children's early academic skills.[10,37–41] Taken together, the research base indicates that teacher training focused on increasing teacher's use of behavior management strategies within the classroom in improving children's behavioral outcomes is well established at OCEBM level 1.

CLINICAL DECISION MAKING
Who Is Most Likely to Respond (eg, Patient Characteristics, Family Variables)?

Research indicates that PT is not equally effective for all children and that the variability in treatment effectiveness has more to do with parent and sociodemographic characteristics than child characteristics.[26] Low income, single parenthood, maternal depression, social isolation, and stress have been identified as parental factors that are likely to reduce the effectiveness of PT to improve child behavior.[42,43] Attrition rates in PT programs are high, with 50% or more parents failing to attend at least half of group PT sessions.[23,44] Teacher training is also not universally effective. Effectiveness depends on the intensity of teacher training, with more evidence supporting the use of ongoing coaching as opposed to one-and-done workshops.[45] In addition, research indicates that effectiveness of ECMHC depends on consultants implementing teacher training of behavior management principles with fidelity.[46]

What Outcomes Are Most Likely to Be Affected by Treatment (eg, ADHD Symptoms, Academic Impairment, Parental Stress)?

Research indicates that parent and teacher training results in improvement in child disruptive behavior as measured by rating scales and independent observations of child behavior.[4,26,35,46,47] In addition, one can also expect to see changes in parent and teacher behavior in terms of increased use of effective behavior management strategies and decreased use of ineffective strategies.[23,26,39] Outcomes for treatment are likely to be at point of performance—one expects to see positive impacts on behavior at the time that the behavior management strategies are being implemented.[48] There is little indication that treatment in one area generalizes to another. This is true both proximally (eg, a teacher's use of praise during circle time will likely improve the child's attention level during circle time but the teacher's use of praise during circle time would likely not extend to seeing improvement in child behavior during small group time) and distally (eg, a parents' use of effective commands is not expected to change the child's behavior in the preschool classroom and vice versa).

What Are the Contraindications for Behavior Management Treatment?

There are no known contraindications for providing behavior management–focused interventions to preschool children who are diagnosed with or who are at risk for ADHD.

What Are Potential Adverse Effects of the Treatment?

There are no adverse effects for providing behavior management–focused interventions to preschool children who are diagnosed with or who are at risk for ADHD.

How Should Behavior Management Treatment Be Sequenced and/or Integrated with Drug Therapy and with Other Nondrug Treatments (eg, Stand Alone, Combination Therapy)

Stimulant medication

The use of stimulant medication for children younger than 6 years, alone or in combination with psychosocial treatments, is not indicated as the first choice of treatment.[26] Results from the Preschool Attention-Deficit/Hyperactivity Disorder Treatment Study, a comprehensive examination of the use of methylphenidate in preschool children with ADHD indicated that the use of stimulant medication was not as effective in reducing symptoms of ADHD or functional impairments as compared with outcomes of school-aged children and that significantly more side effects were reported for preschool children as compared with older, school-aged children.[1,26] In addition, parents do not prefer medication as a first line of treatment of young children and report significant concerns regarding side effects.[26,49]

Comprehensive treatment

The treatments that have been shown to be effective in improving behavioral outcomes across contexts (ie, home and school) for young children at high risk for ADHD tend to be intensive and comprehensive in nature. For example, the parent and teacher training portions of Webster-Stratton's Incredible Years Program were summarized previously. Although each of these programs in isolation is effective at significantly reducing young children's externalizing problems, the effects on children's outcomes are enhanced when these programs are used in combination.[13,50]

In addition, the PT and/or teacher training can also be combined with social skills training for children. There is evidence that group-based social skills programs are effective in decreasing the social, cognitive, and behavioral deficits that often accompany disruptive behavior problems[47,51–53] if the programs

1. Explicitly teach children targeted and specific social and emotional management skills
2. Are implemented within the actual environments where children have to interact with other children
3. Teach and coach skills in vivo
4. Have children practice in the actual settings in which the skills need to be used

Key to these interventions is that the social skills training is delivered by teachers directly to children within the classroom, the context in which children are struggling in their interactions with their peers. In addition, these interventions share an emphasis on the importance of enhancing children's ability to regulate their emotions, which has been found to mediate the relationship between implementation of multimodal interventions and improvements in child outcomes.[54]

Example: Chicago School Readiness Project
The Chicago School Readiness Project (CSRP) is an example of an effective multicomponent treatment that combines the use of several evidence-based treatments to be delivered largely through mental health consultation.[55] The project was targeted to children in preschool Head Start classrooms and intended to improve the emotional and behavioral regulation of students living in poverty. MHCs helped teachers form positive relationships with their students through classroom management and engagement techniques. The intervention occurred across an entire school year and consisted of 4 components.

1. The first part of the intervention was based on the Incredible Years,[13] which specifically targets teachers' effective classroom management.
2. The second component of the intervention involved teachers and consultants working together to implement strategies learned in the training.
3. The third component of the intervention focused on teacher stress reduction and personalized discussions between consultants and teachers on ways to cope with difficult situations.
4. The final component of the intervention occurred during the final 10 weeks of the program. At this time, consultants provided individual and group therapy to children identified as evidencing high levels of behavior problems.

Results
The results from the initial trial of CSRP indicated that the program increased positive teacher practices and reduced children's behavior problems. Teachers in the intervention condition showed increases in teacher sensitivity and were more likely to demonstrate improved behavior management skills relative to controls.[56] The intervention was also effective in improving student behaviors; students in treatment sites showed significant reductions in behavior problems according to both teacher report and classroom behavioral observations.[55] CSRP has been replicated in 2 larger trials (now known as the Foundations of Learning Project) that also evidenced improvements in positive child outcomes.[57] In both trials, participation in the intervention resulted in teachers providing more effective classroom management, children displaying fewer problem behaviors, children displaying improved cognitive regulation skills (ie, attention, working memory, inhibitory control), and increased classroom task engagement.

FUTURE DIRECTIONS

The research summarized in this article highlights the need for combined approaches (PT, teacher training, child social skills training) to positively affect children's behaviors across home and school contexts.[13,50] In addition, behavior management treatment of young children at high risk for ADHD, like child intervention in general, needs additional focus and research on understanding and addressing those factors that serve as barriers to accessing the effective strategies outlined in this article.[58]

Even though well-validated approaches to support children's social-emotional competence are available, teachers continue to indicate that addressing challenging behaviors is the area in which they most need additional training.[59] Thus, additional research is needed on how to increase the uptake of these strategies by parents of young children and early childhood teachers. For example, the new emphasis on ECMHC and the availability of research-informed but easily accessible materials such as those found at the CSEFEL and TACSEI technical assistance Web sites may help increase the likelihood that behavior management strategies will be used by parents and teachers to improve the behavior outcomes for young children who are at high risk for ADHD and associated disruptive behaviors. There is some evidence that this approach is having a positive impact on children's behavioral outcomes.[36,41]

SUMMARY

This article reviewed parent and teacher training as behavior management treatments to improve the behavioral outcomes of preschool children at high risk for ADHD. Both PT and teacher training are backed by substantial research evidence such that their effectiveness can be identified at OCEBM level 1. In addition, multimodal treatments that include some combination of PT, teacher training, and social skills training would also classify as OCEBM level 1 in terms of their effectiveness in improving child behavior outcomes. These interventions are delivered to the adults that the child interacts with during the day. Parents and teachers are provided with training and guidance on how to alter the child's environment to increase the child's behavioral success. Both parent and teacher training emphasize the need for a strong adult–child relationship combined with proactive behavior management strategies to prevent the display of negative child behavior and thus limit the need for more harsh and punitive strategies. The addition of social skills training provided in the classroom context has been shown to be beneficial improving children's skills to initiate and maintain appropriate peer interactions.

RECOMMENDATIONS FOR CLINICIANS

- PT should be considered as a first treatment choice for preschool children who are at high risk for ADHD and whose behaviors need to be addressed within the home context.
- If the child is struggling in the preschool or child care context, teacher training on the use of behavior management strategies in the classroom should be implemented.
- Combining PT with ECMHC to early childhood education teachers is a strong approach to increasing young children's behavioral outcomes across contexts.
- Parent and teacher training of behavior management strategies can be supplemented with social skills training to facilitate initiation and maintenance of adaptive peer interactions.

REFERENCES

1. Riddle MA, Yershova K, Lazzaretto D, et al. The preschool attention-deficit/hyperactivity disorder treatment study (PATS) 6-year follow-up. J Am Acad Child Adolesc Psychiatry 2013;52(3):264–78. http://dx.doi.org/10.1016/j.jaac.2012.12.007.
2. Egger H, Angold A. Common emotional and behavioral disorders in preschool children: presentation, nosology, and epidemiology. J Child Psychol Psychiatry 2006;47(3–4):313–37. http://dx.doi.org/10.1111/j.1469-7610.2006.01618.x.
3. Qi C, Kaiser A. Behavior problems of preschool children from low-income families: review of the literature. Top Early Child Spec Educ 2003;23(4):188–216.
4. Comer JS, Chow C, Chan PT, et al. Psychosocial treatment efficacy for disruptive behavior problems in very young children: a meta-analytic examination. J Am Acad Child Adolesc Psychiatry 2013;52(1):26–36. http://dx.doi.org/10.1016/j.jaac.2012.10.001.

5. Campbell SB, editor. Behavior problems in preschool children: clinical and developmental issues. New York: Guilford Press; 2006.
6. Masten AS, Cicchetti D. Developmental cascades. Dev Psychopathol 2010; 22(03):491–5.
7. Weisz JR, Kazdin AE, editors. Evidence-based psychotherapies for children and adolescents. New York: Guilford Press; 2010.
8. Sonuga-Barke EJ, Koerting J, Smith E, et al. Early detection and intervention for attention-deficit/hyperactivity disorder. Expert Rev Neurother 2011;11(4): 557–63. http://dx.doi.org/10.1586/ERN.11.39.
9. OCEBM Levels of Evidence Working Group. The Oxford 2011 levels of evidence. Oxford Centre for Evidence-Based Medicine; 2011. Available at: http://www.cebm.net/index.aspx?o=5653.
10. Pelham WE Jr, Fabiano GA. Evidence-based psychosocial treatments for attention-deficit/hyperactivity disorder. J Clin Child Adolesc Psychol 2008; 37(1):184–214. http://dx.doi.org/10.1080/15374410701818681.
11. Barkley RA. Defiant children. New York: Guilford press; 1987.
12. Brinkmeyer MY, Eyberg SM. Parent-child interaction therapy for oppositional children. In: Kazdin AE, Weisz JR, editors. Evidence-based psychotherapies for children and adolescents. New York: Guilford Press; 2003. p. 204–23.
13. Webster-Stratton C, Reid MJ. The Incredible Years parents, teachers, and children training series: a multifaceted treatment approach for young children with conduct disorders. In: Weisz J, Kazdin A, editors. Evidence-based psychotherapies for children and adolescents. 2nd edition. New York: Guilford; 2010. p. 194–210.
14. Ainsworth MD, Bell SM, Stayton DF. Infant-mother attachment and social development: Socialization as a product of reciprocal responsiveness to signals. New York: Cambridge University Press; 1974. p. 99–135.
15. Gardner F, Shaw DS, Dishion TJ, et al. Randomized prevention trial for early conduct problems: effects on proactive parenting and links to toddler disruptive behavior. J Fam Psychol 2007;21(3):398.
16. Van Zeijl J, Mesman J, Van IJzendoorn MH, et al. Attachment-based intervention for enhancing sensitive discipline in mothers of 1- to 3-year-old children at risk for externalizing behavior problems: a randomized controlled trial. J Consult Clin Psychol 2006;74(6):994.
17. Chamberlain P, Patterson GR. Discipline and child compliance in parenting. In: Bornstein MH, editor. Handbook of parenting: applied and practical parenting, vol. 4. Mahwah (NJ): Erlbaum; 1995. p. 205–25.
18. Sonuga-Barke EJ, Brandeis D, Cortese S, et al. Nonpharmacological interventions for ADHD: systematic review and meta-analyses of randomized controlled trials of dietary and psychological treatments. Am J Psychiatry 2013;170(3): 275–89. http://dx.doi.org/10.1176/appi.ajp.2012.12070991.
19. McGilloway S, Mhaille GN, Bywater T, et al. A parenting intervention for childhood behavioral problems: a randomized controlled trial in disadvantaged community-based settings. J Consult Clin Psychol 2012;80(1):116–27. http://dx.doi.org/10.1037/a0026304.
20. Sonuga-Barke E, Thompson M, Abikoff H, et al. Nonpharmacological interventions for preschoolers with ADHD - the case for specialized parent training. Infants Young Child 2006;19(2):142–53.
21. Hood K, Eyberg S. Outcomes of parent-child interaction therapy: mothers' reports of maintenance three to six years after treatment. J Clin Child Adolesc Psychol 2003;32(3):419–29. http://dx.doi.org/10.1207/S15374424JCCP3203_10.

22. Axelrad ME, Butler AM, Dempsey J, et al. Treatment effectiveness of a brief behavioral intervention for preschool disruptive behavior. J Clin Psychol Med Settings 2013;20(3):323–32. http://dx.doi.org/10.1007/s10880-013-9359-y.

23. Williford AP, Shelton TL. Using mental health consultation to decrease disruptive behaviors in preschoolers: adapting an empirically supported intervention. J Child Psychol Psychiatry 2008;49(2):191–200. http://dx.doi.org/10.1111/j.1469-7610.2007.01839.x.

24. LaForett DR, Murray DW, Kollins SH. Psychosocial treatments for preschool-aged children with attention-deficit hyperactivity disorder. Dev Disabil Res Rev 2008;14(4):300–10.

25. Eyberg SM, Nelson MM, Boggs SR. Evidence-based psychosocial treatments for children and adolescents with disruptive behavior. J Clin Child Adolesc Psychol 2008;37(1):215–37. http://dx.doi.org/10.1080/15374410701820117.

26. Charach A, Carson P, Fox S, et al. Interventions for preschool children at high risk for ADHD: a comparative effectiveness review. Pediatrics 2013;131(5): E1584–604. http://dx.doi.org/10.1542/peds.2012-0974.

27. Snyder TD, Dillow SA, editors. Digest of education statistics 2011. Washington, DC: National Center for Education Statistics; 2012.

28. Gilliam W, Shahar G. Preschool and child care expulsion and suspension - rates and predictors in one state. Infants Young Child 2006;19(3):228–45.

29. Hemmeter ML, Ostrosky M, Fox L. Social and emotional foundations for early learning: a conceptual model for intervention. Sch Psychol Rev 2006;35(4): 583–601.

30. Buyse E, Verschueren K, Doumen S, et al. Classroom problem behavior and teacher-child relationships in kindergarten: the moderating role of classroom climate. J Sch Psychol 2008;46(4):367–91.

31. Ramani GB, Brownell CA, Campbell SB. Positive and negative peer interaction in 3- and 4-year-olds in relation to regulation and dysregulation. J Genet Psychol 2010;171(3):218–50.

32. Bulotsky-Shearer RJ, Fernandez V, Dominguez X, et al. Behavior problems in learning activities and social interactions in head start classrooms and early reading, mathematics, and approaches to learning. Sch Psychol Rev 2011; 40(1):39–56.

33. Conroy M, Sutherland K, Haydon T, et al. Preventing and ameliorating young children's chronic problem behaviors: an ecological classroom-based approach. Psychol Sch 2009;46(1):3–17.

34. Fox L, Carta J, Strain PS, et al. Response to intervention and the pyramid model. Infants Young Child 2010;23(1):3–13.

35. Jones HA, Chronis-Tuscano A. Efficacy of teacher in-service training for attention-deficit/hyperactivity disorder. Psychol Sch 2008;45(10):918–29. http://dx.doi.org/10.1002/pits.20342.

36. Perry DF, Linas K. Building the evidence base for early childhood mental health consultation: where we've been, where we are, and where we are going. Infant Ment Health J 2012;33(3):223–5. http://dx.doi.org/10.1002/imhj.21331.

37. Park KL, Scott TM. Antecedent-based interventions for young children at risk for emotional and behavioral disorders. Behav Disord 2009;34(4):196–211.

38. Vo AK, Sutherland KS, Conroy MA. Best in class: a classroom-based model for ameliorating problem behavior in early childhood settings. Psychol Sch 2012; 49(5):402–15. http://dx.doi.org/10.1002/pits.21609.

39. Reinke WM, Stormont M, Webster-Stratton C, et al. The Incredible Years teacher classroom management program: using coaching to support generalization to

real-world classroom settings. Psychol Sch 2012;49(5):416–28. http://dx.doi.org/10.1002/pits.21608.

40. Gilliam W. Effects of a statewide early childhood mental health consultation system in three random-controlled evaluations. Infant Ment Health J 2011;32(3):226–7.

41. Perry DF, Allen MD, Brennan EM, et al. The evidence base for mental health consultation in early childhood settings: a research synthesis addressing children's behavioral outcomes. Early Educ Dev 2010;21(6):795–824. http://dx.doi.org/10.1080/10409280903475444.

42. Fernandez MA, Eyberg SM. Predicting treatment and follow-up attrition in parent–child interaction therapy. J Abnorm Child Psychol 2009;37(3):431–41.

43. Beauchaine T, Webster-Stratton C, Reid M. Mediators, moderators, and predictors of 1-year outcomes among children treated for early-onset conduct problems: a latent growth curve analysis. J Consult Clin Psychol 2005;73(3):371–88. http://dx.doi.org/10.1037/0022-006X.73.3.371.

44. Reid MJ, Webster-Stratton C, Hammond M. Enhancing a classroom social competence and problem-solving curriculum by offering parent training to families of moderate- to high-risk elementary school children. J Clin Child Adolesc Psychol 2007;36(4):605–20.

45. Conners-Burrow N, McKelvey L, Sockwell L, et al. Beginning to "unpack" early childhood mental health consultation: types of consultation services and their impact on teachers. Infant Ment Health J 2013;34(4):280–9. http://dx.doi.org/10.1002/imhj.21387.

46. Webster-Stratton C, Reinke WM, Herman KC, et al. The Incredible Years teacher classroom management training: the methods and principles that support fidelity of training delivery. Sch Psychol Rev 2011;40(4):509–29.

47. Webster-Stratton C, Reid MJ, Beauchaine TP. One-year follow-up of combined parent and child intervention for young children with ADHD. J Clin Child Adolesc Psychol 2013;42(2):251–61. http://dx.doi.org/10.1080/15374416.2012.723263.

48. Abikoff H. ADHD psychosocial treatments generalization reconsidered. J Atten Disord 2009;13(3):207–10. http://dx.doi.org/10.1177/1087054709333385.

49. Williford AP, Graves KN, Shelton TL, et al. Contextual risk and parental attributions of children's behavior as factors that influence the acceptability of empirically supported treatments. Vulnerable Child Youth Stud 2009;4(3):226–37.

50. Foster EM, Olchowski AE, Webster-Stratton CH. Is stacking intervention components cost-effective? An analysis of the Incredible Years program. J Am Acad Child Adolesc Psychiatry 2007;46(11):1414–24. http://dx.doi.org/10.1097/chi.0b013e3181514c8a.

51. Webster-Stratton C, Reid MJ, Beauchaine T. Combining parent and child training for young children with ADHD. J Clin Child Adolesc Psychol 2011;40(2):191–203. http://dx.doi.org/10.1080/15374416.2011.546044. Available at: http://search.ebscohost.com/login.aspx?direct=true&db=ehh&AN=59165344&site=ehost-live.

52. Webster-Stratton C, Reid MJ, Stoolmiller M. Preventing conduct problems and improving school readiness: evaluation of the Incredible Years teacher and child training programs in high-risk schools. J Child Psychol Psychiatry 2008;49(5):471–88. http://dx.doi.org/10.1111/j.1469-7610.2007.01861.x.

53. Domitrovich CE, Cortes RC, Greenberg MT. Improving young children's social and emotional competence: a randomized trial of the preschool "PATHS" curriculum. J Prim Prev 2007;28(2):67–91.

54. Jones SM, Bub KL, Raver CC. Unpacking the black box of the Chicago School Readiness Project intervention: the mediating roles of teacher-child relationship quality and self-regulation. Early Educ Dev 2013;24(7):1043–64. http://dx.doi.org/10.1080/10409289.2013.825188.
55. Raver CC, Jones SM, Li-Grining C, et al. Targeting children's behavior problems in preschool classrooms: a cluster-randomized controlled trial. J Consult Clin Psychol 2009;77(2):302–16. http://dx.doi.org/10.1037/a0015302.
56. Raver CC, Jones SM, Li-Grining CP, et al. Improving preschool classroom processes: preliminary findings from a randomized trial implemented in head start settings. Early Child Res Q 2008;23(1):10–26. http://dx.doi.org/10.1016/j.ecresq.2007.09.001.
57. Morris P, Millenky M, Raver CC, et al. Does a preschool social and emotional learning intervention pay off for classroom instruction and children's behavior and academic skills? Evidence from the foundations of learning project. Early Educ Dev 2013;24(7):1020–42. http://dx.doi.org/10.1080/10409289.2013.825187.
58. Domitrovich CE, Gest SD, Jones D, et al. Implementation quality: lessons learned in the context of the head start REDI trial. Early Child Res Q 2010; 25(3):284–98. http://dx.doi.org/10.1016/j.ecresq.2010.04.001.
59. Hemmeter ML, Corso R, Cheatham G. Issues in addressing challenging behaviors in young children: a national survey of early childhood educators. Presented at the Conference on Research Innovations in Early Intervention. San Diego, 2006.

Behavior Management for School-Aged Children with ADHD

Linda J. Pfiffner, PhD[a],*, Lauren M. Haack, PhD[b]

KEYWORDS

- Attention-deficit/hyperactivity disorder • Children • Parent training
- Behavior management • Evidence-based treatment

KEY POINTS

- Behavior management treatments are well-established, evidence-based treatments for school-age children with attention-deficit/hyperactivity disorder (ADHD) and should be widely recommended to families.
- Behavioral parent training can be augmented with classroom-based intervention or child components to extend results across home, school, and social settings.
- Combined behavior management and stimulant medication often produce the most potent outcomes and when used in combination may reduce the dose needed for each, although family/cultural preferences for treatment modalities should also be considered.
- Continued research is needed to better tailor treatment to families with multiple stressors, parent mental health concerns (eg, ADHD, depression), and those from varied family structures and cultures.
- Translation and dissemination of evidence-based behavioral treatments to school and community settings are sorely needed to increase accessibility. Feasible, cost-effective models for treatment and training of school-based and community-based providers are crucial.

INTRODUCTION/BACKGROUND
Target of Treatment

School-aged children with attention-deficit/hyperactivity disorder (ADHD) show a range of inattentive, hyperactivity, and impulsivity symptoms that translate into serious

Disclosures: Work on this article was supported, in part, by grants from the National Institute of Mental Health R01 MH077671 (L.J. Pfiffner) and F32MH101971 (L.M. Haack) and Institute of Education Sciences, US Department of Education, R324A120358 (L.J. Pfiffner).
[a] Department of Psychiatry, University of California, San Francisco, 401 Parnassus Avenue, Box 0984, San Francisco, CA 94143, USA; [b] Department of Psychiatry, University of California, San Francisco, 401 Parnassus Avenue, G06, San Francisco, CA 94143, USA
* Corresponding author.
E-mail address: lindap@lppi.ucsf.edu

1056-4993/14/$ – see front matter © 2014 Elsevier Inc. All rights reserved.

Abbreviations	
BPT	Behavioral parent training
CLAS	Child life and attention skills
CLS	Collaborative life skills
DRC	Daily report card
EBT	Evidence-based treatment

academic and social/interpersonal impairment at home, at school, and in other settings as well (eg, public places, sporting events, camps). Behavior management interventions primarily target functional impairments rather than ADHD symptoms per se.[1] At home, common problems targeted for behavior management treatment may include:

- Noncompliance and lack of independence in completing daily chores and routines (eg, getting ready in the morning and going to bed at established times)
- Homework problems (eg, unrecorded assignments, forgotten materials, need for frequent reminders to start and complete homework, disorganization, and lack of attention to details/careless mistakes)
- Co-occurring aggression and defiance toward parents or siblings

Dysfunctional parenting is usually a key target of behavior management interventions. Parents of children with ADHD show more negative and ineffective parenting (eg, power assertive, punitive, inconsistent) and less positive or warm parenting, relative to parents of children without ADHD,[2,3] and family conflict tends to be high. Behavior management interventions, such as behavioral parent training (BPT), directly target these parenting styles to improve child behaviors and family relationships and to reduce overall family conflict.

At school, students with ADHD are often inattentive, disorganized, off-task, and disruptive, which often leads to low rates of work completion both in class and at home.[4,5] Children with ADHD also show a variety of peer-related problems, including overly intrusive and negative peer interactions,[6] which can be further exacerbated by associated aggression, argumentativeness, disruptiveness, and lack of self-control.[7] Behavior management interventions at school target behaviors across all of these domains.

Need for the Treatment

The need for treating children with ADHD during the school-age years is crucial. The short-term consequences of ADHD symptoms and organizational impairments include poor scores on class tests, report cards, or academic achievement tests.[8] The short-term consequences of these children's social interaction problems include conflicted family relationships and few friendships, as well as frequent rejection or neglect from peer groups.[7] Prospective follow-up studies show that children with ADHD are at considerable risk for interpersonal and educational problems as they grow older, as shown by frequent placement in special education classrooms, grade retention, school failure, early dropout, and juvenile delinquency[9,10] and girls in particular are at risk for self-harm and suicide.[11]

Several behavioral treatments are available that target the multiple impairments and risk factors for ADHD across settings. This article focuses on behavior management treatments developed for the home setting, known as BPT (also variously referred to as parent management training, parent training, or behavioral family therapy), as well as those home-focused treatments that include additional components to enhance generalization to other settings (eg, schools). Readers are referred to other articles in this issue for coverage on social skills training (Mikami, Jia, Na), summer treatment programs (Fabiano, Schatz), and school-based interventions (Evans, Langberg, Egan, Molitor).

BEHAVIOR MANAGEMENT INTERVENTIONS
Theoretic Overview

The theoretic underpinnings for the practices taught to parents and teachers in behavior management treatment are grounded in contingency theory.[12] Consistent with this theory, child behavior can be increased by following it with rewarding stimuli (ie, positive reinforcement) or by removing aversive stimuli (ie, negative reinforcement). Alternatively, behavior can be decreased by following it with aversive stimuli (ie, punishment) or by removing rewarding stimuli (ie, extinction). With consistent use of contingency management over time, the child's behavior can be shaped to achieve desired goals. Behavior management treatment is also grounded in social learning theory,[13] which considers contingency theory principles alongside other factors, including modeling and imitation of observed behaviors (eg, parent behaviors) as well as cognitive factors (eg, parental appraisals and attributions of child behavior).

Functional behavioral analysis

The first step in designing a behavior management intervention involves conducting a functional behavior analysis, which includes identifying target behaviors to increase (ie, positive behaviors) or decrease (ie, negative behaviors) and then identifying factors in the child's environment related to the occurrence of the target behavior. Specifically, factors in the child's environment occurring immediately before and after the behavior (ie, antecedents and consequences, respectively) that may be precipitating or maintaining the likelihood of the behavior are identified. In this way, the function of the behavior can be determined (eg, to gain attention or avoid work). Target behaviors typically represent areas of functional impairment affecting the child in their everyday life and sometimes, but not always, map directly onto the symptoms of ADHD defined in the *Diagnostic and Statistical Manual of Mental Disorders*.[14,15] Behaviors, as well as their antecedents and consequences, are defined so as to be objective and measurable. Based on this analysis, a behavior plan can be developed that changes the antecedents and consequences that have been maintaining the target behavior, thereby modifying the likelihood of the behavior in the desired direction (eg, increases positive behavior and reduces negative behavior).

Parent-child interaction alterations

In addition to using functional behavior analysis, behavior management treatment focuses specifically on altering negative parent-child interaction patterns, which are often present in families with a child with problem behavior, including ADHD. These interaction patterns, referred to as the coercive process, are cycles in which parents and children control one another's behavior via negative reinforcement.[12] An example of this process occurs when children show problem behaviors (eg, noncompliance to a parent request) and parents respond negatively, creating a cycle, each time escalating in severity or emotional tone. Either the child or parent complies with the other's demand, ending the cycle, and reinforcing the escalated negative behavior pattern.

Many of the functional impairments and related conduct problems shown by children with ADHD become reinforced through this process. Thus, although not a cause of ADHD, the coercive parent-child interaction cycle predicts poor educational outcomes, peer relations, social skills, and aggressive behavior.[16,17] Furthermore, parenting styles associated with the coercive cycle mediate the effects of contextual risk factors, such as stress, parental depression, and social disadvantage, on child behavior problems.[18] Behavior management training directly targets these dysfunctional parenting practices by teaching families how to modify antecedents and consequences to reduce the likelihood of the coercive process and improve child behaviors and family relationships.

The usefulness of behavioral approaches with ADHD is supported by studies showing that ADHD is associated with neurally based motivational systems that respond poorly to the kinds of contingencies commonly used by parents and teachers. Specifically, children with ADHD relative to those without ADHD are less responsive to inconsistent, delayed, and weak reinforcement and are less responsive to cues of punishment or nonreward.[19,20] Integral to behavior management interventions is a focus on modifying parent-delivered and teacher-delivered rewards and consequences. These practices, together with the additional external structure provided by behavioral interventions, can also help address the executive weaknesses that are a part of ADHD.

Intervention Description: How Is the Treatment Delivered?

BPT is the predominant mode of behavior management treatment targeting home-based problems for school-age youth with ADHD.[15,21] BPT typically includes 8 to 12 group or individual sessions focused on 3 main objectives:

1. Providing psychoeducation about ADHD and the behavioral framework for treatment
2. Teaching effective parenting skills for improving desired behavior and decreasing problem behavior through altering antecedents and consequences, as discussed earlier
3. Practicing/troubleshooting effective implementation of such skills

To accomplish these goals, each session is usually structured to include a didactic portion, in which new material is presented, as well as an interactive portion, in which parents discuss the implementation of parenting skills. A crucial aspect of the treatment is the homework assignments, in which the parents apply the newly learned skills at home and track child improvement for discussion and troubleshooting in the next session.

Parenting skills

BPT programs tend to cover a set of similar topics. Psychoeducation about ADHD and the behavioral model for treatment is often covered first. Thereafter, most BPT programs begin with teaching parents positive attending skills to improve the parent-child relationship and promote a positive family climate, as well as contingent positive consequences (eg, praise, activity rewards, token economies/point systems) to encourage appropriate child behavior. Positive strategies are discussed first, because they can interrupt the coercive cycle often shown in families of children with ADHD. In addition, parents often find it easier to implement reward rather than punishment programs consistently and effectively, and the initial use of reward programs may result in substantial improvement, reducing the need for negative consequences. BPT also emphasizes setting the stage for child compliance and independence by teaching parents to provide clear, specific commands (eg, effective vs ineffective instructions), to establish consistent routines and expectations, and to implement when/then contingency systems (eg, when you complete your homework, then you can have screen time). BPT programs also cover effective use of negative consequences for rule violations (eg, noncompliance or aggression). For example, time-out and response cost (eg, loss of desired activity or tokens) as well as extinction strategies for attention-seeking behavior (eg, planned ignoring) are commonly taught. Information about school accommodations and advocacy and troubleshooting future problem behaviors are also a part of BPT.

Teacher involvement

BPT can be expanded to include adjunctive empirically supported behavioral interventions to address a broader range of problem behavior and enhance generalization of treatment gains across settings. Many BPT programs add school-based interventions, such as a daily report card (DRC) system (see article on middle school–based and high school–based interventions for adolescents with ADHD by Evans and colleagues elsewhere in this issue for full description of school-based interventions). DRCs are individually designed for each child and include target problem behaviors in academic or social domains (eg, turning in schoolwork, following directions, getting along with others) shown in the classroom. Teachers provide a rating for each target behavior on the DRC, which is sent home daily, and the child is provided with home-based rewards based on the ratings at school. This system provides the child with frequent and immediate feedback on their classroom behavior and facilitates regular communication between the parents and teachers. In BPT programs that include DRCs, parents are taught how to work with teachers to support the program at home. In addition, the clinician may provide support and guidance for establishing, implementing, and troubleshooting the DRC through conjoint consultation meetings with the teacher, parent, and child.[22–25]

Peer involvement

BPT has also been combined with child treatments including behavioral peer interventions (eg, summer treatment program; see article on summer treatment programs for youth with attention-deficit/hyperactivity disorder by Fabiano and Schatz elsewhere in this issue) and child skills training. These treatments generally focus on improving social interactions or study/organizational skills. For example, Pfiffner and colleagues[24,25] combined BPT and school consultation (including a DRC) with child training in executive/organizational and social interaction skills in an integrated program for the inattentive presentation of ADHD (child life and attention skills [CLAS] program). CLAS uses BPT adapted for inattentive-related target behaviors and executive function problems through rehabilitation psychology techniques. Child training modules focus on skills for independence (academic, study, and organizational skills; self-care and daily living skills) and social skills (eg, good sportsmanship, assertion, conversational skills, dealing with teasing, friendship making, playdate skills). These skills are taught to children in a group setting through a combination of didactic instruction, modeling of skills by group leaders, behavioral rehearsal, corrective feedback, and in vivo practice in the context of a reward-based contingency management program. An important feature of the group is that it serves as a vehicle to introduce and support/reinforce behavioral programs at home and school. Crucially, parents and teachers are taught the same skills and coached to effectively reinforce their child's use outside the group to promote generalization.

Nontraditional caregiver adaptations

Recently, BPT has been adapted for use with caregiver populations underrepresented or less responsive to traditional programs, such as single mothers,[26] depressed mothers,[27] and fathers.[28] These treatments largely follow the structure and topics described earlier but modify certain aspects of program delivery or content. For example, the strategies to enhance positive parenting program, designed for single mothers of children with ADHD, uses an enhanced intake procedure to increase parental motivation and to troubleshoot potential barriers to treatment adherence and also uses group problem-solving activities to encourage development of social support networks. Integrated parent intervention for ADHD is an adaptation of BPT for depressed mothers of children with ADHD, which integrates mood monitoring, cognitive restructuring, and behavioral activation through pleasant activities and relaxation into the standard BPT curriculum.[27] BPT has also been adapted for fathers of children with ADHD.[28] The adapted intervention integrates standard BPT with a recreational sports activity (ie, soccer game) for fathers to practice newly learned parenting skills with their children.

Specific child problems

BPT has also been tailored to specific child profiles and problems. For example, Mikami and colleagues[29] modified the scope of BPT to target friendship problems, a commonly associated impairment domain for children with ADHD. This treatment, called parental friendship coaching, teaches parents strategies for encouraging and reinforcing their children in the practice of successful peer interactions.[29] In another case, Abikoff and colleagues[30] used a modified BPT approach focused on improving children's organizational problems. Treatment involved training parents and teachers to reinforce children contingently for meeting end-point target goals for improving organizational, homework, and school performance and included a DRC, token economy for achieving home goals, and homework rules and structure. In addition, Pfiffner and colleagues[24,25] adapted BPT for the inattentive presentation of ADHD (CLAS), as described earlier.

Improved accessibility

Recent efforts have been made to improve accessibility and feasibility of behavior management interventions by delivering treatment via convenient, trusted, and cost-effective environments and modalities. For example, a more practical alternative to clinic-based BPT has been developed relying on handbooks, videos, and weekly telephone sessions for intervention delivery.[31] The collaborative life skills (CLS) program[32] trains public elementary school social workers to deliver a school-home treatment incorporating BPT with school-based treatment and child skills training entirely within the school setting.

Empirical Support

Several systematic reviews and meta-analyses of behavioral interventions, based on more than 40 years of research with more than 3500 youth, have been published in recent years.[33] In the most comprehensive meta-analysis of behavioral interventions to date, Fabiano and colleagues[34] reported large between-group effect sizes (ES = 0.83) for behavioral interventions when collapsed across outcome measures. The largest effects were seen for parent-rated functional impairment, teacher-rated ADHD symptoms, and academic productivity. Large ES were also found across pre-post (ES = 0.7), within-subject (ES = 2.64), and single-subject designs (ES = 3.78). These ES are in the same range as those for stimulant medication.[35] Although a different meta-analysis reported smaller effects for behavioral interventions,[36] the criteria for study inclusion in the latter review were restricted (eg, only randomized clinical trials with an ADHD symptom outcome), and the review focused exclusively on ADHD symptom outcomes, with an emphasis on blinded measures of ADHD. As a result, much of the literature supporting behavioral intervention effects on functional impairment, a crucial clinical outcome, was not considered in that review.

Evidence-based treatment validation

Of particular relevance to this discussion, BPT has been confirmed as a well-established treatment based on strict evidence-based treatment (EBT) evaluation criteria for evaluating psychosocial treatments in 3 separate reviews since 1998.[1,33,37] Combined behavioral treatments, which add school or child components to BPT, also meet criteria as well-established treatments based on the most recent review.[37] Furthermore, numerous studies of BPT alone and combined with other behavioral treatments meet evidence criteria based on What Works Clearinghouse standards (Institute of Education Sciences), and are categorized as type 1 and 2 controlled studies that use rigorous scientific methodology using Nathan and Gorman categorization criteria.[33] Outcomes from these studies include improvements in child compliance, conduct problems and parenting as measured through blinded observations and ratings and improvements in parent-rated ADHD and oppositional defiant disorder symptoms, disruptive and aggressive behaviors, homework problems, and overall functional impairment compared with alternative treatment, waitlist, or usual care controls. Reduced parenting stress and increased parenting self-confidence are also reported. Evidence exists for maintenance of treatment gains for several months after treatment ends. Based on these multiple systematic reviews of randomized clinical trials, BPT alone and combined with other behavioral interventions meets the criteria for level 1 (most stringent level) regarding treatment benefits in the levels of evidence framework specified by the Oxford Center for Evidence-Based Medicine guidelines.

Benefits of therapy adaptations

The recent adaptations of BPT to reach fathers, single mothers, and depressed mothers all show benefit in terms of better engaging the families in treatment,[26–28] and father involvement may enhance treatment maintenance.[28] Adding cognitive-behavioral treatment of maternal depression to BPT results in additional reductions in maternal depressive symptoms. Adaptations of BPT to include school-based interventions through home-school partnerships have been successful in improving the quality of family-school relationships and homework relative to psychoeducational support.[23] When BPT and home-school interventions are combined with child skills training for the inattentive presentation of ADHD, greater improvement is found on a broad array of school-based measures (inattention symptoms, organizational and social skills, global impairment) and parent report of organizational skills than BPT alone or usual care.[25] Additional adaptations of BPT focused on specific child problems have been successful in improving children's social skills and friendship quality on playdates,[29] as well as organization and academic skills.[30] Initial findings examining interventions designed to be more accessible and feasible show promising effects on ADHD symptom reduction,[31] academic and organizational skills, social behavior, and classroom engagement[32]; a randomized trial comparing the latter intervention (CLS) with usual school services is under way.

Limitations of therapy

Several important limitations in behavioral treatment effects have been reported.

1. Outcomes from behavioral interventions tend to be setting specific, so that behavioral interventions implemented in one setting (eg, home) often do not generalize to another setting (eg, school) without behavioral intervention in that setting as well.[25,38]
2. Although treatment effects can persist for at least several months after treatment ends, beyond that time, periodic treatment may be necessary.
3. Although they are large, the effects from behavioral treatments may not achieve full normalization.

CLINICAL DECISION MAKING
Who Is Most Likely to Respond

Several parent factors affect response to behavioral interventions, because parents serve such a critical role in provision of treatment. As might be expected, families who are able to attend treatment sessions regularly and consistently implement the interventions at home tend to have the most favorable outcomes.[39,40] Families with sufficient resources tend to be able to follow through more consistently. Such resources might include finance/health care, transportation, time available to attend sessions, and caretaking for siblings while they attend sessions. Two-parent families, those with social support, and those with low levels of parental stress and psychopathology (eg, ADHD, depression) tend to have more favorable outcomes.[33] Behavioral interventions tend to be successful across races and ethnicities,[41] although there may be a need for some cultural adaptations.[42] In addition, positive parental expectations and beliefs about the child's capacity for change can improve engagement in BPT and child outcomes,[43] and including a child component can reduce premature termination in BPT,[44] suggesting that including the child in treatment may exert a positive effect on parents' motivation for treatment.

The severity of child symptoms and impairments can also influence outcomes. For example, Langberg and colleagues[45] found that, at 24-month follow-up in the Multisite Treatment Study for ADHD (MTA) study, the benefits of the combined intervention on homework problems were strongest for children with moderate (rather than severe) parent-rated ADHD symptoms. Behavioral interventions seem to be equally effective for those with or without co-occurring oppositional or conduct problems or comorbid anxiety, and both boys and girls through the school-age range (age 6–12 years) respond well to behavioral interventions.[46]

Which Outcomes Are Most Likely Affected by Treatment

Treatment-related gains are found across several child, family, and parent outcomes, with the greatest impact occurring in treated settings. For BPT, effects are reliably observed on parent report of their child's ADHD symptoms, oppositional and conduct problems, homework problems, and overall functional impairment.[33,34] Increased compliance and reductions in problem behavior are also observed on blinded observations of child behavior during parent-child interactions in the clinic or home.[47] Changes in child behaviors are often a direct result of improvements in parenting, which is the most immediate target of BPT. Parenting outcomes include increased use of positive parenting strategies (eg, praise, attending) and effective commands and decreased negative and ineffective discipline, as reported by parents and as observed in blinded observations of parent-child interaction.[16,47] Parents also report less stress and depression and an increased confidence in their ability to manage their child's behavior after participation in BPT, as well as generalized improvement in parent-child and family relationships, and report high satisfaction with treatment.[48,49]

When BPT is combined with school-focused or child-focused interventions, a broader range of risk factors and settings contributing to child problems are targeted, and as a result, a broader array of improvements is expected. For example, combined BPT and school-based interventions show improvements that extend to family-school relationships[23] and child outcomes at school, as shown by reductions in teacher-reported ADHD symptoms and externalizing behaviors.[24,25] When BPT is combined with a child component, improvements occur in outcome domains addressed in the child component, such as in organizational or social skills and academic performance.[25]

Contraindications for Treatment

Behavioral treatments are effective across a broad population of families and children with ADHD. However, traditional BPT may be contraindicated for those parents unable to meet the varied demands of this intervention, most notably, the time and effort to attend weekly sessions and implement behavioral plans between sessions at home. For example, parents with significant psychopathology (such as anger management problems, ADHD, depression, substance abuse), limited cognitive capacity, or those in highly conflicted marital/partner relationships may be unlikely to participate in the treatment.[50] In these cases, alternative formats, such as a more graduated and tailored introduction of skills, may be successful or adjunctive treatment such as anger management, individual counseling, or couples therapy may be indicated concurrently or before initiation of BPT.

Potential Adverse Effects of the Treatment

Adverse effects from behavioral interventions tend to be low. The most common adverse effects are likely related to frustration that children may feel if they are not successful (eg, in earning the rewards) or that parents may feel if the program is not working as well as they would like. Modifying the program in some way (eg, revising the behavioral requirements or changing rewards) is usually effective in mitigating these problems. More serious complications may occur in the case of a parent who is overly critical or potentially violent and misuses or overuses punishment or a child who is aggressive toward a parent when punished. An errorless learning approach,[51] which minimizes child noncompliance by using a success-based gradual introduction of more demanding requests or reward-only programs, may be beneficial in these cases.

Misuse of rewards may also lead to untoward effects. Studies show that rewarding behaviors that already have intrinsic value decreases their intrinsic value.[52] Also, as discussed earlier, rewarding the termination of a problem behavior may inadvertently increase that behavior through negative reinforcement (eg, "If you stop the tantrum, you can have dessert" or in the case of children demanding rewards to complete tasks). In addition, recent studies have shown that children who receive ability-focused praise are more likely to become discouraged and give up during challenging tasks; whereas effort-focused praise is best for improving motivation and persistence on challenging tasks.[53] These studies highlight the need to carefully design and judiciously use praise and other reward-based programs.

How Should the Treatment Be Sequenced or Integrated with Drug Therapy and with Other Nondrug Treatments (eg, Stand Alone, Combination)

Behavioral interventions are often applied in tandem with medication treatment of optimal effects. In the large-scale multisite MTA study[54] comparing the separate and combined effects of behavioral interventions and stimulant medication, combined treatment showed incremental benefit on composite measures of parent and teacher behavior ratings. Consistent with the respective targets of these 2 treatment modalities, medication seems to have greater impact on ADHD symptom reduction,[22] whereas behavioral intervention seems to have greater impact on some areas of functional impairment, including homework success[45] and parenting.[47] Professional practice guidelines often recommend multimodal approaches for school-age youth.[55] The decision about whether to use 1 or both interventions is based on a variety of factors. Child symptom severity is an important consideration, and severe levels of ADHD symptoms and impairment often dictate combined treatment approaches.[55]

Parent preferences and cultural factors are also important to take into account, because adherence to treatment regimens is a requirement for the success of either approach. Most parents favor the use of behavioral interventions over medication, and an initial trial of behavior modification before medication use is supported by the literature. For example, the MTA study found that approximately 75% of children assigned to the behavior modification alone condition were successfully treated without medication, and nearly two-thirds of this group were maintained without medication for the 1-year and 2-year follow-ups.[1] In addition, previous use of behavior modification has been shown to reduce the optimal dose needed for medication.[56,57]

In general, optimal sequencing and integration of behavior management and medication requires taking into account the dose or intensity of each treatment. Based on recent studies of varying doses/intensities of behavioral and medication treatments, fewer benefits of combined treatments are observed when the dosage of either treatment is high.[56,57] Therefore, the optimal dose needed for medication is less when behavioral interventions are in place and the combination of low doses of each intervention is equivalent to a high dose of either treatment alone. Given the interactive effects of behavioral interventions and medication, it is imperative that treatment providers closely collaborate to optimize outcomes.[8]

Clinical Vignette

The following case vignette shows processes involved in behavior management treatment, including the application of functional behavior analysis, description of treatment strategies, and common outcomes associated with implementation.

CLINICAL VIGNETTE: BEHAVIOR MANAGEMENT TREATMENT PROCESSES

Mr and Ms Jones brought Ethan, their 8-year-old son, to an outpatient child mental health clinic because of concerns about their son's behavior at home. During the initial assessment, Mr and Ms Jones described that their primary concern was getting Ethan to school on time each morning. According to the family, Ms Jones typically needed to wake Ethan multiple times before he got out of bed, and often his parents had to physically go in his room to get him up. Once up, Ethan would become easily distracted from what he was supposed to be doing and required frequent parental reminders to brush his teeth, get dressed, and pack his backpack. In addition, Mr and Ms Jones reported that they were getting into daily power struggles with Ethan about taking healthy food in his lunch. As a result of these behaviors, Ethan had been arriving late to school almost every day. In addition, Mr and Ms Jones felt frustrated and deflated, describing the climate of their house in the morning as "an angry circus." At the end of the interview, Mr Jones disclosed, "Sometimes I wonder if Ethan even has the capability of being independent and I worry that I will be getting him out of bed until he's 40. Other times, it's like he's doing these things on purpose to drive us crazy!"

A functional behavior analysis identified the following problem behaviors:

- *Daily noncompliance to parental instructions to get out of bed*

- *Frequent distraction during task completion*

- *Daily arguing/negotiating with parents about his lunch*

The lack of a structured morning routine was identified as an antecedent reinforcing the problem behaviors. Ethan's staying in bed despite multiple warnings, parental attention/assistance given to Ethan in the form of constant reminders to stay on task, and Ethan's failing to take recommended food for lunch were all identified as consequences unintentionally increasing the likelihood of the problem behaviors. A coercive cycle in which Ethan and his parents were reinforcing this pattern was also identified. Specifically, the more noncompliance, distraction, and negotiation Ethan showed, the more nagging, supervision, and giving in his parents showed. Thus, Ethan had learned that he could wait through his parent's multiple instructions, and if he avoided and complained long enough, he could get out of tasks altogether. Mr and Ms Jones learned that they either needed to give multiple instructions/reminders for Ethan to comply with requests, or they needed to give in and forget about the tasks altogether to get out of the house on time.

After this analysis, Ethan's independent compliance with a structured morning routine program was set as the main treatment goal. Ethan's parents altered their antecedents and consequences by creating a structured morning routine incentive program in which Ethan was rewarded for independently getting out of bed, getting dressed, brushing his teeth, and packing a healthy lunch, without whining or arguing (described on a checklist displayed in his bedroom). If Ethan completed all steps of his morning routine with 2 or fewer parental reminders, he was allowed to play on Ms Jones' tablet or build with Lego until they left the house at 7:45 AM (rewards that he chose to maximize motivation). Mr and Ms Jones made a concerted effort to ignore all whining/negotiating and praise Ethan each time a task was completed. Within a few days of consistently implementing the new system, Mr and Ms Jones reported that Ethan was completing all steps of his routine by 7:15 AM, with 1 or no reminders. They also noticed a dramatic decrease in his whining/negotiating and an improvement in their parent-child relationships and overall family climate. By the end of the treatment, Mr Jones proclaimed, "Now I know he can do it. It's just a little harder for him to be independent, and we as his parents need to work a little harder to be organized and structured, but it's much more manageable than I ever thought it would be!"

FUTURE DIRECTIONS

Strong support exists for the efficacy of behavior management interventions for ADHD during the school-age years. Despite this situation, not all families and youth show a similarly positive response. Continued research on mechanisms of change and moderators of response is needed to inform treatment adaptations tailored to individual family needs. Strategies to improve parents' and teachers' implementation of behavior management approaches are especially important, given the association between these factors and treatment outcome.[39,40] In addition, questions persist about optimal methods for combining and sequencing various behavioral treatment components as well as behavioral treatments and medication for individual children and families. These areas of study are especially crucial given the limitations of each approach in addressing the long-term adverse outcomes for ADHD.

There is a pressing need to improve accessibility, feasibility, and acceptability of empirically supported behavioral treatments, especially for broad, high-risk populations. Interventions are seldom implemented in other settings such as schools or community clinics and are therefore not reaching many of those in greatest need.[58] The extent to which these interventions can be directly exported to the community is not known, although recent efforts have suggested that with some minor modifications and focused training for providers, this should be possible.[31,32] Issues of training requirements and intervention cost-effectiveness are critical for successful translation and dissemination into community settings. To this end, innovative approaches may include greater use of existing community resources and emerging technologies (eg, interactive Web-based treatment and training). Culturally modified treatment programs may be necessary to encourage participation, engagement, and optimal treatment outcomes across diverse ethnicities and cultures.[42,59]

SUMMARY

Behavior management treatments in the form of BPT for school-age children with ADHD are well-established, EBTs meeting rigorous criteria for level 1 in the levels of evidence framework specified by the Oxford Center for Evidence-Based Medicine guidelines. These approaches can be combined with empirically supported school-based and child treatments to enhance potency and generalization of effects.

Recommendations for clinicians

- Behavior management treatments are recommended for most caregivers of children with ADHD. Many parent training programs are available for school-age youth with ADHD or related conduct problems.[60–63]

- Families with multiple stressors, including parent mental health problems, may be less responsive to BPT and require adjunctive treatment (eg, stress management, cognitive-behavioral therapy for depression, couples therapy) either before or concurrent with BPT.

- When both home and school impairments are present, clinicians should partner school personnel to implement home-school interventions (eg, DRC), because generalization of child gains from BPT to school settings should not be expected without direct intervention in the school.

- Multicomponent treatments, which include parents, teachers, and child components, provide the most comprehensive approach and likely result in the greatest yield across all domains of difficulty for youth with ADHD.

- Combined behavior management and medication often produce the most potent outcomes and may be especially important for cases with more severe ADHD symptoms and related problems. However, when behavioral interventions are sufficiently intensive, there may be less need for medication, or lower doses of medication may be sufficient. Similarly, the intensity of the behavioral intervention needed is less when medication is simultaneously delivered.[56,57]

- Parent preferences should also be considered when making decisions about medication use and sequencing with behavioral interventions to maximize treatment engagement and adherence.

- Periodically reinitiating treatment during school-age years and adolescence may be needed, especially during periods of developmental transitions, given the chronic and pervasive nature of ADHD.

REFERENCES

1. Pelham WE Jr, Fabiano GA. Evidence-based psychosocial treatments for attention-deficit/hyperactivity disorder. J Clin Child Adolesc Psychol 2008; 37(1):184–214.
2. Gerdes AC, Hoza B, Pelham WE. Attention-deficit/hyperactivity disordered boys' relationships with their mothers and fathers: child, mother, and father perceptions. Dev Psychopathol 2003;15(2):363–82.
3. Johnston C, Mash EJ. Families of children with attention-deficit/hyperactivity disorder: review and recommendations for future research. Clin Child Fam Psychol Rev 2001;4(3):183–207.
4. Langberg JM, Molina BS, Arnold LE, et al. Patterns and predictors of adolescent academic achievement and performance in a sample of children with

attention-deficit/hyperactivity disorder. J Clin Child Adolesc Psychol 2011;40(4): 519–31.

5. Power TJ, Werba BE, Watkins MW, et al. Patterns of parent-reported homework problems among ADHD-referred and non-referred children. Sch Psychol Q 2006;21(1):13–33.

6. Mikami AY. The importance of friendship for youth with attention-deficit/ hyperactivity disorder. Clin Child Fam Psychol Rev 2010;13(2):181–98.

7. Pfiffner LJ, Calzada E, McBurnett K. Interventions to enhance social competence. Child Adolesc Psychiatr Clin N Am 2000;9(3):689–709.

8. DuPaul GJ, Stoner GD. ADHD in the schools. 3rd edition. New York: Guilford Press; 2014.

9. Barkley RA, Fischer M, Edelbrock CS, et al. The adolescent outcome of hyperactive children diagnosed by research criteria: I. An 8-year prospective follow-up study. J Am Acad Child Adolesc Psychiatry 1990;29(4):546–57.

10. Fischer M, Barkley RA, Fletcher KE, et al. The stability of dimensions of behavior in ADHD and normal children over an 8-year followup. J Abnorm Child Psychol 1993;21(3):315–37.

11. Hinshaw SP, Owens EB, Zalecki C, et al. Prospective follow-up of girls with attention-deficit/hyperactivity disorder into early adulthood: continuing impairment includes elevated risk for suicide attempts and self-injury. J Consult Clin Psychol 2012;80(6):1041–51.

12. Patterson GR. Coercive family process. Eugene (OR): Castalia; 1982.

13. Bandura A, McClelland DC. Social learning theory. New York: General Learning Press; 1977.

14. Pelham J, William E, Fabiano GA, et al. Evidence-based assessment of attention deficit hyperactivity disorder in children and adolescents. J Clin Child Adolesc Psychol 2005;34(3):449–76.

15. Pfiffner L, Kaiser N. Behavioral parent training. Dulcan's textbook of child and adolescent psychiatry. Washington, DC: Am Psychiatric Assoc; 2010. p. 845–68.

16. Hinshaw SP, Owens EB, Wells KC, et al. Family processes and treatment outcome in the MTA: negative/ineffective parenting practices in relation to multimodal treatment. J Abnorm Child Psychol 2000;28(6):555–68.

17. Kaiser NM, McBurnett K, Pfiffner LJ. Child ADHD severity and positive and negative parenting as predictors of child social functioning: evaluation of three theoretical models. J Atten Disord 2011;15(3):193–203.

18. Patterson CJ, Griesler PC. Family economic circumstances, life transitions, and children's peer relationships. In: Parke RD, Ladd GW, editors. Family-peer relationships: modes of linkage. Hillsdale (NJ): Lawrence Erlbaum; 1992. p. 385–429.

19. Pfiffner LJ. More rewards or more punishment? In: McBurnett K, Pfiffner LJ, editors. Attention deficit/hyperactivity disorder: concepts, controversies, new directions. New York: Informa Health Care; 2008. p. 293–300.

20. Sonuga-Barke EJ. Causal models of attention-deficit/hyperactivity disorder: from common simple deficits to multiple developmental pathways. Biol Psychiatry 2005;57(11):1231–8.

21. Anastopoulos AD, Farley SE. A cognitive-behavioral training program for parents of children with attention-deficit/hyperactivity disorder. In: Kazdin AE, Weisz JR, editors. Evidence-based psychotherapies for children and adolescents. New York: Guilford Press; 2003. p. 187–203.

22. MTA Cooperative Group. A 14-month randomized clinical trial of treatment strategies for attention-deficit/hyperactivity disorder. Arch Gen Psychiatry 1999; 56(12):1073–86.

23. Power TJ, Mautone JA, Soffer SL, et al. A family–school intervention for children with ADHD: results of a randomized clinical trial. J Consult Clin Psychol 2012; 80(4):611–23.

24. Pfiffner LJ, Yee Mikami A, Huang-Pollock C, et al. A randomized, controlled trial of integrated home-school behavioral treatment for ADHD, predominantly inattentive type. J Am Acad Child Adolesc Psychiatry 2007;46(8):1041–50.

25. Pfiffner LJ, Hinshaw S, Owens E, et al. A two-site randomized clinical trial of integrated psychosocial treatment for ADHD-inattentive type. J Consult Clin Psychol 2014. [Epub ahead of print].

26. Chacko A, Wymbs BT, Wymbs FA, et al. Enhancing traditional behavioral parent training for single mothers of children with ADHD. J Clin Child Adolesc Psychol 2009;38(2):206–18.

27. Chronis-Tuscano A, Clarke TL, O'Brien KA, et al. Development and preliminary evaluation of an integrated treatment targeting parenting and depressive symptoms in mothers of children with attention-deficit/hyperactivity disorder. J Consult Clin Psychol 2013;81(5):918–25.

28. Fabiano GA, Pelham WE, Cunningham CE, et al. A waitlist-controlled trial of behavioral parent training for fathers of children with ADHD. J Clin Child Adolesc Psychol 2012;41(3):337–45.

29. Mikami AY, Lerner MD, Griggs MS, et al. Parental influence on children with attention-deficit/hyperactivity disorder: II. Results of a pilot intervention training parents as friendship coaches for children. J Abnorm Child Psychol 2010; 38(6):737–49.

30. Abikoff H, Gallagher R, Wells KC, et al. Remediating organizational functioning in children with ADHD: immediate and long-term effects from a randomized controlled trial. J Consult Clin Psychol 2013;81(1):113–28.

31. McGrath PJ, Lingley-Pottie P, Thurston C, et al. Telephone-based mental health interventions for child disruptive behavior or anxiety disorders: randomized trials and overall analysis. J Am Acad Child Adolesc Psychiatry 2011;50(11):1162–72.

32. Pfiffner LJ, Villodas M, Kaiser N, et al. Educational outcomes of a collaborative school–home behavioral intervention for ADHD. Sch Psychol Q 2013;28(1):25.

33. Pfiffner LJ, Haack LM. Nonpharmacological treatments for childhood ADHD and their combination with medication. In: Nathan PE, Gordon JM, editors. A guide to treatments that work. 4th edition. New York: Oxford University Press; 2014.

34. Fabiano GA, Pelham WE Jr, Coles EK, et al. A meta-analysis of behavioral treatments for attention-deficit/hyperactivity disorder. Clin Psychol Rev 2009;29(2): 129–40.

35. Wolraich ML. Pharmacological interventions for individuals with attention deficit hyperactivity disorder. In: Evans SW, Hoza B, editors. Treating ADHD: assessment and intervention in developmental context. Kingston: Civic Research Institute; 2011. p. 8.2–8.14.

36. Sonuga-Barke EJ, Brandeis D, Cortese S, et al. Nonpharmacological interventions for ADHD: systematic review and meta-analyses of randomized controlled trials of dietary and psychological treatments. Am J Psychiatry 2013;170(3): 275–89.

37. Evans SW, Owens JS, Bunford N. Evidence-based psychosocial treatments for children and adolescents with attention-deficit/hyperactivity disorder. J Clin Child Adolesc Psychol 2014;43(4):527–51.

38. Owens JS, Murphy CE, Richerson L, et al. Science to practice in underserved communities: the effectiveness of school mental health programming. J Clin Child Adolesc Psychol 2008;37(2):434–47.

39. Clarke AT, Marshall SA, Mautone JA, et al. Parent attendance and homework adherence predict response to a family–school intervention for children with ADHD. J Clin Child Adolesc Psychol 2013. [Epub ahead of print].
40. Villodas MT, McBurnett K, Kaiser N, et al. Additive effects of parent adherence on social and behavioral outcomes of a collaborative school–home behavioral intervention for ADHD. Child Psychiatry Hum Dev 2014;45(3):348–60.
41. Jones HA, Epstein JN, Hinshaw SP, et al. Ethnicity as a moderator of treatment effects on parent–child interaction for children with ADHD. J Atten Disord 2010; 13(6):592–600.
42. Lee SS, Humphreys KL. Assessment of attention deficit hyperactivity disorder in young children. In: Evans SW, Hoza B, editors. Treating attention deficit hyperactivity disorder. Kingston (NJ): Civic Research Institute; 2011. p. 2–24.
43. Kaiser NM, Hinshaw SP, Pfiffner LJ. Parent cognitions and behavioral parent training: engagement and outcomes. The ADHD Report 2010;18(1):6–12.
44. Miller GE, Prinz RJ. Enhancement of social learning family interventions for childhood conduct disorder. Psychol Bull 1990;108(2):291–307.
45. Langberg JM, Arnold LE, Flowers AM, et al. Parent-reported homework problems in the MTA study: evidence for sustained improvement with behavioral treatment. J Clin Child Adolesc Psychol 2010;39(2):220–33.
46. MTA Cooperative Group. Moderators and mediators of treatment response for children with attention-deficit/hyperactivity disorder: the Multimodal Treatment Study of children with attention-deficit/hyperactivity disorder. Arch Gen Psychiatry 1999;56(12):1088–96.
47. Wells KC, Chi TC, Hinshaw SP, et al. Treatment-related changes in objectively measured parenting behaviors in the multimodal treatment study of children with attention-deficit/hyperactivity disorder. J Consult Clin Psychol 2006;74(4): 649–57.
48. Gerdes AC, Haack LM, Schneider BW. Parental functioning in families of children with ADHD: evidence for behavioral parent training and importance of clinically meaningful change. J Atten Disord 2012;16(2):147–56.
49. Karpenko V, Owens JS, Evangelista NM, et al. Clinically significant symptom change in children with attention-deficit/hyperactivity disorder: does it correspond with reliable improvement in functioning? J Clin Psychol 2009;65(1):76–93.
50. Chronis AM, Chacko A, Fabiano GA, et al. Enhancements to the behavioral parent training paradigm for families of children with ADHD: review and future directions. Clin Child Fam Psychol Rev 2004;7(1):1–27.
51. Ducharme JM, Atkinson L, Poulton L. Success-based, noncoercive treatment of oppositional behavior in children from violent homes. J Am Acad Child Adolesc Psychiatry 2000;39:995–1004.
52. Deci EL, Koestner R, Ryan RM. A meta-analytic review of experiments examining the effects of extrinsic rewards on intrinsic motivation. Psychol Bull 1999; 125(6):627–68.
53. Dweck C. Mindset: the new psychology of success. New York: Random House; 2006.
54. Swanson J, Arnold LE, Kraemer H, et al. Evidence, interpretation, and qualification from multiple reports of long-term outcomes in the Multimodal Treatment Study of Children with ADHD (MTA) Part II: supporting details. J Atten Disord 2008;12(1):15–43.
55. American Academy of Pediatrics (AAP), Subcommittee on Attention-Deficit/ Hyperactivity Disorder, Steering Committee on Quality Improvement and Management. ADHD: clinical practice guideline for the diagnosis, evaluation and

treatment of attention deficit/hyperactivity disorder in children and adolescents. Pediatrics 2011;128(5):1007–22.

56. Fabiano GA, Pelham WE Jr, Gnagy EM, et al. The single and combined effects of multiple intensities of behavior modification and methylphenidate for children with attention deficit hyperactivity disorder in a classroom setting. Sch Psychol Rev 2007;36(2):195–216.

57. Pelham WE, Burrows-MacLean L, Gnagy EM, et al. A dose-ranging study of behavioral and pharmacological treatment in social settings for children with ADHD. J Abnorm Child Psychol 2014;42(6):1019–31.

58. Hoagwood K, Kelleher KJ, Feil M, et al. Treatment services for children with ADHD: a national perspective. J Am Acad Child Adolesc Psychiatry 2000; 39(2):198–206.

59. Huey SJ Jr, Polo AJ. Evidence-based psychosocial treatments for ethnic minority youth. J Clin Child Adolesc Psychol 2008;37(1):262–301.

60. Barkley RA. Defiant children: a clinician's manual for assessment and parent training. New York: Guilford Press; 1997.

61. Kazdin AE. Parent management training: evidence, outcomes, and issues. J Am Acad Child Adolesc Psychiatry 1997;36(10):1349–56.

62. Sanders MR, Turner KM, Markie-Dadds C. The development and dissemination of the Triple P–positive parenting program: a multilevel, evidence-based system of parenting and family support. Prev Sci 2002;3(3):173–89.

63. Webster-Stratton C, Reid MJ. The incredible years parents, teachers, and children training series: a multifaceted treatment approach for young children with conduct disorders. New York: Guilford Press; 2010.

Family Therapy for Adolescents with ADHD

Arthur L. Robin, PhD

KEYWORDS

- Family therapy • Defiant teens • Individuation • Behavior management
- Problem solving • Communication training • Attention deficit hyperactivity disorder

KEY POINTS

- Adolescents with attention deficit hyperactivity disorder have increased family conflict because their diminished self-control impedes individuation from their parents and handling responsibility in an age-appropriate manner.
- The intervention in this article improves family relationships by (1) educating families about attention deficit hyperactivity disorder, (2) providing principles for parenting an adolescent with attention deficit hyperactivity disorder, (3) fostering realistic beliefs about the parent-teen relationship, (4) preparing the adolescent for medication, (5) breaking negativity through one-on-one time and praise, (6) teaching parents to use positive incentives before punishments, (7) teaching parents and adolescents the steps of problem solving for resolving disagreements, and (8) replacing negative with positive communication.
- Research supports the effectiveness of the original version of this intervention in reducing family conflict, but the clinical significance of the results is modest.

INTRODUCTION/BACKGROUND

Adolescence is a developmental period of exponential change as teenagers individuate from their parents, establish their identities, explore deeper same- and opposite-sex relationships, and make career and higher-education plans. All families experience increased parent-adolescent conflict, coercive interchanges, negative communication, and extreme thinking as adolescents pursue these developmental tasks. Because of the neurobiologically based executive function deficits inherent in attention deficit hyperactivity disorder (ADHD) and the common comorbid conditions such as oppositional defiant disorder (ODD) and conduct disorder (CD), these conflicts

There are no disclosures for the author.
Child Psychiatry and Psychology Department, Children's Hospital of Michigan, 3901 Beaubien Boulevard, Detroit, MI 48201, USA
E-mail address: arobin@med.wayne.edu

Child Adolesc Psychiatric Clin N Am 23 (2014) 747–756
http://dx.doi.org/10.1016/j.chc.2014.06.001
1056-4993/14/$ – see front matter © 2014 Elsevier Inc. All rights reserved.

Abbreviations	
ADHD	Attention deficit hyperactivity disorder
BMT	Behavior management training
CD	Conduct disorder
DT	Defiant teen
MTA	Multimodal treatment study of ADHD
ODD	Oppositional defiant disorder
PSCT	Problem solving communication training
SFT	Structural family therapy

are more intense and frequent for teenagers with ADHD and their parents than for teenagers without psychiatric problems and their parents.[1] Their conflicts take the form of seemingly endless cycles of coercive interchanges regarding a variety of issues—homework, chores, sibling and peer relationships, family responsibilities, and several other topics. In a typical coercive interchange, the parent commands the adolescent to engage in a particular behavior (eg, "turn off the video game and start your homework"), but the adolescent ignores the command and continues playing video games. The parent escalates the intensity of the command ("You turn that game off now or else!") while the teenager escalates his or her defiant behavior ("In a moment," or "you can't make me"). Eventually, 1 of 2 outcomes occurs: (1) the parent makes the teenager turn off the video game and get started on the homework, or (2) the adolescent makes the parent back off and avoids homework. A lot of shouting, arguing, name calling, negative communication, and ineffective problem solving accompany such coercive interchanges. These negative interactions pervade the daily lives of families with adolescents who have ADHD, impairing family relationships, interfering with the developmental tasks of the adolescents, and spurring rage, hopelessness, and depression.

Coercive interchanges and the associated parent-adolescent conflicts are the primary treatment targets of the intervention described in this article.

INTERVENTIONS
Theoretic Overview

The defiant teen (DT) family intervention[2,3] is the approach used by this author to change coercive interactions between parents and adolescents with ADHD. It follows from Barkley's 4-factor model of family interactions,[2] which explains how the normal coercive interchanges that most families sometimes experience escalate to clinical proportions. The 4 factors are the adolescent's characteristics, the parents' characteristics, the family environment/stresses, and parenting practices. The adolescent's characteristics refer to genetics, temperament, psychiatric diagnoses such as ADHD, ODD, CD, mood disorders, substance use, chronic illnesses, or physical disabilities. The parents' characteristics include all of the items listed for the adolescents, with particular emphasis on depression, substance use, personality disorders and parental ADHD. The environment/stresses refer to items such as financial stresses, socioeconomic status, single versus 2-parent status, family structure problems, joblessness, unsafe neighborhood, the available peer group for the adolescent. Parenting practices include warmth/hostility, structure/chaos, monitoring the adolescent, consistency in administering rules, and behavior management skills. To these parenting practices are added problem-solving communication skills and belief systems.

Negative extremities on one or more of these factors can combine to spur clinically significant coercive interchanges and parent-adolescent conflict. Although it is difficult to change adolescent characteristics, parent characteristics, or family environment/ stresses, parents can change their parenting practices and in return get a reciprocally positive change from the adolescents. The therapist explains this model to parents and guides them in changing their parenting practice to those proven to work with teens who have ADHD.

How is the treatment delivered?
Before starting treatment, the clinician needs to conduct a comprehensive assessment of individual and family problems, following the approach outlined by Barkley and Robin.[2] Interviews, observations, and standardized self-report inventories are administered to help the clinician paint a picture of the problems in the parent-adolescent relationship as well as individual domains and marital functioning. This clinician uses the Parent Adolescent Relationship Questionnaire[4] completed separately by parents and adolescents, to construct a comprehensive profile of family problems in the areas of global distress, problem solving communication, school and sibling conflict, extreme belief systems, and family structure. These profile graphs are shared with the family as a way of helping them pinpoint their problems, establish the need for family intervention, and develop goals for change.

After completing the assessment, the therapist introduces the steps of the DT intervention, which are a modified version of the original 18-step manual. Some steps are completed in a single session, and others are completed in several sessions, but all in the order outlined in **Box 1**. As each step is described, it will be noted who attends the sessions. The therapist does not proceed to the next step until the family has successfully completed the homework assignments associated with the previous step. Parents are asked to obtain a copy of *Your Defiant Teen*[3] and read the chapters relevant to each step of this intervention. A more detailed discussion of each step can be found in the references to this article.[1,2,5]

Step 1: educating families I: ADHD, coercion, 4-factor model The parents and adolescent attend this session but are seen separately. During the first part of the session, the therapist explains to the parents the Diagnostic and Statistical Manual of Mental

---

Box 1
Steps of family intervention

Step 1. Educating families I: ADHD, coercive interchanges, 4-factor model

Step 2. Educating families II: parenting principles

Step 3. Fostering realistic beliefs and expectations

Step 4. Preparing families for medication

Step 5. Breaking the negativity cycle: one-on-one time

Step 6. Praise, ignoring, commands

Step 7. Implementing positive incentive systems

Step 8. Implementing punishment systems

Step 9. Problem-solving negotiable issues

Step 10. Improving communication

Step 11. Putting it all together

Disorders, Fifth Edition definition of ADHD[6] and the enhanced executive function definition of ADHD.[7] Next, the therapist explains the coercive interchange, the 4-factor model, and problem-solving communication skills. This discussion ends with the therapist emphasizing that if the parents change their parenting style and problem-solving communication techniques, they will get back a positive change from their adolescent. During the second part of the session, the therapist gives the adolescent a brief definition of ADHD and its treatments, listens to the adolescent's reactions, and uses cognitive restructuring to correct myths about ADHD and instill a positive coping attitude toward treatment for ADHD. The discussion with the adolescent is informal and highly interactive, with short statements from the therapist and flexible responses to whatever concerns the adolescent expresses and is done in an upbeat, humorous manner.

Step 2: educating families II: parenting principles The parents attend this session without the adolescent. The therapist distributes and reviews a handout with the principles for parenting an adolescent with ADHD.[1,5] The therapist instructs the parents to base all of their parenting techniques on these principles. Although all of the principles cannot be reviewed in this article, 3 have been selected to illustrate the process.

1. *Divide the world of issues with your adolescent into those that can be negotiated and those that cannot.* Nonnegotiable issues are bottom line rules for teens living in a civilized society, such as "no drugs," "no violence," "use respectful language," "you will attend school and do homework," "you will contribute to the family by doing chores." The therapist coaches the parents to develop such a list and reassures them that consequences will be established for compliance with them. All other issues are negotiable.
2. *Involve the adolescent in decision making regarding negotiable issues.* Adolescents are more likely to comply with rules that they helped establish. The therapist explains that the family will learn the steps of mutual problem solving as a means to deal with negotiable issues (step 9).
3. *Use incentives before punishments.* Parents often give out so many punishments that the teenager has nothing to lose by misbehaving, leading to angry, entrenched negative interactions. It is much more effective to use positive incentives for appropriate behavior and then judiciously add punishments if incentives prove insufficient (steps 7 and 8).

Step 3: fostering realistic beliefs Extreme beliefs and inappropriate expectations interfere with improving parent-adolescent relationships. The therapist sees the parents for one session and the adolescent for a second session regarding beliefs and expectations. The therapist gives the parents a crash course in adolescent development, emphasizing individuation from parents as a primary task for adolescents and normalizing increased conflict as part of individuation. Noting how ADHD characteristics exponentially increase the normative conflicts of individuation, the therapist introduces 4 extreme belief themes, reviews the extent to which the parents adhere to them, and provides alternative, more reasonable beliefs: (1) obedience: teenagers should always obey their parents and behave perfectly; (2) ruination: giving teenagers too much freedom will cause them to ruin their lives; (3) malicious intent: teenagers misbehave on purpose to anger their parents; and (4) love/appreciation: teenagers should always show gratitude for what their parents do for them.

Analogously, in the beliefs session with the adolescent, the therapist introduces the injustice triad of extreme beliefs and uses cognitive restructuring to help teenagers develop more reasonable beliefs: (1) ruination: parents' rules will ruin the teenager's life; (2) unfairness: parents' rules are intrinsically unfair; and (3) autonomy: teenagers should have total freedom.

Step 4: preparing families for medication Medication is an effective intervention for ameliorating the core symptoms of ADHD. In this session, the therapist describes ADHD medications to the parents, answers their questions, and provides them with the resources they need to make an informed decision about it. Then, the therapist provides the adolescent with information about medication, carefully listens to his or her concerns, and addresses them. Common adolescent concerns include (1) medication will change their personalities, (2) their parents will use medication to control them, (3) their friends will treat them differently if they take medication, and (4) they will experience stigma because of ADHD. The session ends with the therapist suggesting reasonable target behaviors that medication is likely to improve and suggesting ways to monitor these behaviors. Medication should be started after this step. The therapist refers the family to a physician who understands how to talk to teenagers about psychoactive medicine.

Step 5: breaking the negativity cycle Before other techniques will work, the therapist needs to introduce tasks that help break the seemingly endless negativity cycle between the parents and the adolescent. "One on one time" is such a task. With the parents alone in the session, the therapist asks them to take turns inviting their adolescent to select a favorite activity that can be done together for 20 to 30 minutes at home without spending money. During the activity, the parents must refrain from directing, ordering, criticizing, or using any other negative comments, simply doing the activity as the adolescent wishes, trying to have fun. For those adolescents who would refuse to do an activity with a parent, the therapist advises them to wait until the adolescent is engaging in an enjoyable activity, stand nearby, and ask to join the activity. The homework for this session is to implement one on one time at least 4 times in the next week, returning to the next session with the adolescent to discuss how it worked. The adolescent and parent describe their experiences, and if one on one time went well, it is continued. If not, the therapist helps them pinpoint the problems and plan to correct them.

Step 6: praise, ignoring, commands With the parents alone in the room, the therapist asks what percentage of their comments to their teenager in the past week was positive. Usually, most comments were negative, leading the therapist to ask how the parent would feel if his or her boss made so many negative comments. Furthermore, the therapist points out that the parents may pay attention to the adolescent mainly when he or she misbehaves. Step 6 is designed to increase the percentage of positive parental comments to the adolescent. The parents are asked to make 10 additional praise statements per day to the adolescent for any behaviors that they like, even very small positive behaviors. If they can't find any praise worthy behaviors, they are to wait until their teenager does nothing offensive for 10 seconds and praise him or her. Pointing out that correcting every negative adolescent behavior might be virtually impossible and would evoke a hostile reaction, the therapist asks the parents to identify several minor misbehaviors that they could ignore. They are asked to start ignoring these behaviors as another way to reduce their percentage of negative comments.

Finally, the therapist models the appropriate way to give commands—short, assertive, statements unambiguously specifying what the teenager should do and when: "Get ready for bed now." "Start your homework now." "Turn off the video games and pick up the stuff in your room." Parents are asked to give commands following this guideline. To lighten the mood and give the parent practice having their teenager do what they ask, the therapist asks the parents to give their adolescent commands to do things that they know the adolescent enjoys: "Go send instagrams to 3 of your friends." "Go text 3 friends." "Have a second dessert." "Go play videogames." "Bring me my purse so I can give you $20 spending money." The adolescent accompanies the parents to the next session, where their experiences with praise, ignoring, and positive commands are discussed.

Step 7: implementing positive incentive systems With the parents alone in the session, the therapist explains how the creative use of positive incentives contingent on behaviors that the parents wish to see the adolescent increase is a highly effective tool. For the 11- to 13-year-old youngsters, parents are taught to use behavior charts and point systems. For the 14- to 18-year-old youngsters, parents are taught to write behavioral contracts specifying privileges earned in return for performance of desired behaviors. Here are the 6 steps for writing a behavioral contract: First, the parents list the behaviors that they want the adolescent to increase, emphasizing positives (talk respectfully, complete homework when asked) rather than negatives (don't curse, don't delay starting homework). Second, parents rank order the behaviors from least to most difficult for the teenager to do. Third, the parents list potential privileges, reviewing and updating this list with the adolescent at home. Fourth, the parents select a low difficulty target behavior and a moderately desirable privilege that lend themselves to a simple contract, for example, "I agree to take the trash from each room to the large trash cans in the garage by 8 PM daily and take the large trash cans to the curb by 8 PM Thursdays; in return, my parents agree to give me $15 per week on Thursdays by 9 PM." Fifth, the parents draft a written contract specifying the exchange of the target behavior for the privilege. Sixth, the parents review the contract with the adolescent at home, obtain the adolescent's input, and finalize the written contract, which everyone signs.

The family implements the contract and returns together to the next session to report on its success. With the parents and adolescent in the room, the therapist praises them for successfully writing and implementing the contract, or if difficulties arose, coaches them to revise the contract and implement it again before the next session. The parents and adolescent attend the next few sessions together, during which the therapist coaches them to write and implement comprehensive contracts for more difficult behaviors. For example, an electronics contract usually includes smart phones, videogames, computer, and internet use; access to each electronic medium contingent on following rules for when these devices can be used; and limits on the maximum amount of use (eg, videogames); and internet and smart phone use during homework time, social media, etc. Because most adolescents want unrestricted access to all forms of electronic media, these contracts are tricky to develop and implement. It is best to write a contract that specifies a small number of hours, which are easily earned (eg, make the bed, pick up the room), and then add additional hours based on behaviors that are more mentally taxing (eg, get homework done, study for examinations).

Step 8: implementing punishment systems In accordance with the parenting principle, incentives before punishments, the therapist only introduces punishments after the parents have had extensive experience with one-on-one time, praise and ignoring, effective commands, and positive incentive systems. In a session with the parents alone, the therapist explains that punishment is needed when positive approaches do not produce sufficient change in serious problem behavior. Taking away privileges and grounding are the 2 primary forms of punishment used with adolescents who have ADHD. Parents can take away texting and internet access on smart phones, video-games, computers, iPad or iPods, TVs; having friends visit; access to sports; privacy (door on the teen's room); driving; and more. Grounding refers to staying at home when the teenager wants to go out with friends. The therapist teaches parents that short duration punishments (1–2 days) are effective; extending them for weeks or months makes them difficult to monitor and ends up punishing the parents. Parents are urged to refrain from corporal punishment. In the session, the parents develop a punishment contingency for a particular behavior that does not changed sufficiently with a positive incentive system. Then, they go home to implement the punishment contingency, returning with the adolescent to the next session to review implementation and make any needed adjustments.

For example, one family wrote a curfew contract for 16-year-old Sally that specified a Friday and Saturday curfew of 11 PM; if she came home by 11 PM on both nights, she earned the right to have the same curfew for the next weekend; if she came home late on either night, her curfew was to be 9 PM for the next weekend. At first Sally came home by her curfew. But then she pushed the limits and started coming home at 11:30 PM or 12 AM. The therapist suggested that Sally be grounded to the house for the entire next weekend if she came home late on one night. After 2 groundings, Sally consistently came home by 11 PM.

Step 9: problem solving negotiable issues The parents and adolescent attend 3 to 4 sessions together to work on problem solving. In step 9 the therapist teaches family members to follow the 4 steps of problem solving to resolve all of the negotiable disagreements between them. The 4 steps are: (1) define the problem, (2) generate a list of solutions, (3) evaluate the solutions and reach an agreement, and (4) plan the implementation details. The therapist uses instructions, modeling, behavior rehearsal, feedback, and shaping to teach the family problem-solving skills. After problem solving one issue per session, the family implements the solution and reports back to the therapist. The therapist helps the family integrate problem solving into their daily routine.

Step 10: improving communication The parents and adolescent attend 2 to 3 sessions together to work on improving communication. Using a handout of communication habits,[2] the therapist and family identify the most common problems in their communication. Accusations, defensive remarks, nasty language, lectures, dredging up the past, sarcasm, interrupting, poor eye contact, silent treatment, and many others are reviewed. The family and therapist agree to work on a small number of pivotal negative communication habits. Assume a family selects accusations and defensive remarks. The therapist asks them to problem solve and stops the action whenever an accusing or defensive remark occurs. Then, the family members are asked to repeat their points using a nonaccusing "I" statement or a nondefensive but assertive statement. This process continues throughout the session followed by practice at home of alternatives to accusations and defensive remarks. Over several sessions, such a specific negative communication habit begins to change.

Step 11: putting it all together Parents and adolescents attend this session together. The therapist reviews steps 1 through 10, particularly interventions that the family has continued to use. The therapist prompts the parents and adolescents to state the changes that they have noticed and the problems that remain to be dealt with. Suggestions for coping with the remaining problems are made, and the therapist also asks for input about how to improve the intervention.

Empirical support

The empirical support for this intervention comes from 2 random assignment studies and meets the criteria for level 2 in the Oxford Center for Evidence Based Medicine criteria.[8] In the first study,[9] 61 adolescents with ADHD and their parents were randomly assigned to 8 to 10 sessions of behavior management training (BMT), problem solving communication training (PSCT), or structural family therapy (SFT). All 3 treatments resulted in significant group mean improvements on several self-report and observational measures of family interactions from preassessment to postassessment along with further improvements from postassessment to follow-up. There were no significant differences between the 3 treatment conditions. However, clinical significance analyses showed that only 10% to 24% of the families made reliable changes and moved into the normal range on the dependent measures.

To boost clinical significance, in the second study Barkley and colleagues[10] doubled the number of therapy sessions and randomly assigned 97 teenagers with ADHD and ODD and their parents to a combination of BMT (9 sessions) and PSCT (9 sessions) or to 18 sessions of PSCT alone. The combined condition is closest to the treatment described in the manual.[2] Both treatments resulted in significant group mean changes on measures of conflict, communication, and specific disputes completed by parents and adolescents. Twenty to 24% of the families made reliable changes, and 34% of 78% of the families moved into the normal range on the dependent measures; thus, the clinical significance rates were higher than those in the first study. Although there were no significant differences between BMT/PSCT and PSCT alone on the dependent measures, there was a substantial difference in dropout rates. By postassessment 18% of the families receiving BMT/PSCT versus 38% of the families receiving PSCT had dropped out. These results demonstrated that PSCT and BMT both produce change in parent-adolescent relationships for some families when adolescents have ADHD or ADHD plus ODD. The combination of BMT plus PSCT maintains the highest number of families completing treatment and would, therefore, be the recommended intervention. The clinical significance data from these 2 studies are sobering but must be understood in the proper context. Traditional family therapy produced even lower clinical significance results than BMT or PSCT.[9] In addition, medication was not standardized in these 2 studies. Many adolescents were not taking medication, and for those taking medication, the study was not designed to maximize or even control medication. In the multimodal treatment study of ADHD (MTA) study with younger children,[11] BMT alone produced much less change than medication alone or medication plus BMT. All of the treatment groups in the 2 Barkley studies[9,10] can be likened to the BMT alone group in the MTA study. Studies comparing medication alone with medication plus BMT/PSCT are needed.

Clinical decision making

1. Who is most likely to respond? Clinical impressions suggest that those who will respond are parents and adolescents from single or 2-parent families of any ethnic background in which the adolescents are diagnosed with ADHD, ODD, CD, or adjustment reactions and there is a high level of parent-adolescent conflict. However, these 2 studies did not formally examine mediators or moderators of treatment efficacy, so there is not yet an evidence-based answer to this question.
2. What outcomes are most likely to be affected by treatment? Parents rate these outcomes to be externalizing adolescent behavior, ODD symptoms, and ADHD symptoms. Parents and adolescents rate these outcomes to be communication frequency and anger intensity level of specific parent-adolescent disputes.

Observers code for positive and negative communication of videotaped parent-adolescent discussions.
3. What are the contraindications for treatment? The studies did not directly collect data on the contraindications for treatment. The investigators a priori excluded adolescents with intellectual ability less than 80, deafness, blindness, severe language delay, cerebral palsy, epilepsy, autism, or psychosis.
4. What are the potential adverse effects of treatment? The investigators did not report any adverse effects of the treatments. Clinically, an increase in conflict between the parents and the adolescent may occur when treatment fails.
5. How should treatment be sequenced or integrated with drug therapy and with other nondrug treatments? Stimulant or nonstimulant medication should be started after step 4 — Preparation for Medication. In those cases in which a parent or adolescent has significant depression or anxiety, individual cognitive behavior therapy might also be indicated.

FUTURE DIRECTIONS

Improving the percentage of families who benefit from DT is the highest priority future direction for clinicians and researchers. As noted earlier, studies comparing DT alone with DT plus medication are sorely needed. In addition, studies are needed comparing the enhanced version of DT described here to the original manualized version. The contribution of various comorbidities (ODD, CD, depression, anxiety, autism spectrum disorders) to the clinical and research outcomes from DT also need to be studied, along with the role of various parental characteristics, particularly parental ADHD (factor 2 in the 4-factor model) and environmental stressors (factor 3 in the 4-factor model). Supplementing DT with individual CBT or behavioral marital therapy for parents is often necessary clinically, but there is not yet any research that addresses the contributions of these therapies to the outcomes with DT.

SUMMARY

This article described a model and intervention for clinicians to use with families in which the adolescents have ADHD and the family is experiencing significant conflict and negative interactions. The first portion of the intervention emphasizes educating families about ADHD, developing reasonable beliefs and teaching parents to break the cycle of negativity and to use effective behavior management techniques to

---

Box 2
Recommendations for clinicians

1. Conduct a comprehensive assessment of the parent adolescent relationship, using interviews, observations, and measures such as the Parent Adolescent Relationship Questionnaire.

2. Provide psychoeducation about ADHD, the 4-factor model, and the importance of changing parenting practices.

3. Systematically follow the 11 steps outlined in this article. Do not move on to the next step until the family has completed the assignments for the previous step.

4. Help the family get to a knowledgeable physician who can appropriately prescribe medication for the adolescent.

5. Understand the implications of the clinical significance data and look for individual adolescent or parental disorders that need to be addressed for DT to work.

improve their interactions with the adolescents. The second portion emphasizes mutual problem solving and communication training to help parents and adolescents negotiate acceptable agreements and talk respectfully to each other. Two research studies support the effectiveness of the original version of this intervention but show limitations in the percentage of families who make clinically meaningful changes. The modified version discussed in this article is expected to help a larger number of families achieve clinically meaningful change. Please see **Box 2** for recommendations for clinicians (level of evidence: step 2).

REFERENCES

1. Robin AL. Training families of adolescents with ADHD. In: Barkley RA, editor. Attention deficit hyperactivity disorder: a handbook for diagnosis and treatment. 4th edition. New York: Guilford Publications; in press.
2. Barkley RA, Robin AL. Defiant teens: a clinicians manual for assessment and family intervention. 2nd edition. New York: Guilford Publications; 2014.
3. Barkley RA, Robin AL, Benton C. Your defiant teen. 2nd edition. New York: Guilford Publications; 2013.
4. Robin AL, Koepke T, Moye AW, et al. Parent adolescent relationship questionnaire professional manual. Lutz (FL): Psychological Assessment Resources; 2009.
5. Robin AL. ADHD in adolescents. New York: Guilford Publications; 1998.
6. American Psychiatric Association. Diagnostic and statistical manual of mental disorders. DSM-5. 5th edition. Arlington (VA): American Psychiatric Association; 2013.
7. Barkley RA. Barkley deficits in executive functioning scale- children and adolescents (DBEFS-CA). New York: Guilford Publications; 2012.
8. Center for evidence based medicine guidelines. Available at: http://www.cebm.net/mod_product/design/files/CEBM-Levels-of-Evidence_2.1.pdf.
9. Barkley RA, Guevremont DG, Anastopoulos AD, et al. A comparison of three family therapy programs for treating family conflict in adolescents with attention-deficit hyperactivity disorder. J Consult Clin Psychol 1992;60:450–62.
10. Barkley RA, Edwards G, Laneri M, et al. The efficacy of problem-solving communication training alone, behavior management training alone, and their combination for parent–adolescent conflict in teenagers with ADHD and ODD. J Consult Clin Psychol 2001;69:926–41.
11. The MTA Cooperative Group. A 14-month randomized clinical trials of treatment strategies for attention- deficit/hyperactivity disorder. Arch Gen Psychiatry 1999; 56:1073–86.

Summer Treatment Programs for Youth with ADHD

Gregory A. Fabiano, PhD[a],*, Nicole K. Schatz, PhD[a],
William E. Pelham Jr, PhD[b]

KEYWORDS

- Attention-deficit/hyperactivity disorder • Summer treatment program
- Behavior modification • Evidence-based treatment • Contingency management
- Parent training

KEY POINTS

- The summer treatment program (STP) is an intensive treatment for youth with attention-deficit/hyperactivity disorder (ADHD). It includes behavioral interventions that support youth in developing adaptive skills and reducing impairing behaviors.
- The STP includes child-focused interventions such as a reward and response-cost token economy and time-out. It also includes behavioral parent management training.
- The STP has been evaluated in 36 independent studies and 2 systematic reviews, making it an exemplar of intensive intervention for the treatment of youth with ADHD.

Attention-deficit/hyperactivity disorder (ADHD) is a chronic, pervasive childhood mental health disorder with a typical onset during early childhood.[1] Hallmark features of ADHD include developmentally inappropriate and excessive levels of inattention, impulsivity, and hyperactivity. These difficulties are present early in development and they persist over time.[2] These behaviors result in impaired functioning in social, academic, and occupational roles.[1] These areas of impairment include being rejected in peer relationships,[3,4] attaining lower levels of academic achievement and academic and occupational status,[5,6] and the families of youth with ADHD are marked by considerable caregiver strain.[7]

Disclosures: Dr G.A. Fabiano has received royalties from Guilford Press and consultation honoraria from Health and Wellness Partners. Dr W.E. Pelham was a coinvestigator on a research grant from Noven Pharmaceuticals from 2012 to 2013.
[a] Department of Counseling, School, and Educational Psychology, University at Buffalo, SUNY, 334 Diefendorf Hall, Buffalo, NY 14214, USA; [b] Department of Psychology, Florida International University, Miami, FL 33199, USA
* Corresponding author.
E-mail address: fabiano@buffalo.edu

Abbreviations	
ADHD	Attention-deficit/hyperactivity disorder
BPT	Behavioral parent training
COPE	Community parent education program
DRC	Daily report card
NREPP	National registry of evidence-based programs and practices
OCEBM	Oxford centre for evidence based medicine
SAMHSA	Substance abuse and mental health services administration
STP	Summer treatment program

The economic costs associated with ADHD are also substantial.[8] Estimates suggest that the lifetime costs of treating ADHD approximate the costs for major depressive disorder and stroke.[8] Costs related to ADHD are accrued within multiple functional domains, and they include medical costs (emergency room visits, pediatric care, medication costs), educational costs (costs for special education, repeating grades, academic accommodations, and tutoring), family costs (lost work time to supervise a child suspended from school or driving a child to school suspended from the bus), and justice-related costs (fines, juvenile detention). Beyond monetary costs, raising a child with ADHD can result in personal costs including higher rates of separation/divorce in families that include a youth with ADHD[9] and greater parental stress[10]; these are costs that are difficult to quantify in economic terms but they are important to consider as part of the burden of the disorder. Because of the short-term and long-term negative outcomes associated with ADHD,[11,12] effective treatment approaches are needed. It is likely that the summer treatment program (STP) is an effective intervention for individuals with ADHD because it is highly intensive, sustained, and targets behaviors within the settings in which impaired functioning is evident.

TARGET OF TREATMENT

As noted earlier, youth with ADHD experience varied and pervasive impairment in functioning. To obtain a diagnosis of ADHD consistent with the Diagnostic and Statistical Manual of Mental Disorders, Fifth Edition (DSM-5) criteria, the individual must have the requisite number of symptoms (ie, at least 6 inattentive and/or hyperactive/impulsive symptoms), the symptoms must cause functional impairment, and the symptoms must be pervasive and long-standing.[1] Thus, although the symptoms provide a criterion for the specific constellation of behaviors that must be present for a diagnosis of ADHD to be made, it is the functional impairment that drives the diagnosis and should be the target of intervention because the symptoms of ADHD are not in themselves abnormal: all people show inattentive, overactive, or impulsive behaviors from time to time; ADHD is only diagnosed if these symptoms are developmentally inappropriate, maladaptive, and dysfunctional, and if they occur over a sustained time period and across settings. Thus, impairment in functioning is the proximal target of intervention for youth with ADHD.

This manner of conceptualizing targets of treatment may run counter to prevailing approaches that prioritize targeting ADHD symptoms as the primary target of treatment and outcome measured. For instance, studies of primary outcome and systematic reviews routinely prioritize symptom ratings.[13] However, impairment is what drives initial treatment-seeking in families,[14] improvement in impaired functional domains are emphasized by parents in their evaluation of intervention components,[15] and improvement in impaired areas (eg, functioning in peer relationships, academic achievement, improvements in family functioning and parenting) are strong predictors of long-term outcome relative to ADHD symptoms.[16] Thus, one reason for the effectiveness of the STP is its explicit targeting of behaviors that are meaningful outcomes for children and families.

NEED FOR THE TREATMENT

ADHD is a disorder that relies on others to implement treatment. The evidence-based, nonpharmacologic interventions for ADHD include behavioral parent training (BPT), school-based contingency management approaches implemented in classrooms, and training interventions that teach the individual adaptive skills.[17–19] There is a large and consistent evidence base that supports the use of these approaches for youth with ADHD. However, these interventions require consistent implementation, considerable implementer effort, and they often need to be sustained over time to realize beneficial outcomes. Further, the targets of treatment that include impaired functioning in recreational settings, academic classrooms, and other situations common in daily living are not able to be treated within clinical office settings. Clinicians attempting to determine how the child behaves in response to social or academic demands have to rely on secondhand or at times third-hand reports that may be inaccurate or biased. STPs bring the treatment to the child rather than waiting for the child to access and engage with treatment. In an STP setting, intensive evidence-based treatment can be implemented, modified, and tailored. For this reason, STP interventions are also an evidence-based approach to ADHD intervention.[18]

THEORETIC OVERVIEW FOR THE STP

The STP represents a packaging of evidence-based interventions for youth with ADHD. Most of the interventions are based on an applied behavior analytical approach using operant conditioning and social learning theory.[20,21] Applied behavior analytical approaches identify the antecedents and consequences of targeted behaviors, and these, along with setting events, are manipulated so as to promote the occurrence of positive behaviors and suppress negative or maladaptive behaviors. This approach relies heavily on individuals (ie, teachers, counselors, parents) who implement strategies in the child's natural environment consistently over time. Social learning theory suggests that learning can also occur through the observation of rewards or punishments directed toward others, even if the individual does not directly experience these consequences. Thus, learning also can occur through vicarious reinforcement and modeling.[22]

Within the context of the STP, antecedents, consequences, and social learning opportunities are embedded within all program activities.[23] As described later, antecedents such as the establishment of clear rules for all activities, the provision of clear commands for expected behaviors, and structured activities support appropriate child behaviors. Consequences include time-out, a token economy supported by rewards, and labeled praise for good behavior and corrective feedback following negative behaviors. Social learning opportunities frequently include modeled social skills during group discussions as well as multiple opportunities for children to observe other youth receive rewards and punishments following clearly labeled targeted behaviors.

TREATMENT DELIVERY

The STP is a 6-week to 9-week program for children and adolescents aged 5 to 16 years. Children are placed in age-matched groups of approximately 12 to 15 children, and counselors implement treatments for each group. Groups stay together throughout the summer so that children receive intensive experience in functioning as a group, in making friends, and in interacting appropriately with adults. A notable aspect of the treatment delivery in the STP is that all interventions occur in the context of typical child and adolescent activities. Further, treatment is implemented by counselors, teachers, and aides, supervised by senior clinical staff (ie, MD or PhD level). It is also important to emphasize that weekly behavioral parent management training sessions[24] are also a component of the STP. These sessions facilitate parents' development of adaptive and effective parenting strategies that can then be applied outside the STP setting. Childcare is typically provided by STP staff 1 evening per week to facilitate parent attendance at these treatment sessions.

Treatment delivery in the STP is also continuous. From the moment the child arrives at the STP each morning until the child departs, best-practice behavioral interventions are interwoven into all daily activities. The intervention is a multicomponent approach that includes several contingency management and training strategies that are evidence based for youth with ADHD.[17–19] A treatment manual and multiple supporting documents describe the program in detail.[23] The multiple aspects of the intervention approach are briefly described later in this article.

Contingency Management

The guiding framework for the STP is a reward and response-cost token economy that assigns points for targeted behaviors within the program setting. These behaviors include adaptive behaviors that children are encouraged to exhibit more frequently (eg, following rules, ignoring provocation) and negative behaviors that children are encouraged to decrease (eg, aggression, interrupting others). Children earn points for appropriate behaviors and lose points if they behave negatively. The points that children earn are exchanged for privileges (ie, field trips), social honors and camp privileges, and home-based rewards.

Supporting the point system is an individualized daily report card (DRC), which is a best practice for youth with ADHD.[25–27] DRCs in the STP include idiographic target behaviors as well as specific criteria for meeting behavioral goals (eg, completing all seatwork assigned within the time provided at 80% accuracy or better; no instances of intentional aggression; interrupting group discussions 2 or fewer times). Target behaviors and criteria for meeting daily goals are set and revised in an ongoing manner. It is important that success on the DRC is rewarded with STP and home-based rewards. In the STP parenting sessions, parents learn how to provide home-based rewards for meeting DRC goals (eg, screen time, special activities).

There is also a need to use consequence control at times following negative behaviors in the STP. Following certain prohibited behaviors (eg, intentional aggression, repeated noncompliance), children receive a time-out from positive reinforcement. Consistent with the positive approach emphasized in the STP, time-outs are designed to be short in duration such that the child can reenter the time-in setting as soon as possible. Children also are rewarded by shorter time-outs if they show self-control and self-management after a time-out is assigned. The time-out program used in the STP assigns children with an initial time-out duration that is long (eg, 10–30 minutes depending on the child's age), but a child may immediately earn a 50% reduction in time for good behavior.[23,28]

Attention to Antecedents and Consequences

Social reinforcement in the form of praise and public recognition (buttons, stickers, and posted charts) is embedded within all activities to provide a positive, supportive atmosphere. This reinforcement begins immediately as a counselor greets the child warmly and with enthusiasm at the car door at drop-off (this can be contrasted with a typical day in other settings in which the first interaction with a child with a disruptive behavior disorder may be a reprimand or criticism). The end of the day also includes a brief conversation between the child, the counselor, and the parent to review the day's success and encourage the child to continue to work toward individual behavioral goals. In addition to the liberal use of praise, staff members attempt to shape appropriate behavior by issuing commands with characteristics (eg, brevity, specificity) that maximize compliance.[23]

Peer Interventions

Current reviews of evidence-based practice emphasize the importance of training children in adaptive functioning.[17] In the STP, social skills training is provided in brief, daily group sessions that are part of the morning meeting with the children. Specific social skills introduced and reviewed with the children include communication, participation, validation, and cooperation.[29] Sessions include instruction, modeling, role-playing, and practice in key social concepts as well as more specific skills when necessary. Throughout daily activities, children's implementation of the social skills training program is reviewed and reinforced using the other treatment components (eg, token economy, DRC). The combination of training reinforced by a contingency management approach has been shown to be necessary for children with externalizing disorders.[4]

An additional peer-focused intervention component within the STP is the emphasis on the development of sports skills and related competencies. Children with ADHD may have low knowledge of the pragmatic and social aspects of sports activities.[30,31] This limitation is concerning because sports activities currently comprise an important setting for typical development. It is estimated that a third of children in kindergarten to eighth grade participate in sports after school at least weekly.[32] Many more children participate in recreational activities informally (eg, board games, sports with neighborhood youth, playing with siblings), and thus these activities are important settings for interventions. The intensive practice and time that are necessary to effect changes in sports skills highlights the value of the STP as a setting for this goal. For instance, in a recent study in which youth were randomly assigned to receive the STP intervention or summer activities as usual, those who participated in a 6-week STP evinced improved sports knowledge and game awareness, sports skills, and improved fine and gross motor skills as measured by a standardized measure of these functional outcomes.[30]

Classrooms

Academic impairments are a key concern for youth with ADHD proximally[33,34] and distally.[5] To deal with these serious academic impairments, several academic accommodations and interventions[35,36] are integrated into the 2 to 3 hours of academic classroom time each day. Children spend 2 hours daily in a classroom modeled after an academic special education classroom, and they spend a further hour in an art class. Behavior in the classrooms is managed using a simple point system that includes both reward (earning points for work completion and accuracy) and response-cost (losing points for rule violations) components.[37–39] The other behavioral intervention strategies (eg, liberal use of labeled praise, time-out) are also integrated into the classroom. The behavior management system in the classroom is designed to be implemented by a single teacher and a classroom aide, which is consistent with the approach in most inclusive and special education settings.

The goal of the STP classroom is to teach children adaptive skills and academic enablers that can be supportive within the authentic classroom setting in the fall. Children engage in independent seatwork tasks in which they are required to persist with academic seatwork for at least 30 minutes, a peer-tutoring period in which they cooperate with a partner on a reading task in a cooperative learning exercise,[40] and a computer class in which additional academic fluency practice is implemented.

Parent Involvement

BPT is an evidence-based treatment of youth with ADHD.[17–19] BPT includes teaching parents how to use strategies similar to those used by counselors and teachers during the STP day. A typical course of BPT includes how to attend to and catch a child behaving appropriately; use planned ignoring for minor, inappropriate behaviors; use effective instructions and commands; use contingency management strategies (eg, DRCs, Premack contingencies, token economies, time-out); and use effective problem-solving strategies for new problems that might occur or new settings in which intervention is needed (eg, school, outside the home). There are several evidence-based parent training programs suitable for youth with ADHD. The parent training program most commonly used within the STP is a large-group problem-solving approach that is designed to improve maintenance of skills learned in parent training, called the Community Parent Education (COPE) program.[24] COPE is appropriate for working with large groups, such as the parents of children with the STP, and it uses an approach that encourages parents to identify parenting errors and then generate personal solutions for managing identified problems. Parents practice parenting strategies through role-play and weekly at-home assignments. The BPT component of the STP is nearly universally attended by parents, with most attending all sessions. This participation rate is considerably greater than that found in community or standalone BPT courses for youth with ADHD,[41] suggesting that one advantage of the STP is the engagement and retention of parents in a course of this effective treatment.

Beyond the formal, weekly BPT classes, there are several other opportunities for parental involvement. Parents have daily contact with staff members and with each other when they drop off or pick up their children. At times based on individual family needs, or for parents who have already completed the foundational BPT course, the children and their parents participate in shared exercises and activities, using in vivo training situations. The STP has also spawned several BPT approaches to target particular groups in need of specialized support, including mothers with depressed mood,[10] fathers,[42,43] and low-income or single-parent families.[44]

Medication Assessment

Stimulant medication is an evidence-based intervention for youth with ADHD.[45] The stimulants prescribed to children with ADHD are generally inadequately assessed and monitored,[46] which may result in the overall poor compliance with, and sustainability of, this intervention.[47] If desired by the child's parent(s), and the child's response to the intensive behavioral treatment within the STP is not sufficient to normalize functioning, a child may undergo a controlled evaluation of the effects of stimulant medication.[23] Data gathered routinely in the STP provide ecologically valid outcome measures of the effects of medication within the child's daily activities. Staff and parents can also provide daily ratings of side effects to determine whether there are any reasons to discontinue medication or adjust doses.

In numerous studies conducted in the STP in which doses of medication have been compared, lower doses of medication (eg, 0.15 mg/kg to 0.30 mg/kg methylphenidate given twice daily) combined with behavior modification are routinely as effective as doses of methylphenidate of 0.60 mg/kg twice a day.[37–39,48,49] Recent studies within the STP have clearly shown that even a modified, less intensive version of the STP procedures can be combined with a low dose (0.15 mg/kg twice a day) of methylphenidate to produce benefits comparable to 0.60 mg/kg twice a day used alone.[38,48]

Developmental Modifications

Most of the description given earlier applies to the STP for elementary-aged children with ADHD. However, the STP has been successfully modified at both ends of the ADHD age spectrum: preschoolers and adolescents. Manuals have been developed for both of these ages, and the data indicate that the program works well for preschool-aged children through the middle school and early high school years.[50–54] The modifications are those that would be expected for use with very young children and with adolescents. For example, the classroom procedures are adapted to resemble preschool and middle/high school classrooms, respectively. The point system and procedures are simplified for younger children, and the program for teens involves more involvement of the teen in treatment (eg, selecting treatment goals).

Individualized Programming

As discussed earlier, the STP is a highly operationalized and rigorous treatment with a set of clearly detailed treatment manuals that describe all aspects of the treatment programming. However, it is also important to note that the STP is a highly flexible intervention that includes clear procedures for determining whether treatment modifications are needed, how to make treatment modifications, and how to evaluate these modifications. Some modifications are made on a group level. For instance, procedures are included in the STP manual for group problem-solving discussions and group contingencies, which are modifications of interventions applied to the entire group of children.

The STP manual also includes an article on how to develop and evaluate individualized behavioral programming for youth who are nonresponsive to the standard STP procedures. There are a multitude of modifications that can be made to the STP procedures, including reducing latency to reward, increasing or modifying feedback on behavior, modifying time-out strategies, and enhancing staff-to-child interactions. Given the standardized STP schedule, procedures, and measurement of outcomes, individualized programming can be rigorously used and evaluated using single-subject research methodology.[55] In addition to providing more effective intervention within the context of the STP, individualized behavioral programs also provide information on effective intervention approaches that might be useful in the child's home or school setting.[56]

Monitoring Treatment Integrity and Fidelity

For any intervention, the integrity and fidelity of implementation are critical constructs to assess and provide feedback to clinicians.[57] Treatment fidelity can be defined as the skill, care, and genuineness with which the intervention is implemented, and integrity refers to the degree to which the intervention was implemented as intended. Multiple procedures have been developed to monitor integrity and fidelity in the STP setting.[23] Integrity materials include both lists of treatment procedures and ratings of the quality of treatment that staff members are providing, and 20 fidelity forms have been developed that cover every intervention and related component parts

Table 1	
Sample daily schedule for the STP	
Time	**Activity**
7:30–8:00 AM	Arrivals
8:00–8:15 AM	Morning discussion/social skills review and training
8:15–8:25 AM	Transition/bathroom break
8:25–9:25 AM	Sports skill drills: soccer
9:25–9:35 AM	Transition/bathroom break
9:35–11:35 AM	Academic classroom (seatwork, classwide peer tutoring, and computer classes)
11:35–11:45 AM	Transition/bathroom break
11:45 AM–12:00 PM	Lunch
12:00–12:15 PM	Recess
12:15–1:15 PM	Recreational activity: soccer game
1:15–1:25 PM	Transition/bathroom break
1:25–2:25 PM	Art classroom
2:25–2:35 PM	Transition/bathroom break
2:35–3:35 PM	Basketball game
3:35–4:45 PM	Swimming
4:45–5:00 PM	Recess
5:00–5:30 PM	Departures

Note: For 1 designated day during each week a parent training class is held from 6:30 to 8:30 PM. Program staff provide childcare while the parents are in the meeting.

used in the STP. **Table 1** includes a sample program day, and integrity and fidelity forms are available for each activity listed.

EMPIRICAL SUPPORT

The STP has been used as an intervention since the early 1980s. It was developed by William E. Pelham, Jr, as a set of activities for children with ADHD participating in a classroom-based medication efficacy study[58] at Florida State University. The recreational and other activities that filled the remainder of the day were so well received by the parents of children in the study they requested that the STP be implemented as an intervention during the next summer. Since that time, the STP has been established in several academic settings (eg, University of Pittsburgh Medical Center; University at Buffalo; Florida International University; New York University Medical Center; The Cleveland Clinic; University of Illinois, Chicago, Medical Center). It was a core component of the psychosocial treatment used by the Multimodal Treatment Study of ADHD (MTA) study.[59] It has been adapted for use in community settings.[60,61] Several community agencies have implemented the STP nationally and internationally.[61–64] Although outside the scope of this article, the STP procedures have also been successfully adapted for use in general education classroom settings,[65] parent training programs designed to engage and intervene with fathers,[42,43] and investigations of medication efficacy.[66,67] The remainder of the review of the evidence for the STP focuses on studies for youth that occurred in the STP model as operationalized in the treatment manual.[23]

Before discussing the specific empirical studies, it is important to describe the results of other systematic reviews of the STP. The Substance Abuse and Mental Health

Services Administration (SAMHSA) has reviewed the STP and includes it in its National Registry of Evidence-based Programs and Practices (NREPP). As an arm of SAMSHA, NREPP individually reviews treatments for mental health and assigns a rating of the strength of the evidence base supporting the intervention as well as a rating of readiness for dissemination. In September 2008 the NREPP review provided a quality of research rating of 3.3 out of 4.0 and a readiness for dissemination rating of 3.8 out of 4.0; these were both favorable scores supporting the STP intervention.

The STP has also been systematically reviewed by 2 independent teams applying the American Psychological Association, Division 53 Clinical Child and Adolescent Psychology criteria for evidence-based treatment. Pelham and Fabiano[18] concluded that the STP meets criteria for a well-established evidence-based treatment based on 2 between-group studies, 5 crossover design studies, and multiple single-case design studies. Evans and colleagues[17] updated the prior review and reached similar conclusions that interventions that provide training opportunities for children to develop and practice adaptive skills are a well-established treatment. This conclusion included the STP as well as other interventions that enhance peer relationship, social skills, and academic skills.

For the present article, the Oxford Centre for Evidence-Based Medicine (OCEBM) guidelines were used to categorize the rigor of the studies conducted to evaluate the STP or component parts. **Table 2** includes each of the studies within the review as well as a classification of study methodology using the guidelines. Overall, 38 studies were identified that evaluated the STP or component parts. **Table 2** shows that there are 2 systematic reviews of the STP evidence base (as described earlier), 15 randomized controlled trials (either between-group or crossover design), 1 quasiexperimental design, and 20 single-subject or case-series design investigations of the STP or component parts. This evidence base is large and includes clear evidence for the STP as an intervention with support for the OCEBM question of "Does the intervention help?" Thus, there is clear and replicated evidence, across the past 30 years and different investigatory teams, that the STP is an efficacious intervention. Based on OCEBM guidelines, the STP is a level 1 intervention.

CLINICAL DECISION MAKING
Who is Most Likely to Respond?

The studies included in **Table 2** include a range of ages from preschoolers[30] to adolescents.[51] The preponderance of evidence within studies has been collected from investigations of the STP with elementary school–aged children (ie, 6–12 years of age). Most participants in these studies are also boys. Although there is no clear indication that girls respond any differently to the STP procedures than boys, this is an empirical question in need of further study (see Babinski and colleagues[68] for an example of how gender may affect treatment response in some domains for adolescents). The STP has been successfully modified for different developmental levels, so the current evidence suggests effectiveness across different age ranges. Analyses of individual differences have routinely shown that children with ADHD with and without conduct problems respond equally well to the STP and that STP response is independent of socioeconomic status.[69]

What Outcomes Are Most Likely to be Affected by Treatment?

Table 2 lists overall domains targeted by the STP intervention. Most studies target academic (eg, seatwork completion, classroom rule following, notetaking skill building), and social outcomes (peer and adult interactions). Additional targets of the STP treatment include sports skill and sportsmanship development (eg, O'Connor and

Table 2
Oxford levels of evidence summary table for STP studies

Study/Year	Target	Design	OCEBM Rating
Evans et al,[17] 2013	Academic and social	Systematic review	1
Pelham & Fabiano,[18] 2008	Academic and social	Systematic review	1
August et al,[71] 2001	Academic and social	Between group	2
Carlson et al,[37] 1992	Academic and social	Within subject	2
Chronis et al,[72] 2004	Academic and social	Within subject	2
Evans et al,[73] 1995	Academic	Within subject	2
Fabiano et al,[28] 2004	Academic and social	Within subject	2
Fabiano et al,[a,38] 2007	Academic and social	Within subject	2
Haas et al,[74] 2011	Social	Within subject	2
Kolko et al,[75] 1999	Academic and social	Within subject	2
Manos et al,[76] 2012	Academic and social	Within subject	2
MTA Cooperative Group,[b,13] 1999	Academic and social	Between group	2
O'Connor et al,[30] 2013	Social and athletics	Between group	2
Pelham et al,[39] 1993	Academic and social	Within subject	2
Pelham et al,[49] 2005	Academic and social	Within subject	2
Pelham et al,[b,77] 2000	Academic and social	Between group	2
Pelham et al,[a,48] 2014	Social	Within subject	2
O'Connor et al,[61] 2012	Academic and social	Between group	3
Chronis et al,[56] 2001	Academic and social	Single subject	4
Coles et al,[55] 2005	Academic and social	Single subject	4
Graziano et al,[50] 2014	Academic and social	Within subject	4
Gulley et al,[78] 2003	Social	Single subject	4
Hoza et al,[79] 1992	Academic and social	Single subject	4
Hupp & Reitman,[80] 1999	Social and athletics	Single subject	4
Hupp et al,[81] 2002	Social	Single subject	4
Miller et al,[82] 2013	Social	Within subject	4
Northup et al,[83] 1997	Social	Single subject	4
Northup et al,[84] 1999	Social	Single subject	4
O'Callaghan et al,[85] 2003	Social	Single subject	4
Pelham & Hoza,[69] 1996	Academic and social	Within subject	4
Reitman et al,[86] 2001	Social	Single subject	4
Sibley et al,[87] 2013	Social	Within subject	4
Sibley et al,[52] 2011	Academic and social	Within subject	4
Sibley et al, (a)[51] 2012	Academic and social	Within subject	4
Sibley et al, (b)[88] 2012	Social	Single subject	4
Waschbusch et al,[89] 1998	Academic and social	Single subject	4
Yamashita et al,[c,63] 2011	Social, academic, cognitive	Within subject	4
Yamashita et al,[c,64] 2010	Academic and social	Within subject	4

Abbreviation: SRP, summer research program.
[a] Indicates reports from the SRP study investigating single and combined effects of behavior therapy and stimulant medication.
[b] Indicates reports from the Multimodal Treatment Study for attention-deficit/hyperactivity disorder.
[c] Overlapping sample from summer treatment programs conducted in Japan.

colleagues[30]). Future work should focus on other positive outcomes from the STP such as modifications in parenting and maintenance of STP treatment gains in the child's natural settings following the program.

What Are the Contraindications or Adverse Effects of Treatment?

There are no identified contraindications or adverse effects of treatment. Some children respond with increased disruptive behaviors because of the behavioral demands present in the STP setting. However, this is typically reduced as the program progresses, or through the implementation of individualized behavioral programs. There was also a concern raised within the larger field regarding whether group treatments for youth with disruptive behavior disorders results in so-called deviancy training.[70] Given its emphasis on delivering the intervention in a group context, the STP could potentially present this adverse effect. However, the extent to which this was a problem in the STP was addressed empirically, and deviancy training occurs rarely and at levels comparable with typically developing children in the context of the STP behavioral intervention(Helseth SA, Waschbusch DA, Gnagy EM, et al: Effects of behavioral and pharmacological therapies on peer reinforcement of deviancy in children with ADHD-only, ADHD and conduct problems, and controls. Submitted for publication). The rates of deviancy training are present to a significant extent if the STP behavioral intervention components are removed. Thus, for individuals conducting group interventions with youth with ADHD, the procedures used in the STP can mitigate the possibility of deviancy training in group-based treatment.

How Should the Treatment be Sequenced with Drug Therapy and Other Nondrug Treatments?

There is no current study investigating the appropriate sequencing of drug therapy with the STP intervention. In the largest study of the STP,[13] the STP occurred for most participants around the same time, after medication was established. Other crossover studies did not address sequencing as an aim. An advantage of the STP is that the daily point system, DRC, and other observational measures provide clear indications of response to intervention and progress. It seems logical to start the child in the STP off medication, in order to determine whether medication is necessary. Studies of the STP intervention, compared with no-STP intervention, indicate that for many children there are sizable treatment effects.[38,48] Adding medication may improve behavior incrementally, but for many children and their parents these improvements are not clinically meaningful. Future study is needed to investigate the interactions between treatment modality, treatment intensity, and outcomes targeted.

FUTURE DIRECTIONS

This article outlines the STP, the components included within the intervention, and the state of the evidence base. Based on the large number of studies, including systematic reviews, clinical trials, and case studies, there is clear and strong evidence in support of the STP as an intervention for youth with ADHD. Future directions include continued study of the STP, and associated programs as implemented in after-school, school, and community settings.[60] Two current projects funded by the Institute of Education Sciences examine the utility of the STP as a summer transition from preschool to kindergarten, from elementary to middle, and from middle to high school. Further, researchers should study various ways of sequencing the STP in the context of a treatment package for individual children, as well as varying intensities of implementation.[38,48] Cost-effectiveness studies are also needed to determine in part whether all children with

ADHD need and benefit from an intervention as intensive as the STP. In addition, investigating the best way to integrate the STP into a multimodal and chronic model of treatment of ADHD is also needed. The STP represents a best-practice intervention for treating the academic and social impairments present in youth with ADHD, and it is a model program for building child and family competencies to alleviate these impairments. Given the strength of these findings, future directions also include problem-solving how to increase access and affordability of this intensive intervention. This problem-solving could be done by reallocating resources from existing community or school district–based summer programs to underwrite an intensive treatment such as the STP. Community agencies and clinics may also find that the start-up costs of the STP are acceptable given the high patient retention, satisfaction, and improved functioning that results from the treatment. Compared with other interventions for ADHD that are not evidence supported (eg, individual counseling with the child) but are widely implemented, dedicating resources to STP interventions instead is justified.

REFERENCES

1. American Psychiatric Association. Diagnostic and statistical manual of mental disorders. 5th edition. Washington, DC: American Psychiatric Association; 2013.
2. American Academy of Pediatrics. ADHD: clinical practice guideline for the diagnosis, evaluation, and treatment of attention-deficit/hyperactivity disorder in children and adolescents. Pediatrics 2011;128:1–9.
3. Hinshaw SP, Melnick SM. Peer relationships in boys with attention-deficit hyperactivity disorder with and without comorbid aggression. Dev Psychopathol 1995;7:627–47.
4. Pelham WE, Bender ME. Peer relationships in hyperactive children: description and treatment. Adv Learn Behav Disabil 1982;1:365–436.
5. Kent KM, Pelham WE, Molina BS, et al. The academic experience of male high school students with ADHD. J Abnorm Child Psychol 2012;39:451–562.
6. Kuriyan AB, Pelham WE, Molina BS, et al. Young adult educational and vocational outcomes of children diagnosed with ADHD. J Abnorm Child Psychol 2013;41:27–41.
7. Anastopoulos AD, Sommer JL, Schatz NK. ADHD and family functioning. Current Attention Disorders Reports 2009;1:167–70.
8. Pelham WE, Foster EM, Robb JA. The economic impact of ADHD in children and adolescents. Ambul Pediatr 2007;7:121–31.
9. Wymbs BT, Pelham WE, Molina BS, et al. Rate and predictors of divorce among parents of youths with ADHD. J Consult Clin Psychol 2008;76:735–44.
10. Chronis AM, Gamble SA, Roberts JE, et al. Cognitive-behavioral depression treatment for mothers of children with attention-deficit/hyperactivity disorder. Behav Ther 2006;37:143–58.
11. Fabiano GA, Pelham WE, Waschbusch D, et al. A practical measure of impairment: psychometric properties of the Impairment Rating Scale in samples of children with attention-deficit/hyperactivity disorder and two school-based samples. J Clin Child Adolesc Psychol 2006;35:369–85.
12. Molina BS, Hinshaw SP, Swanson JM, et al. MTA at 8 years: prospective follow-up of children treated for combined type ADHD in a multisite study. J Am Acad Child Adolesc Psychiatry 2009;48:484–500.
13. MTA Cooperative Group. A 14-month randomized clinical trial of treatment strategies for attention-deficit/hyperactivity disorder. Arch Gen Psychiatry 1999;56: 1073–86.

14. Angold A, Costello EJ, Farmer EM, et al. Impaired but undiagnosed. J Am Acad Child Adolesc Psychiatry 1999;38:129–37.
15. Waschbusch DA, Cunningham CE, Pelham WE, et al. A discrete choice conjoint experiment to evaluate parent preferences for treatment of young, medication naïve children with ADHD. J Clin Child Adolesc Psychol 2011;40:546–61.
16. Pelham WE, Fabiano GA. Treatment of attention-deficit hyperactivity disorder: the impact of comorbidity. J Clin Psychol Psychother 2001;8:315–29.
17. Evans SW, Owens JS, Bunford N. Evidence-based psychosocial treatment for children and adolescents with attention-deficit/hyperactivity disorder. J Clin Child Adolesc Psychol 2013. http://dx.doi.org/10.1080/15374416.2013.850700.
18. Pelham WE, Fabiano GA. Evidence-based psychosocial treatment for ADHD: an update. J Clin Child Adolesc Psychol 2008;37:184–214.
19. Pelham WE, Wheeler T, Chronis A. Empirically supported psychosocial treatments for attention deficit hyperactivity disorder. J Clin Child Psychol 1998;27:190–205.
20. Martin G, Pear J. Behavior modification: what it is and how to do it. New York: Pearson; 2010.
21. O'Leary KD, O'Leary SG. Classroom management: the successful use of behavior modification. New York: Pergamon Press; 1972.
22. Bandura A, Ross D, Ross SA. Imitation of film-mediated aggressive models. J Abnorm Soc Psychol 1963;66:3–11.
23. Pelham WE, Greiner AR, Gnagy EM. Children's summer treatment program manual. Unpublished Treatment Manual. Miami (FL): Florida International University; 2012.
24. Cunningham CE, Bremner R, Secord M. The Community Parent Education (COPE) program: a school based family systems oriented course for parents of children with disruptive behavior disorders. Unpublished manual. Hamilton (ON): COPE Works; 1998.
25. Fabiano GA, Vujnovic R, Pelham WE, et al. Enhancing the effectiveness of special education programming for children with ADHD using a daily report card. Sch Psychol Rev 2010;39:219–39.
26. O'Leary KD, Pelham WE, Rosenbaum A, et al. Behavioral treatment of hyperkinetic children. Clin Pediatr 1976;15:510–5.
27. Volpe R, Fabiano GA. Daily behavior report cards: an evidence-based system of assessment and intervention. New York: The Guilford Press; 2013.
28. Fabiano GA, Pelham WE, Manos M, et al. An evaluation of three time out procedures for children with attention-deficit/hyperactivity disorder. Behav Ther 2004;35:449–69.
29. Oden S, Asher SR. Coaching children in social skills for friendship making. Child Dev 1977;48:495–506.
30. O'Connor BC, Fabiano GA, Waschbusch DA, et al. Effects of a summer treatment program on functional sports outcomes in young children with ADHD. J Abnorm Child Psychol 2013. http://dx.doi.org/10.1007/s10802-013-9830-0.
31. Pelham WE, McBurnett K, Harper GW, et al. Methylphenidate and baseball playing in ADHD children: who's on first? J Consult Clin Psychol 1990;58:130–3.
32. Wirt J, Choy S, Rooney P, et al. The condition of education 2006 (NCES 2006-071). Washington, DC: US Department of Education, National Center for Educational Statistics; 2006.
33. McConaughy SH, Volpe RJ, Antshel KM, et al. Academic and social impairments in elementary school children with attention deficit hyperactivity disorder. Sch Psychol Rev 2011;40:200–25.

34. Pfiffner LJ, Villodas M, Kaiser N, et al. Educational outcomes of a collaborative school-home behavioral intervention for ADHD. Sch Psychol Q 2013;28:25–36.
35. DuPaul GJ, Stoner GD. ADHD in the schools: assessment and intervention strategies. New York: The Guilford Press; 2003.
36. Raggi VL, Chronis AM. Interventions to address the academic impairment of children and adolescents with ADHD. Clin Child Fam Psychol Rev 2003;9: 85–111.
37. Carlson CL, Pelham WE, Milich R, et al. Single and combined effects of methylphenidate and behavior therapy on the classroom performance of children with attention-deficit hyperactivity disorder. J Abnorm Child Psychol 1992;20: 213–32.
38. Fabiano GA, Pelham WE, Gnagy EM, et al. The single and combined effects of multiple intensities of behavior modification and multiple intensities of methylphenidate in a classroom setting. Sch Psychol Rev 2007;36:195–216.
39. Pelham WE, Carlson C, Sams SE, et al. Separate and combined effects of methylphenidate and behavior modification on boys with attention deficit-hyperactivity disorder in the classroom. J Consult Clin Psychol 1993;61:506–15.
40. Fuchs D, Fuchs LS, Mathes PG, et al. Peer assisted learning strategies: making classrooms more responsive to diversity. American Educational Research Journal 1997;34:174–206.
41. Chronis AM, Chacko A, Fabiano GA, et al. Enhancements to the behavioral parent training paradigm for families of children with ADHD: review and future directions. Clin Child Fam Psychol Rev 2004;7:1–27.
42. Fabiano GA, Chacko A, Pelham WE, et al. A comparison of behavioral parent training programs for fathers of children with attention-deficit/hyperactivity disorder. Behav Ther 2009;40:190–204.
43. Fabiano GA, Pelham WE, Cunningham CE, et al. A waitlist-controlled trial of behavioral parent training for fathers of children with attention-deficit/hyperactivity disorder. J Clin Child Adolesc Psychol 2012;41:337–45.
44. Chacko A, Wymbs BT, Wymbs FA, et al. Enhancing traditional behavioral parent training for single mothers of children with ADHD. J Clin Child Adolesc Psychol 2009;38:206–18.
45. Conners CK. Forty years of methylphenidate treatment in attention-deficit/hyperactivity disorder. J Atten Disord 2002;6(Suppl 1):S17–30.
46. Pelham WE. Pharmacotherapy for children with attention deficit hyperactivity disorder. Sch Psychol Rev 1993;22:199–227.
47. Swanson JM. Compliance with stimulants for attention-deficit/hyperactivity disorder: issues and approaches for improvement. CNS Drugs 2003;17:117–31.
48. Pelham WE, Burrows-MacLean L, Gnagy EM, et al. A dose-ranging study of behavioral and pharmacological treatment in social settings for children with ADHD. J Abnorm Child Psychol 2014. http://dx.doi.org/10.1007/s10802-013-9843-8.
49. Pelham WE, Burrows-MacLean L, Gnagy EM, et al. Transdermal methylphenidate, behavioral, and combined treatment for children with ADHD. Exp Clin Psychopharmacol 2005;13:111–26.
50. Graziano PA, Slavec J, Hart K, et al. Improving school readiness in preschoolers with behavior problems: results from a summer treatment program. J Psychopathol Behav Assess 2014. http://dx.doi.org/10.1007/s10862-014-9418-1.
51. Sibley MH, Smith BH, Evans SW, et al. Treatment response to an intensive summer treatment program for adolescents with ADHD. J Atten Disord 2012;16: 443–8.

52. Sibley MH, Pelham WE, Evans SW, et al. Evaluation of a summer treatment program for adolescents with ADHD. Cognit Behav Pract 2011;18:530–44.
53. Sibley MH, Pelham WE, Evans SW, et al. Summer treatment program for adolescents treatment manual. Unpublished Treatment Manual. Miami (FL): Florida International University; 2014.
54. Hart KC, Pelham WE, Graziano P, et al. Summer Treatment Program for PreKindergarteners (STP-PreK). Unpublished treatment manual. Miami (FL): Florida International University; 2014.
55. Coles EK, Pelham WE, Gnagy EM, et al. A controlled evaluation of behavioral treatment with children with ADHD attending a summer treatment program. J Emot Behav Disord 2005;13:99–112.
56. Chronis AM, Fabiano GA, Gnagy EM, et al. Comprehensive, sustained behavioral and pharmacological treatment for attention-deficit/hyperactivity disorder: a case study. Cognit Behav Pract 2001;8:346–59.
57. Waltz J, Addis ME, Koerner K, et al. Testing the integrity of a psychotherapy protocol: assessment of adherence and competence. J Consult Clin Psychol 1993; 61:620–30.
58. Pelham WE, Bender ME, Caddell J, et al. Methylphenidate and children with attention deficit hyperactivity disorder: dose effects on classroom academic and social behavior. Arch Gen Psychiatry 1985;42:948–52.
59. Wells KC, Pelham WE, Kotkin RA, et al. Psychosocial treatment strategies in the MTA study: rationale, methods, and critical issues in design and implementation. J Abnorm Child Psychol 2000;28:483–505.
60. Frazier SL, Chacko A, Van Gessel C, et al. The summer treatment program meets the south side of Chicago: bridging science and service in urban afterschool programs. Child Adolesc Ment Health 2012;17:86–92.
61. O'Connor BC, Tresco KE, Pelham WE, et al. Modifying an evidence-based summer treatment program for use in a summer school setting: a pilot effectiveness evaluation. School Mental Health 2012;4:143–54.
62. Pelham WE, Fabiano GA, Gnagy EM, et al. The role of summer treatment programs in the context of comprehensive treatment for ADHD. In: Hibbs E, Jensen P, editors. Psychosocial treatments for child and adolescent disorders: empirically based strategies for clinical practice. 2nd edition. Washington, DC: APA Press; 2005. p. 377–410.
63. Yamashita Y, Mukasa A, Anai C, et al. Summer treatment program for children with attention deficit hyperactivity disorder: Japanese experience in 5 years. Brain Dev 2011;33:260–7.
64. Yamashita Y, Mukasa A, Honda Y, et al. Short-term effect of American summer treatment program for Japanese children with attention deficit hyperactivity disorder. Brain Dev 2010;32:115–22.
65. Pelham WE, Massetti GM, Wilson T, et al. Implementation of a comprehensive schoolwide behavioral intervention: the ABC program. J Atten Disord 2005;9: 248–60.
66. Pelham WE, Gnagy EM, Burrows-Maclean L, et al. Once-a-day Concerta™ methylphenidate versus t.i.d. methylphenidate in laboratory and natural settings. Pediatrics 2001;107:e105. Available at: http://www.pediatrics.org/cgi/content/full/107/6/e105.
67. Pelham WE, Gnagy EM, Chronis AM, et al. A comparison of morning, midday, and late-afternoon methylphenidate with morning and late-afternoon Adderall in children with attention-deficit/hyperactivity disorder. Pediatrics 1999;104(6): 1300–11.

68. Babinski DE, Sibley MH, Ross JM, et al. The effects of single versus mixed gender treatment for adolescent girls with ADHD. J Clin Child Adolesc Psychol 2013;42:243–50.

69. Pelham WE, Hoza B. Intensive treatment: a summer treatment program for children with ADHD. In: Hibbs ED, Jensen PS, editors. Psychosocial treatments for child and adolescent disorders: empirically based strategies for clinical practices. Washington, DC: American Psychological Association; 1996. p. 311–40.

70. Dishion TJ, Spracklen KM, Andrews DW, et al. Deviancy training in male adolescent friendships. Behav Ther 1996;27:373–90.

71. August GJ, Realmuto GM, Hektner JM, et al. An integrated components preventive intervention for aggressive elementary school children: the Early Risers Program. J Consult Clin Psychol 2001;69:614–26.

72. Chronis AM, Fabiano GA, Gnagy EM, et al. An evaluation of the summer treatment program for children with attention-deficit/hyperactivity disorder using a treatment withdrawal design. Behav Ther 2004;35:561–85.

73. Evans SW, Pelham W, Grudberg MV. The efficacy of notetaking to improve behavior and comprehension of adolescents with attention-deficit hyperactivity disorder. Exceptionality 1995;5:1–17.

74. Haas SM, Waschbusch DA, Pelham WE, et al. Treatment response in CP/ADHD children with callous/unemotional traits. J Abnorm Child Psychol 2011;39: 541–52.

75. Kolko DJ, Bukstein OG, Barron J. Methylphenidate and behavior modification in children with ADHD and comorbid ODD and CD: main and incremental effects across settings. J Am Acad Child Adolesc Psychiatry 1999;38:578–86.

76. Manos MJ, Caserta DA, Short EJ, et al. Evaluation of the duration of action and comparative effectiveness of lisdexamfetamine dimesylate and behavioral treatment in youth with ADHD in a quasi-naturalistic setting. J Atten Disord 2012. http://dx.doi.org/10.1177/1087054712452915.

77. Pelham WE, Gnagy EM, Greiner AR, et al. Behavioral versus behavioral and pharmacological treatment in ADHD children attending a summer treatment program. J Abnorm Child Psychol 2000;28:507–25.

78. Gulley V, Northup J, Hupp S, et al. Sequential evaluation of behavioral treatments and methylphenidate dosage for children with attention deficit hyperactivity disorder. J Appl Behav Anal 2003;36:375–8.

79. Hoza B, Pelham WE, Sams SE, et al. An examination of the "dosage" effects of both behavior therapy and methylphenidate on the classroom performance of two ADHD children. Behav Modif 1992;16:164–92.

80. Hupp SD, Reitman D. Improving sports skills and sportsmanship in children diagnosed with attention-deficit/hyperactivity disorder. Child Fam Behav Ther 1999;21:35–51.

81. Hupp SD, Reitman D, Northup J, et al. The effects of delayed rewards, tokens, and stimulant medication on sportsmanlike behavior with ADHD-diagnosed children. Behav Modif 2002;26:148–62.

82. Miller NV, Haas SM, Waschbusch DA, et al. Behavior therapy and callous-unemotional traits: effects of a pilot study examining modified behavioral contingencies on child behavior. Behav Ther 2013. http://dx.doi.org/10.1016/j.beth.2013.10.006.

83. Northup J, Jones K, Broussard C, et al. A preliminary analysis of interactive effects between common classroom contingencies and methylphenidate. J Appl Behav Anal 1997;30:121–5.

84. Northup J, Fusilier I, Swanson V, et al. Further analysis of the separate and interactive effects of methylphenidate and common classroom contingencies. J Appl Behav Anal 1999;32:35–50.
85. O'Callaghan PM, Reitman D, Northup J, et al. Promoting social skills generalization with ADHD-diagnosed children in a sports setting. Behav Ther 2003;34: 313–30.
86. Reitman D, Hupp SD, O'Callaghan PM, et al. The influence of a token economy and methylphenidate on attentive and disruptive behavior during sports with ADHD-diagnosed children. Behav Modif 2001;25:305–23.
87. Sibley MH, Ross JM, Gnagy EM, et al. An intensive summer treatment program for ADHD reduces parent-adolescent conflict. Journal Psychopathology Behavioral Assessment 2013;35:10–9.
88. Sibley MH, Pelham WE, Mazur A, et al. The effect of video feedback on the social behavior of an adolescent with ADHD. J Atten Disord 2012;16:579–88.
89. Waschbusch DA, Kipp HL, Pelham WE. Generalization of behavioral and psychostimulant treatment of attention-deficit/hyperactivity disorder (ADHD): discussion and examples. Behav Res Ther 1998;36:675–94.

Social Skills Training

Amori Yee Mikami, PhD*, Mary Jia, BSc, Jennifer Jiwon Na, BSc

KEYWORDS

- Social skills • Social competency • Peer relationships • Social behavior • ADHD

KEY POINTS

- Social impairment among youth with attention-deficit/hyperactivity disorder (ADHD) is common, and often persists after administration of interventions documented to reduce the core symptoms of the disorder (eg, medication, behavioral contingency management).
- Traditional SST is an intervention intended to target social impairment, which focuses on increasing children's knowledge of skilled behaviors and in-session practice. However, traditional SST approaches may have difficulty with encouraging treated children's generalization of knowledge to out-of-session contexts and with changing peers' negative biases toward children with ADHD.
- Alternative SST approaches that heavily involve parents and teachers to provide children with in vivo reminders during real-world peer interactions, and to help alter peers' behaviors toward children with ADHD, may hold promise.

INTRODUCTION/BACKGROUND

Although social problems are not part of the diagnostic criteria of attention-deficit/hyperactivity disorder (ADHD), impairment in social functioning is a prominent associated feature of this condition.[1] Social impairment can be displayed in multiple ways,[2] but a common manifestation is the poor, unskilled behaviors that children with ADHD display in social situations.[3,4] Specifically, children with ADHD are likely to engage in aggressive and disruptive behaviors with peers, such as intruding into ongoing conversations, breaking rules in games, and being a sore loser.[5] Children with ADHD also may be less likely than their typically developing peers to display prosocial behaviors, such as helpfulness, consideration, or leadership.[6] However, the differences between children with ADHD and typically developing children may predominantly lie in the presence of disruptive/offensive social behavior and less in the absence of prosocial behavior.[6,7] At least partially as a result of these poor social behaviors, children with ADHD are likely to be rejected (disliked) by their peer group and tend to have fewer, or no, reciprocated friendships,[8] problems referred to as poor regard by peers.

None of the authors has any conflict of interest to disclose.
Department of Psychology, University of British Columbia, 2136 West Mall, Vancouver, British Colombia V6T 1Z4, Canada
* Corresponding author.
E-mail address: mikami@psych.ubc.ca

Abbreviations	
ADHD	Attention-deficit/hyperactivity disorder
SST	Social skills training

Poor peer regard is another commonly considered indication of social impairment in this population.[2]

These social problems are concerning because they incrementally increase the likelihood that children with ADHD will experience subsequent emotional/behavioral maladjustment. Several studies find that if children with ADHD had social impairment, this augmented the risk associated with ADHD diagnostic status for depression/anxiety, delinquency, academic problems, eating pathology, and substance abuse in adolescence[9–11]; note that these effects have been found regardless of whether measures of unskilled social behavior or peer rejection were used to index social impairment. Poor social behavior and negative peer regard may compound one another, leading to cascading negative effects of peer problems over time. In one study, the extent to which classroom peers disliked the participant in childhood predicted children lacking socially skilled behavior, which in turn predicted exacerbated peer rejection and maladjustment in adolescence.[12]

Another reason why social impairment is concerning is because treatments that reduce the core symptoms of ADHD are less successful in improving the associated feature of social impairment. In the Multimodal Treatment Study of Children with ADHD (MTA),[13] intensive pharmacotherapy and the combination of pharmacotherapy and behavioral management were efficacious at reducing inattentive and hyperactive/impulsive symptoms. However, although the combination treatment yielded improvement in adult informant reported social skills, no study treatment resulted in improvements in children's peer regard, as assessed via liking and friendship nominations from classroom peers.[14] Taken together, these reasons underscore the need for specific treatments targeting the associated feature of social impairment in ADHD populations.

SOCIAL SKILLS TRAINING INTERVENTIONS

Social skills training (SST) has proliferated in the past 2 decades to address the prevalent social impairment among children with ADHD,[15,16] although it also has been used to treat children who have social problems but do not have ADHD.[17] The traditional form of SST is based on the logic that children lack the core skills to enact prosocial, positive behaviors, and therefore they resort to displaying disruptive, offensive behaviors in peer situations. According to the theory behind SST, the reason why medication and behavioral management interventions may remediate ADHD symptoms but fail to reduce social impairment is because these treatments focus on suppressing children's disruptive/offensive behavior as opposed to teaching children skills to enact positive behaviors.[18,19]

Consistent with this logic, the predominant focus of traditional SST is on providing direct instruction (and practice opportunities) to children in how to enact prosocial, socially skilled behaviors. Traditional SST does not attempt to directly affect the child's positive regard by peers. The assumption is that if children with ADHD increase their display of skilled behaviors, then peers will respond naturally with more liking and friendship[18]; as will be discussed in this article, however, this logic may be faulty.

Description

Although a variety of different SST curricula have been used with children with ADHD, these curricula contain some common factors.[5,16] One consistent factor across curricula is that traditional SST is provided directly to the child by a clinician. Many clinicians prefer to deliver SST in a group format so that children have the opportunity to practice their social skills with one another, although some clinicians may administer SST to children individually when it is impractical to conduct SST in a group. Children may attend 60-minute to 90-minute SST sessions once per week for a prescribed period, such as 8 to 12 weeks, although variability exists among SST curricula.

The topic of instruction in a traditional SST curriculum may change each week, but topics typically focus on providing children with knowledge about (and supervised in-session practice with) key social skills that children are thought to be lacking. Social skills taught in SST for children with ADHD include sharing, making conversation, joining new groups of peers, following rules when playing games, taking turns, calming down when upset, and identifying emotions.[20] Commonly, clinicians introduce the social skills to children in a didactic fashion, but also include discussion and role plays within session for the purpose of allowing children to practice the skills. During this in-session practice, the clinician also may correct children's behaviors, as well as reinforce children's successful displays of the skills.

Some clinicians make greater efforts than others to encourage generalization of socially skilled behaviors outside of the therapeutic context. For example, some traditional SST programs attempt to promote generalization by informing parents and teachers of the social behaviors targeted in session. However, there are many traditional, clinic-based SST programs that do little to encourage generalization, which has been referred to as a "train and hope" strategy.[17] Regardless of the extent to which clinicians may consider generalization, in traditional SST the predominant focus of the intervention generally remains on in-session instruction of the child in social skills by the clinician.

Empirical Support

The empirical support for traditional, clinic-based SST for children with ADHD differs somewhat depending on the outcome being assessed. Traditional SST holds most promise for increasing children's demonstration of prosocial, socially skilled interactions while in the treatment group setting.[21] For example, this outcome variable might be tested via analog role play situations in session, which was successfully increased by clinic-based SST in one study.[22] Another positive result was found in a study by Pfiffner and McBurnett,[23] who reported that 8 weeks of a traditional clinic-based SST group for children with ADHD resulted in children's ability to generate more appropriate ideas about how to behave in hypothetical social situations.

However, the evidence is considerably more mixed regarding the efficacy of traditional SST on increasing children's use of socially skilled behaviors in naturalistic situations outside of session. Results have varied depending on the study. On the one hand, Pfiffner and McBurnett[23] found that SST resulted in children's improved behavior at home based on parents' reports (who were aware that their children were receiving treatment), but largely failed to generalize to the school context based on teachers' reports. As well, in the MTA study, the combination of pharmacotherapy and behavioral treatment (which included an SST component) was superior to the other conditions in increasing parent-reported and teacher-reported social skills.[13]

On the other hand, several studies have failed to find generalization of socially skilled behaviors as a result of traditional clinic-based SST. For example, Abikoff and colleagues[24] enrolled 103 children with ADHD (all of whom were medicated) who were randomized to 1 of 3 conditions: (1) intensive SST (with weekly meetings for 1 year and then monthly meetings for the second year), (2) an attention control group where children played with peers but received no instruction, or (3) no intervention. Notable about this study was the extensiveness of the SST condition, which not only taught key social skills (eg, getting along with others, conversational skills, resolving difficult interpersonal situations), but also involved some additional components intended to foster generalization. Specifically, the clinicians provided (1) out-of-session homework assignments to practice the social skills; (2) explanation to parents and teachers about the skills the child was learning in SST, with encouragement to the parents and teachers to reinforce the children's displays of skilled behaviors; and (3) inclusion of the social skills being learned on the Daily Report Card that teachers completed to inform parents about how the child had behaved at school. Nonetheless, results suggested *no* benefit of receiving SST on any outcome measure collected, which included parent report, teacher report, and observations of children's positive (prosocial/socially skilled) and negative (disruptive/offensive) behaviors in social interactions.[24]

Another notable study involved 120 children with ADHD, all of whom were medicated.[25] Participants were randomly assigned to receive SST in 8, 90-minute group sessions, or to a no-treatment condition. For the most part, there were no demonstrated benefits of SST as assessed via parent and child self-report ratings of social skills.[25] Other studies have assessed the efficacy of SST with unmedicated participants and similarly reported few benefits of SST on children's social behavior; this is especially the case when outcome measures are collected from impartial informants who are unaware of which participants have received SST.[26,27]

Measures of peer regard (particularly sociometric measures, in which peers nominate the classmates whom they like/dislike and are friends with) are difficult to collect, which may explain why they are rarely included in efficacy trials of SST. Therefore, the efficacy of traditional, clinic-based SST on peers' actual regard remains largely unknown in ADHD populations. However, traditional SST is unlikely to have beneficial effects on peer regard, for 2 reasons. First, the rationale behind SST is that if children with ADHD increase their socially skilled behaviors, then peers will observe these changes and respond with liking and friendship.[18,28,29] However, given that SST in general fails to result in demonstrated improvements in the social behaviors of children with ADHD in naturalistic settings,[24] changes in children's peer regard as a result of SST is therefore unlikely. Second and potentially more concerning are doubts regarding the assumption that increases in socially skilled behavior on the part of the child with ADHD will directly result in improvements in peer regard.[30] Recall that pharmacotherapy and behavioral management (which included an SST component) in the MTA study resulted in some improvements in actual social behaviors as rated by parents and teachers,[13] yet failed to have effects on peer regard of the children with ADHD.[14] As such, SST may not lead to improvements in peer regard even if it does positively affect social behaviors.

Using the Oxford Center for Evidence Based Medicine (OCEBM) guidelines, traditional clinic-based SST may have efficacy at a level 2 for increasing children's demonstration of positive, prosocial behaviors in session (in role plays or when presented with hypothetical situations). However, the efficacy drops considerably for the outcome variables of socially skilled behavior that generalizes to outside of session, as well as positive peer regard; thus, traditional SST cannot be considered efficacious for these outcomes using OCEBM guidelines. For this reason, 2 recent major reviews of psychosocial treatments for children with ADHD have concluded that SST is ineffective for ADHD populations, at least as is provided in traditional clinic-based settings.[31,32]

Reasons for Lack of Efficacy of Traditional SST Approaches

There are some theoretic reasons why SST, at least how it has been traditionally provided in clinical settings, may not be efficacious. The first reason relates to the nature of the social impairment commonly displayed in ADHD. Recently, researchers have postulated that children's deficient social behaviors occur because of reasons other than a lack of knowledge about the correct action to take (eg, not knowing what to do). Rather, the deficient social behaviors are attributable to factors such as impulsivity or poor emotional regulation that impede the actual performance of the social behaviors they know they should do (eg, not doing what they know).[19,33] Paradoxically, traditional clinic-based SST programs focus largely, if not exclusively, on the provision of social knowledge. If the problem for children with ADHD is not a lack of social knowledge but rather the generalization of that knowledge to real-world peer situations, then the target of traditional SST approaches is misdirected.

The second potential reason for the poor efficacy of traditional SST is that an exclusive focus on training children with ADHD to change their social behaviors, without attention to the peers who interact with the children with ADHD, may be misguided.[30] Peer relationships do not occur in a vacuum where the behavior of the child with ADHD occurs independently from the perceptions, overtures, and reactions of peers.[34] Importantly, peers' stigma about ADHD may negatively bias their actions toward children with this condition, which then elicit socially unskilled behaviors by children with ADHD in response. For instance, Harris and colleagues[35,36] paired previously unacquainted boys together for play sessions. For some of the pairs (randomly selected), researchers told one of the boys that the partner with whom he was about to interact had ADHD; other pairs were given no such expectation. Independent observers (unaware of the experimental manipulation) judged boys to be less friendly to their partner if they expected their partner to have ADHD. Crucially, observers also judged the boys who were thought to have ADHD by their partners to have poorer social skills relative to the boys whose partners were not given this expectation.[35,36] These findings suggest that peers' negative overtures toward children with ADHD (which may relate to preexisting assumptions and stigma peers hold about an ADHD diagnosis) may contribute, at least in part, to eliciting the poor social behaviors demonstrated by children with ADHD.

Also, there is evidence that even if a child with ADHD improves in social behaviors, peers will not necessarily notice this improvement, be willing to change their preexisting negative perceptions of children with ADHD, and respond with liking and friendship.[37] In fact, peers carry many cognitive biases against children whom they dislike, where they will selectively remember the negative behaviors displayed by such children and interpret ambiguous behaviors as having hostile intent; cognitive biases are reversed to favor well-liked children.[38,39] Collectively, results suggest that peers may be resistant to changing their impressions of children with ADHD, even in the face of disconfirming evidence, such as improved socially skilled behavior on the part of the child with ADHD.

Alternative SST Approaches

Researchers in the past decade have moved away from testing traditional SST for ADHD (at least how it has been historically provided via clinician-led instruction to children with a predominant focus on teaching skills in session as opposed to generalization of skills to out-of-session interactions), and instead toward testing alternative SST approaches. Many of these alternative approaches specifically attempt to address impediments to traditional, clinic-based SST in the hopes of augmenting efficacy. One promising strategy has been to heavily involve in the treatment those adults (eg, parents and teachers) who will be present in the child's naturalistic social interactions.[23,40–42] In contrast to traditional SST, which operates on the presumption that children with ADHD have knowledge deficits, this strategy is meant to target performance deficits in this population. The logic is that clinicians cannot realistically accompany the child into their naturalistic peer interactions; therefore, the parents and teachers who will be present are best suited to provide children with the in vivo reminders and incentives that children with ADHD need to carry out socially skilled behaviors with real peers.

Empirical evidence suggests that intensive involvement of parents or teachers in SST may increase the likelihood that children will generalize positive social behaviors to real-world peer situations. For example, Pfiffner and McBurnett[23] randomly assigned families of children with ADHD to 1 of 3 intervention conditions: (1) children received SST, (2) children received SST while their parents attended a simultaneous treatment group in which parents learned to reinforce their child's display of competent social behaviors outside of session, and (3) a no-intervention control group. The condition in which parents received simultaneous treatment with their children resulted in children's incrementally better improvement over the other 2 conditions, particularly in terms of generalization on teacher reports of children's social behaviors in the school setting.[23]

In a more recent study (although involving only children with ADHD-Inattentive Type, who may be more responsive to SST relative to the other ADHD subtypes, as discussed later in this article), a program involving simultaneous child SST and parent groups to encourage the child's generalization of social skills performed better than a no-treatment control group for the outcome of parent and teacher reports of children's socially skilled behaviors.[42] As well, Frankel and colleagues[41,43] have found positive effects of an SST program for children with ADHD involving concurrent child and parent groups, where parents are explicitly taught to reinforce their child's display of socially competent behavior outside of session, on parent and teacher ratings of social behavior.

Other empirical work has documented beneficial effects of SST on children's social behavior (teacher-reported and observations) when the SST is provided in the context of an immersive intervention for children with ADHD, the Summer Treatment Program.[44] Children participate in the Summer Treatment Program for approximately 8 hours per day for 8 weeks. SST is a core part of the program, whereby a target social skill is chosen each day and children receive instruction in the skill, discuss uses of the skill, and engage in role plays to practice the skill. The crucial aspect of the Summer Treatment Program is that the counselors engage in intensive reinforcement and response cost throughout the day to shape children's behaviors. As such, the same counselors teach the SST curriculum and remain with the children all day while they reinforce the children's displays of the social skills taught. Thus, the counselors are present to provide the repeated reminders and reinforcements, in vivo, that children with ADHD need to overcome their performance deficits.[45] Although it can be difficult to isolate the effects of SST from the rest of the interventions provided in the Summer Treatment Program, research suggests that indeed, children who participate in the Summer Treatment Program demonstrate counselor-rated and observed increases in positive social behaviors, as well as reductions in negative social behaviors with peers.[27]

Another example of a new SST approach is the Parental Friendship Coaching intervention, which consists solely of parent groups where instruction is provided about how parents can become "friendship coaches" for their children with ADHD.[40] Unlike the aforementioned interventions, Parental Friendship Coaching has no child treatment component and focuses solely on training the parents to administer the instruction in social skills knowledge and to provide the environmental contingencies and structure needed to facilitate children's generalization of skills to real-world peer situations. A pilot study involved families of 62 children with ADHD, randomly assigned to receive Parental Friendship Coaching or to be in a no-treatment control group. Children whose parents received Parental Friendship Coaching were reported by parents to show better social behaviors, and were reported by teachers (who were unaware of whether the family was provided the intervention) to be more accepted and less rejected by their peers, relative to children whose parents were in the control group.[40] Observations of warm, noncritical, and instructive parental coaching behaviors were more frequent among parents who had received Parental Friendship Coaching, and these parental behaviors partially mediated the effect of the intervention on children's peer relationships, providing support for the theoretic model of change.[40]

A final example of a new SST approach is Making Socially Accepting Inclusive Classrooms (MOSAIC), which is administered by teachers.[46] In MOSAIC, similar to the Summer Treatment Program, teachers administer SST and also remain with children in their naturalistic peer environment to reinforce children's displays of socially skilled behaviors. However, unlike the Summer Treatment Program, MOSAIC contains an additional component in which teachers are trained to encourage peers to be inclusive and welcoming toward children with ADHD, which is meant to address the negative cognitive biases that peers frequently possess toward children with ADHD. In a small randomized pilot study, 24 children with ADHD participating in a summer day camp with 113 typically developing peers, were assigned using a repeated measures crossover design to classrooms where the teacher was trained to deliver either (1) MOSAIC, or (2) the behavioral management and SST components of MOSAIC without the component to increase peers' inclusiveness toward children with ADHD. Results suggested that children with ADHD were better liked and less disliked by peers, and had more reciprocated friendships, as assessed via sociometric measures, when they were in classrooms where MOSAIC was added to behavioral management and SST.[46] These results were supported by observations of peers behaving more positively toward children with ADHD in classrooms where MOSAIC was present.[46]

In summary, alternative SST approaches that heavily train adults in the child's natural environment (parents, teachers, counselors) to instruct their child in SST and to administer contingencies, reminders, and reinforcements to the child to display socially skilled behaviors in naturalistic peer settings, has empirical support on the OCEBM guidelines at a level 2 for increasing children's demonstration of socially skilled behaviors. There have been multiple studies finding positive effects, such that this approach has been referred to as efficacious in recent reviews.[31,32] It is crucial to underscore the high level of involvement required of parents/teachers in these SST approaches, extending far beyond the clinician simply meeting with the parent or teacher periodically to keep them informed about the child's progress. In fact, in these alternative SST approaches, the adults typically receive as much treatment attention as, if not more than, the children themselves so as to learn how to train and reinforce social skills in the children with ADHD.

By contrast, the evidence is weaker that these alternative SST approaches with high parent/teacher involvement will be efficacious on the dependent variable of peer regard. Most of the interventions reviewed previously did not assess peer sociometric measures as a dependent variable. The one exception is MOSAIC, which did demonstrate effects on peer regard, albeit in a very small initial pilot study.[46] For this reason, support is currently a level 3 for the outcome measure of peer regard on the OCEBM guidelines, although the hope is that the empirical support for this outcome may increase as more research is conducted.

The main limitation of these alternative SST approaches, which may prevent them from reaching a level 1 of efficacy at this time, is uncertainty regarding how long intervention effects will persist after the discontinuation of treatment. Pfiffner and colleagues[42] demonstrated maintenance of gains 3 months after intervention discontinuation, but longer follow-up periods are needed. Another issue is that none of these approaches, with the exception of the small pilot study of MOSAIC,[46] have compared the study treatment against an active attention control condition to match participants' expectations for improvement. Finally, demonstration of efficacy on sociometric measures of peer regard, in addition to efficacy on measures of social behaviors, is important. In an attempt to address these gaps in the existing literature, a new trial of Parental Friendship Coaching is currently being undertaken that contains a longer follow-up period, an active attention control treatment condition, and sociometric outcome measures.

CLINICAL DECISION MAKING
Most Likely Responders

SST, even as traditionally provided in clinics, may be more efficacious for populations of children with internalizing problems or social withdrawal relative to those with disruptive behavior problems, such as ADHD.[17,47,48] Among children with ADHD, it is possible that those who have socially withdrawn behaviors and/or comorbid anxiety may be more responsive than children with ADHD alone to psychosocial treatment in general, which would potentially include SST.[49–51]

As well, children with the Inattentive subtype of ADHD (ADHD-I) may be more responsive to SST than children with the Combined (ADHD-C) or Hyperactive/Impulsive subtypes (ADHD-HI).[52] In the study conducted by Antshel and Remer,[25] SST resulted in relatively greater improvements for children with ADHD-I relative to those with ADHD-C, specifically on parent reports of the social skill of assertion. Researchers have theorized that the social deficits in children with ADHD-I are more attributable to a lack of knowledge, whereas the social deficits in ADHD-C may result from performance problems; therefore, children with ADHD-I may be more responsive to traditional forms of SST that focus on social skills knowledge instruction.[52,53]

Interestingly, the efficacy of traditional SST does not seem to differ for boys versus girls.[23,50] Nor has moderation by gender occurred in the alternative SST approaches,[40,42] with one exception that MOSAIC may be more efficacious for boys than for girls.[46] However, these preliminary findings bear replication.

Given the high reliance in the alternative SST approaches on parents to deliver the interventions to their children, parental psychopathology may be an unsurprising impediment to the efficacy of SST. Specifically, in Parental Friendship Coaching, parents' ADHD symptoms predicted their children receiving less benefit from this intervention.[54] The negative impact of parental psychopathology (ADHD and depression) may extend beyond SST to impede parents' ability to carry out any behavioral treatment with their children with ADHD.[55,56]

Outcomes Most Likely Affected

As discussed previously, children's social behavior is the most likely outcome to be positively affected by SST. Traditional clinic-based SST has limited efficacy for improving this outcome in real-world peer situations (as opposed to in the treatment setting), but the recent adaptations of SST have increased likelihood for affecting socially skilled behavior in naturalistic peer interactions. SST may have larger challenges in improving the outcome of peer regard. This may be because socially skilled behavior on the part of the child with ADHD may be a necessary but not sufficient condition for increasing peers' liking and friendship. Without procedures to help peers notice the behavior change among children with ADHD and overcome their negative cognitive biases toward children with this disorder, there may be no positive results on peer regard as a result of SST.[30]

Contraindications for Treatment

The Antshel and Remer[25] study suggested that children with ADHD and comorbid Oppositional Defiant Disorder (ODD) benefited less from SST relative to children with ADHD and no disruptive behavior comorbidities. One reason for this finding may be that children with ODD resist taking direction about their behavior from any adult, including clinicians.[21] Children with ADHD and comorbid ODD also are more likely to deny that they have impaired peer relationships,[57] and it has been suggested these positive self-illusions make children with ADHD unmotivated to change and therefore resistant to any psychosocial treatment, including SST.[58] On the other hand, some of the alterative SST approaches with heavy parent and teacher involvement have not found that the comorbid ODD moderated results.[41,46]

Potential Adverse Effects

Negative peer contagion effects occur when children encourage one another to maintain or increase problem behaviors through active means (eg, laughing, egging on other group member's displays of poor behavior) or passive means (eg, contributing to a social norm of problem behavior).[59] Such peer contagion effects are possible in any SST intervention in which children are selected because they have problem behaviors and treatment is provided to the children in groups.[60] Antshel and Remer,[25] for instance, found that 15% of the children with ADHD-I got worse after SST, and that this nearly always occurred when these children were in SST groups with peers who had ADHD-C, who were thought to have encouraged children with ADHD-I to display disruptive behavior.

Integration of Treatment with Drug Therapy

Many children with ADHD require pharmacotherapy to manage the core symptoms of their disorder. Whereas pharmacotherapy alone typically fails to normalize peer relationships such that there is no longer a need for adjunctive treatment,[61] it is unclear whether children's medication status influences the efficacy of SST. For instance, the lack of efficacy of traditional SST has been documented in samples in which children were medicated and not medicated.[31,32] In 2 large studies reviewed previously involving participants being administered intensive medication and SST by study personnel, there was no incremental benefit of receiving SST, suggesting that, at the least, medication does not appear to facilitate the uptake of social skills during SST.[24,25] Additionally, receipt of medication has largely failed to moderate the efficacy of the new SST approaches that heavily involve parents and teachers in intervention provision.[40,46]

SUMMARY AND FUTURE DIRECTIONS

Social problems are a persistent and treatment-refractory area of impairment for children with ADHD. Currently there is *no* SST intervention that normalizes the social functioning of children with ADHD, even if the intervention is associated with improvement. As such, there remains a clear and persistent need for better interventions for social problems in this population. Because nearly all existing SST approaches focus on changing the problem behaviors of children with ADHD, an exciting future direction may be to further investigate approaches aimed at helping the typically developing peer group to reduce stigma about ADHD behaviors and enhance acceptability of individual differences.[46,62] Perhaps a combination of interventions targeting the unskilled behaviors of children with ADHD with interventions to increase the inclusiveness of the peer group will be most likely to normalize social functioning in ADHD populations.

RECOMMENDATIONS FOR CLINICIANS

- Clinicians working with ADHD populations should be certain to assess social impairment. Even though parents may not bring it directly to clinicians' attention, particularly when children are young, social impairment is important to ask about (and treat) because it tends to persist and augment emotional/behavioral maladjustment over time.
- Clinicians should not assume that treating the core symptoms of ADHD will naturally be sufficient to remediate social impairment. Rather, if clinicians adopt a primary strategy to reduce the core symptoms of ADHD first, they might check with the family about whether there have been any improvements in the associated peer impairments.
- Additional, targeted psychosocial interventions for social impairment may be warranted. However, traditional clinic-based SST approaches have limited generalization outside of session into real-world peer interactions.
- Clinicians might consider alternative approaches to address the problem of generalization, such as heavily involving parents or teachers in administering in vivo reminders and reinforcements to the child about performing socially skilled behavior. The level of evidence for this approach is higher than for traditional, clinic-based SST.
- Approaches might also be undertaken to change peers' biases against children with ADHD, which may be necessary to affect the outcome of peer regard.

REFERENCES

1. American Psychiatric Association. Diagnostic and statistical manual of mental disorders. 5th edition. Arlington (VA): American Psychiatric Publishing; 2013.
2. Dirks MA, Treat TA, Weersing VR. Integrating theoretical, measurement, and intervention models of youth social competence. Clin Psychol Rev 2007;27(3): 327–47.
3. Hoza B. Peer functioning in children with ADHD. Ambul Pediatr 2007;7(Suppl 1): 101–6.
4. Gardner DM, Gerdes AC. A review of peer relationships and friendships in youth with ADHD. J Atten Disord 2013. [Epub ahead of print].
5. Landau S, Milich R, Diener MB. Peer relations of children with attention-deficit hyperactivity disorder. Read Writ Q 1998;14(1):83–105.
6. Erhardt D, Hinshaw SP. Initial sociometric impressions of attention-deficit hyperactivity disorder and comparison boys: predictions from social behaviors and from nonbehavioral variables. J Consult Clin Psychol 1994;62(4):833–42.

7. Ronk MJ, Hund AM, Landau S. Assessment of social competence of boys with attention-deficit/hyperactivity disorder: problematic peer entry, host responses, and evaluations. J Abnorm Child Psychol 2011;39(6):829–40.

8. Hoza B, Mrug S, Gerdes AC, et al. What aspects of peer relationships are impaired in children with attention-deficit/hyperactivity disorder? J Consult Clin Psychol 2005;73(3):411–23.

9. Mikami AY, Hinshaw SP. Resilient adolescent adjustment among girls: buffers of childhood peer rejection and attention-deficit/hyperactivity disorder. J Abnorm Child Psychol 2006;34(6):823–37.

10. Greene RW, Biederman J, Faraone SV, et al. Adolescent outcome of boys with attention-deficit/hyperactivity disorder and social disability: results from a 4-year longitudinal follow-up study. J Consult Clin Psychol 1997;65(5):758–67.

11. Mikami AY, Hinshaw SP, Patterson KA, et al. Eating pathology among adolescent girls with attention-deficit/hyperactivity disorder. J Abnorm Psychol 2008;117(1): 225–35.

12. Murray-Close D, Hoza B, Hinshaw SP, et al. Developmental processes in peer problems of children with attention-deficit/hyperactivity disorder in the Multi-modal Treatment Study of Children with ADHD: developmental cascades and vicious cycles. Dev Psychopathol 2010;22(4):785–802.

13. MTA Cooperative Group. A 14-month randomized clinical trial of treatment strategies for attention-deficit/hyperactivity disorder. Arch Gen Psychiatry 1999; 56(12):1073–86.

14. Hoza B, Gerdes AC, Mrug S, et al. Peer-assessed outcomes in the multimodal treatment study of children with attention deficit hyperactivity disorder. J Clin Child Adolesc Psychol 2005;34(1):74–86.

15. Landau S, Moore LA. Social skill deficits in children with attention-deficit hyperactivity disorder. Sch Psychol Rev 1991;20(2):235–51.

16. Nixon E. The social competence of children with attention deficit hyperactivity disorder: a review of the literature. Child Adolesc Ment Health 2001;6(4):172–80.

17. DuPaul GJ, Eckert TL. The effects of social skills curricula: now you see them, now you don't. Sch Psychol Q 1994;9(2):113–32.

18. de Boo GM, Prins PJ. Social incompetence in children with ADHD: possible moderators and mediators in social-skills training. Clin Psychol Rev 2007; 27(1):78–97.

19. Gresham FM, Cook CR, Crews SD, et al. Social skills training for children and youth with emotional and behavioral disorders: validity considerations and future directions. Behav Disord 2004;30(1):32–46.

20. Pfiffner LJ. Social skills training. In: McBurnett K, Pfiffner LJ, editors. Attention-deficit/hyperactivity disorder: concepts, controversies, new directions. New York: Informa Healthcare; 2008. p. 179–90.

21. Pfiffner LJ, Calzada E, McBurnett K. Interventions to enhance social competence. Child Adolesc Psychiatr Clin N Am 2000;9(3):689–709.

22. Fenstermacher K, Olympia D, Sheridan SM. Effectiveness of a computer-facilitated interactive social skills training program for boys with attention deficit hyperactivity disorder. Sch Psychol Q 2006;21(2):197–224.

23. Pfiffner LJ, McBurnett K. Social skills training with parent generalization: treatment effects for children with attention deficit disorder. J Consult Clin Psychol 1997;65(5):749–57.

24. Abikoff HB, Hechtman L, Klein RG, et al. Social functioning in children with ADHD treated with long-term methylphenidate and multimodal psychosocial treatment. J Am Acad Child Adolesc Psychiatry 2004;43(7):820–9.

25. Antshel KM, Remer R. Social skills training in children with attention deficit hyperactivity disorder: a randomized-controlled clinical trial. J Clin Child Adolesc Psychol 2003;32(1):153–65.
26. Abikoff HB. Efficacy of cognitive training interventions in hyperactive children: a critical review. Clin Psychol Rev 1985;5(5):479–512.
27. Pelham WE, Wheeler T, Chronis A. Empirically supported psychosocial treatments for attention deficit hyperactivity disorder. J Clin Child Psychol 1998; 27(2):190–205.
28. Ladd GW, Mize J. A cognitive–social learning model of social-skill training. Psychol Rev 1983;90(2):127–57.
29. Mize J, Ladd GW. A cognitive-social learning approach to social skill training with low-status preschool children. Dev Psychol 1990;26(3):388–97.
30. Mikami AY, Lerner MD, Lun J. Social context influences on children's rejection by their peers. J Clin Child Psychol 2010;4(2):123–30.
31. Pelham WE, Fabiano GA. Evidence-based psychosocial treatments for attention-deficit/hyperactivity disorder. J Clin Child Adolesc Psychol 2008; 37(1):184–214.
32. Evans SW, Owens JS, Bunford N. Evidence-based psychosocial treatments for children and adolescents with attention-deficit/hyperactivity disorder. J Clin Child Adolesc Psychol 2014;43(4):527–51.
33. Maedgen JW, Carlson CL. Social functioning and emotional regulation in the attention deficit hyperactivity disorder subtypes. J Clin Child Psychol 2000;29(1):30–42.
34. Nesdale D, Lambert A. Effects of experimentally manipulated peer rejection on children's negative affect, self-esteem, and maladaptive social behavior. Int J Behav Dev 2007;31(2):115–22.
35. Harris MJ, Milich R, McAninch CB. When stigma becomes self-fulfilling prophecy: expectancy effects and the causes, consequences, and treatment of peer rejection. In: Brophy J, editor. Advances in research on teaching. Greenwich (CT): JAI Press; 1998. p. 243–72.
36. Harris MJ, Milich R, Corbitt EM, et al. Self-fulfilling effects of stigmatizing information on children's social interactions. J Pers Soc Psychol 1992;63(1):41–50.
37. Hymel S, Wagner E, Butler LJ. Reputational bias: view from the peer group. In: Asher SR, Coie JD, editors. Peer rejection in childhood. New York: Cambridge University Press; 1990. p. 156–86.
38. Peets K, Hodges EV, Kikas E, et al. Hostile attributions and behavioral strategies in children: does relationship type matter? Dev Psychol 2007;43(4):889–900.
39. Peets K, Hodges EV, Salmivalli C. Affect-congruent social-cognitive evaluations and behaviors. Child Dev 2008;79(1):170–85.
40. Mikami AY, Lerner MD, Griggs MS, et al. Parental influence on children with attention-deficit/hyperactivity disorder: II. Results of a pilot intervention training parents as friendship coaches for children. J Abnorm Child Psychol 2010; 38(6):737–49.
41. Frankel F, Myatt R, Cantwell DP, et al. Parent-assisted transfer of children's social skills training: effects on children with and without attention-deficit hyperactivity disorder. J Am Acad Child Adolesc Psychiatry 1997;36(8):1056–64.
42. Pfiffner LJ, Mikami AY, Huang-Pollock C, et al. A randomized, controlled trial of integrated home-school behavioral treatment for ADHD, predominantly inattentive type. J Am Acad Child Adolesc Psychiatry 2007;46(8):1041–50.
43. Frankel F, Myatt R, Cantwell DP. Training outpatient boys to conform with the social ecology of popular peers: effects on parent and teacher ratings. J Clin Child Psychol 1995;24(3):300–10.

44. Pelham WE, Hoza B. Intensive treatment: a summer treatment program for children with ADHD. In: Hibbs E, Jensen PS, editors. Psychosocial treatments for child and adolescent disorders: empirically based strategies for clinical practice. New York: APA Press; 1996. p. 311–40.

45. Pelham WE, Bender ME. Peer relationships in hyperactive children: description and treatment. In: Gadow KD, Bailer I, editors. Advances in learning and behavioral disabilities, vol. 1. Greenwich (CT): JAI Press; 1982. p. 365–436.

46. Mikami AY, Griggs MS, Lerner MD, et al. A randomized trial of a classroom intervention to increase peers' social inclusion of children with attention-deficit/hyperactivity disorder. J Consult Clin Psychol 2013;81(1):100–12.

47. Beelmann A, Pfingsten U, Lösel F. Effects of training social competence in children: a meta-analysis of recent evaluation studies. J Clin Child Psychol 1994; 23(3):260–71.

48. Antshel KM, Polacek C, McMahon M, et al. Comorbid ADHD and anxiety affect social skills group intervention treatment efficacy in children with autism spectrum disorders. J Dev Behav Pediatr 2011;32(6):439–46.

49. Schatz DB, Rostain AL. ADHD with comorbid anxiety: a review of the current literature. J Atten Disord 2006;10(2):141–9.

50. MTA Cooperative Group. Moderators and mediators of treatment response for children with attention-deficit/hyperactivity disorder: the multimodal treatment study of children with attention-deficit/hyperactivity disorder. Arch Gen Psychiatry 1999;56(12):1088–96.

51. Jensen PS, Hinshaw SP, Kraemer HC, et al. ADHD comorbidity findings from the MTA Study: comparing comorbid subgroups. J Am Acad Child Adolesc Psychiatry 2001;40(2):147–58.

52. Pfiffner LJ. Psychosocial treatment for ADHD-inattentive type. The ADHD Report 2003;11(5):1–8.

53. Milich R, Balentine AC, Lynam DR. ADHD combined type and ADHD predominantly inattentive type are distinct and unrelated disorders. Clin Psychol 2001; 8(4):463–88.

54. Griggs MS, Mikami AY. Parental ADHD predicts child and parent outcomes following parental friendship coaching treatment. J Am Acad Child Adolesc Psychiatry 2011;50(12):1236–46.

55. Chronis-Tuscano A, O'Brien KA, Johnston C, et al. The relation between maternal ADHD symptoms and improvement in child behavior following brief behavioral parent training is mediated by change in negative parenting. J Abnorm Child Psychol 2011;39(7):1047–57.

56. Chronis-Tuscano A, Clarke TL, O'Brien KA, et al. Development and preliminary evaluation of an integrated treatment targeting parenting and depressive symptoms in mothers of children with attention-deficit/hyperactivity disorder. J Consult Clin Psychol 2013;81(5):918–25.

57. Hoza B, Gerdes AC, Hinshaw SP, et al. Self-perceptions of competence in children with ADHD and comparison children. J Consult Clin Psychol 2004;72(3): 382–91.

58. Mikami AY, Calhoun CD, Abikoff HB. Positive illusory bias and response to behavioral treatment among children with attention-deficit/hyperactivity disorder. J Clin Child Adolesc Psychol 2010;39(3):373–85.

59. Dishion TJ, Dodge KA. Peer contagion in interventions for children and adolescents: moving towards an understanding of the ecology and dynamics of change. J Abnorm Child Psychol 2005;33(3):395–400.

60. Lavallee KL, Bierman KL, Nix RL. The impact of first-grade "friendship group" experiences on child social outcomes in the fast track program. J Abnorm Child Psychol 2005;33(3):307–24.

61. Hinshaw SP, Henker B, Whalen CK, et al. Aggressive, prosocial, and nonsocial behavior in hyperactive boys: dose effects of methylphenidate in naturalistic settings. J Consult Clin Psychol 1989;57(5):636–43.

62. Mikami AY, Reuland MM, Griggs MS, et al. Collateral effects of a peer relationship intervention for children with ADHD on typically developing classmates. School Psychology Review 2013;42(4):458–76.

Neurofeedback for ADHD
A Review of Current Evidence

Martin Holtmann, MD[a],*, Edmund Sonuga-Barke, PhD[b,c],
Samuele Cortese, MD, PhD[d,e], Daniel Brandeis, PhD[f,g]

KEYWORDS

- ADHD • Treatment • Neurofeedback • Slow cortical potentials • Frequency bands
- Reward

KEY POINTS

- Among alternative treatment approaches for attention-deficit/hyperactivity disorder (ADHD), neurofeedback has gained empirical support in recent years.
- Via neurofeedback, children with ADHD are trained to regulate their neurophysiologic profile or to bring it closer to that of nonaffected children; learning of self-regulation is thus a key mechanism.
- According to recent meta-analytic evidence, neurofeedback leads to significant decreases of ADHD core symptoms; however, if only probably blinded ratings are applied, these effects were reduced to a statistical trend. The evidence remains inconclusive because subsequent studies could demonstrate neither learning of self-regulation nor significant effects for the best blinded assessments.
- There is a strong need for more evidence from well-blinded, methodologically sound, and sensitive trials demonstrating also learning of self-regulation, before neurofeedback can be assigned the highest level of evidence as a front-line treatment of ADHD.
- Future research should focus on testing different types of neurofeedback techniques, establishing the quality of the intervention, the long-term stability of effects, and predictors and mediators of response.
- Neurofeedback may be used within a multimodal treatment setting.

See last page of the article.
[a] LWL-University Hospital for Child and Adolescent Psychiatry, Ruhr University Bochum, Heithofer Allee 64, D 59071 Hamm, Germany; [b] Developmental Brain-Behaviour Laboratory, Psychology, Institute for Disorders of Impulse & Attention, University of Southampton, University Road SO17 1BJ, Southampton, UK; [c] Department of Experimental Clinical & Health Psychology, Ghent University, Henri Dunantlaan 2. B-9000, Ghent, Belgium; [d] Department of Child Psychiatry, Cambridge University Hospitals NHS Foundation Trust, Hills Road, Cambridge PE29 2BQ, UK; [e] Division of Psychiatry, Institute of Mental Health, University of Nottingham, Triumph Road, NG7 2TU Nottingham, UK; [f] Department of Child and Adolescent Psychiatry, University of Zürich, Neumünsterallee 9/Fach, CH-8032 Zürich, Switzerland; [g] Department of Child and Adolescent Psychiatry and Psychotherapy, Central Institute of Mental Health, Medical Faculty Mannheim, Heidelberg University, J5, D-68159 Mannheim, Germany
* Corresponding author.
E-mail address: martin.holtmann@wkp-lwl.org

Child Adolesc Psychiatric Clin N Am 23 (2014) 789–806
http://dx.doi.org/10.1016/J.chc.2014.05.006
1056-4993/14/$ – see front matter © 2014 Elsevier Inc. All rights reserved.

childpsych.theclinics.com

Abbreviations	
ADHD	Attention-deficit/hyperactivity disorder
CNV	Contingent negative variation
EEG	Electroencephalography
ERP	Event-related potential
fMRI	Functional magnetic resonance imaging
NICE	National Institute for Health and Clinical Excellence
QEEG	Quantitative electroencephalography
SCP	Slow cortical potential
SMR	Sensorimotor rhythm

INTRODUCTION/BACKGROUND
Target of Treatment

Attention-deficit/hyperactivity disorder (ADHD) is the most common psychiatric disorder of childhood with an estimated prevalence of about 5% in school-aged children.[1] Core symptoms include impaired attention and/or hyperactivity/impulsivity. ADHD often has a chronic course with up to 65% of affected children displaying ADHD symptoms in adulthood.[2] ADHD is associated with high levels of externalizing (eg, oppositional-defiant and conduct disorders) and internalizing (eg, depression and anxiety) comorbidity as well as learning disorders and leads to impairment in various domains, including poor academic performance, lower occupational success, poor social relationships, and higher risk-taking behavior.

Need for the Treatment

Because of the significant impact of ADHD on children's functioning, considerable effort has been directed at developing effective treatments. Although treatment with psychostimulant and non-psychostimulant medication is efficacious[3] and widely used, it has several limitations: a considerable minority of children treated with stimulants either fail to show an improvement in ADHD symptoms or suffer adverse effects on sleep, appetite, growth, and, less commonly, the cardiovascular system.[4,5] In addition, normalization is rare, and long-term effectiveness remains to be established. Some parents, patients, and/or clinicians have a preference for nonpharmacologic treatments. In summary, these limitations highlight the need for therapeutic innovation in ADHD to develop effective nonpharmacologic interventions that can improve short-term and long-term outcomes.

A range of nonpharmacologic interventions is available to treat ADHD (eg, psychological interventions, dietary elimination strategies, nutritional supplements, and herbal and homeopathic treatments). Evidence for the efficacy of some of these approaches has been partly supported in systematic reviews and meta-analyses, for example, Refs.[6–10] Because of the inclusion of nonrandomized controlled trials designs, non-ADHD samples, and/or non-ADHD outcomes, current meta-analyses allow only limited conclusions to be drawn regarding the effect of these interventions on core ADHD symptoms.[11] Among nonpharmacologic treatment approaches, neurofeedback has emerged as a promising noninvasive treatment for children with ADHD. Neurofeedback is a form of biofeedback, which itself is based on behavior therapy. It may be best described as a training of self-regulation aiming to achieve control over brain activity patterns or to normalize them and thereby reduce the symptoms of ADHD. Neurofeedback with electroencephalography (EEG) (EEG-biofeedback) has been used as a treatment strategy since the 1970s.[12] Initially, the lack of suitably controlled large-scale studies inhibited the acceptance of neurofeedback within the wider psychological, psychiatric, and educational communities. Neurofeedback over time has gained more empirical support.[6] This article reviews the underlying theory and empirical research on the use of neurofeedback in children and adolescents with ADHD.

INTERVENTIONS
Theoretic Overview: Why Does Theory Suggest the Treatment Should Work?

The growing acceptance of neurofeedback can be understood against the backdrop of an increased understanding of the neurodevelopmental basis of ADHD. The rationale for using neurofeedback as an intervention in ADHD derives from the consistent observation of altered brain activation in many children with ADHD detected in EEG and imaging studies. By repeated training of improved cortical (or subcortical) self-regulation, neurofeedback aims to address these deficits by making use of the brain's plasticity. Available treatment protocols mainly address 2 different kinds of deviant cortical activity in ADHD children: although EEG frequency band training is directed at the modification of oscillatory brain activity (eg, the reduction of slow wave activity and increase of faster activity), the training of slow cortical potentials (SCPs) addresses the regulation of phasic cortical activity to optimize allocation of cortical resources. Key findings of EEG studies in ADHD are summarized in the following paragraphs to clarify the theoretic background for the choice of electrophysiologic treatment targets.

EEG frequency band studies

EEG research dating back 80 years has established the presence of various abnormalities of oscillatory brain activity in children with ADHD (then named "behavior problem children"). These early cross-sectional studies used visual evaluation of paper recordings of EEG; the most common finding was an increase in slow-wave activity, often in frontal regions.[13,14] Findings of "cortical slowing" have been replicated by a variety of studies applying quantitative electroencephalography (QEEG). QEEG applies computerized mathematical algorithms (typically spectral analysis using fast Fourier transformation) to convert raw EEG data into frequency bands of interest for statistical comparisons between conditions and groups or against norms. Traditionally, 5 wide frequency bands have been studied, typically defined as delta (1.5–3.5 Hz), theta (3.5–7.5 Hz), alpha (7.5–12.5 Hz), beta (12.5–30 Hz), and finally, also gamma (30–70 Hz). The absolute and relative power (ie, percentage of total power) in each frequency band is then calculated. Pediatric EEG differs from adult EEG because of developmental maturation. Decreases in the lower frequency bands are most prominent during the first years of life but continue until adulthood and parallel decreases in hemodynamic fluctuations,[15] whereas increases in relative alpha and beta typically continue until adolescence or adulthood.[16] Most EEG and QEEG studies have initially reported that a substantial group of ADHD children show elevated levels of slow wave (delta and theta) activity in comparison with healthy children and psychiatric controls.[17,18] The most reliable measures of this have been increased relative theta power, whereas reduced amounts of relative alpha and beta 18 are less consistent. In addition, the theta/alpha and theta/beta ratios have been claimed to be reliable measures differentiating ADHD and control children.[19] Meanwhile, several studies using cluster analysis have reported distinct EEG-defined subgroups within their ADHD samples,[20,21] comprising among others a cortical hypoarousal subtype (increased relative theta and theta/beta ratio), a subtype indicative of a maturational lag, and a hyperarousal subtype (excess of beta activity). Because of more recent results, however, doubt has been cast on claims that the theta and beta ratio may serve as simple and reliable QEEG markers for ADHD, which has led to a major paradigm shift toward neurophysiologic subtyping. Indeed, increasing evidence across clinical groups and studies now indicates that the theta or theta/beta increase is not a specific marker of ADHD[22,23] and may also be more closely related to impaired activation following task demands rather than to hypoarousal,[24] thus implicating somewhat different regulation mechanisms.[25] As a consequence, subgrouping or clustering approaches to QEEG deviance characterization may better characterize ADHD as a heterogeneous disorder.[26] The longitudinal stability of alterations in EEG frequency bands due to ADHD from childhood into adulthood has also been questioned in recent years.[22,27]

Studies of event-related SCP

Event-related potentials (ERPs) are small voltage fluctuations in the EEG resulting from evoked brain activity. ERP components reflect, with high temporal resolution, the patterns of neuronal activity in response to stimuli. ERPs in ADHD allow the examination of electrical representations of preparatory and preattentive processes, auditory and visual attention systems, the frontal inhibition system, and time processing. With regard to ADHD, the most replicated and robust findings in early components are a lower amplitude, longer latency, and different topography of the P300 in affected children compared with healthy controls.[28] However, neurofeedback of ERPs almost exclusively addresses changes in later, slower, or sustained components, which are registered in a latency range of 500 to 1000 ms after cue presentation (SCPs). SCPs represent changes of cortical direct current electrical activity and have been related to the level of excitation of underlying cortical regions. Negative SCP shifts may reflect the depolarization of large cortical cell assemblies leading to higher excitability and the allocation of more neuronal resources; positive shifts reflect reduced excitability or even inhibition.[29] Experimental evidence from animals and humans supports the idea that the contingent negative variation (CNV) of the typical SCP is closely related to cognitive preparation, decision-making, and time estimation. Larger CNV amplitudes reveal greater activation in sets of neurons involved in time processing.[30] Although alterations of some faster cognitive and inhibitory ERP components such as P300 in ADHD patients diminish in early adulthood (partly compatible with the developmental lag model), decreased CNV amplitudes remain detectable even in young adult ADHD subjects, regardless of their remission status.[31] These results seem to indicate residual attentional dysfunctions and timing deficits even in young adults with clinically remitted ADHD.

Description: How Is the Treatment Delivered?

The aim of neurofeedback training can be thought of in 1 of 2 related ways: first, to teach ADHD children to adapt their neurophysiologic profile to more closely approximate that of typically developing children. Second, to help them learn to regulate attentional states and brain functions better on demand, resulting in subsequent improvements of symptoms. The self-regulation of cortical activity is realized through a process of operant learning using real-time representation of EEG parameters. Many different animated feedback presentations that are suited for children and adolescents are now available. EEG measures of interest are converted into visual or acoustic signals and fed back in real time. In some feedback animations, the cortical activity is, for example, represented by the height or speed of a feedback object (eg, a ball, plane, or cartoon character moving across the screen). If the EEG activity is regulated in the desired way, the object rises, falls, or advances more quickly. In other animations, the patient must try to view a movie, or change the color of an object on the screen by generating the neural activity of interest. To date, no studies directly assessed the effects of feedback modality (visual or auditory or combined) on outcome measures.[32] Successful trials are immediately rewarded by a tone, a "smiley," or points. Therefore, neurofeedback may be regarded as "a fine-grained form of cognitive behavior modification."[33] Individual parameter thresholds are typically adjusted throughout the course of the training so that an encouraging amount of positive feedback is guaranteed. Like other operant training approaches, neurofeedback requires a transfer from the training context to the everyday life of the patient. Therefore, some training trials without feedback can be incorporated to catalyze generalization.

Training protocols
Based on the above-mentioned alterations of electrophysiologic parameters (QEEG and ERPs) in ADHD, clinicians utilize 2 basic types of training protocols. In neurofeedback, the term "protocol" also refers to a wide range of details that form a part of the overall training paradigm (eg, a specific selection of reinforcement and inhibitory parameters), and the EEG-montage to deliver the training.[32] In ADHD, a conventional QEEG neurofeedback protocol for reducing inattention and impulsivity consists of operant suppressing of theta activity and enhancement of beta activity.[34] To reduce hypermotoric symptoms, enhancement of sensorimotor rhythm (SMR; low beta 12–15 Hz activity) is sometimes used in addition to this theta-beta protocol. Based on the electrophysiologic evidence of altered SCPs in ADHD, a different protocol has emerged aiming at the modifications of SCPs to regulate cortical excitation thresholds.[35,36]

Empirical Support

The quality of study design and reporting regarding the effectiveness of neurofeedback on ADHD have both clearly improved in recent years.[37,38] Several controlled studies produced evidence of short-term improvements in core symptoms, neuropsychological functions, and electrophysiologic correlates of ADHD; for overviews, see Refs.[39–42] Meanwhile, meta-analyses have been published on the effects of neurofeedback on ADHD symptoms. The first meta-analysis on the effects of neurofeedback on ADHD core symptoms[6] included data on 467 subjects from 10 prospective, controlled trials. Control conditions comprised waiting list groups, interventions like EMG-feedback, and computerized cognitive training and stimulant pharmacotherapy. Mean effect sizes (Cohen's δ) for neurofeedback were 0.81 for inattention, 0.39 for hyperactivity (both assessed via rating scales), and 0.68 for impulsivity as measured by continuous performance tests. No differential improvement was observed between the 2 basic protocols (QEEG and SCP), in line with direct comparisons.[43,44] Some of the studies included in this meta-analysis have, however, been criticized for lacking appropriate controls and follow-up, failing to randomly allocate participants to treatment conditions, using poor diagnostic criteria, and using subjective and unblinded outcome measures.[37,40] In addition, they failed to take into account the influence of the training setting provided during extensive biofeedback.

A subsequent meta-analysis from the European ADHD Guidelines Group,[11] using a more rigorous and selective approach, included 8 studies meeting high methodological standards (**Table 1**). Neurofeedback yielded a significant ($P<.0001$) treatment effect (effect size [ES] = 0.59; 95% CI: 0.31–0.87) using ADHD scores from raters (often unblinded) closest to the therapeutic setting. These effects were substantially reduced to a statistical trend ($P = .07$) when probably blinded ratings were applied (ES = 0.30; 95% CI: −0.02–0.61). Because blinded assessments were only available from 4 of the 8 included studies, the authors concluded that better "evidence of efficacy from blinded assessments is required before Neurofeedback is likely to be supported as ADHD treatment."[11] Since then, and by March 2014 (when this article was finalized), several neurofeedback studies targeting children with ADHD meeting similar rigorous inclusion criteria and using at least partly blinded measures have been published (**Table 2**). Although these recent studies were well controlled, most used partly innovative but nonstandard protocols or equipment and none demonstrated systematic learning of cortical control (considered a prerequisite for specificity, see later discussion). Although only the largest study found a significant advantage for neurofeedback over control treatment on any primary outcome, the nonsignificant advantage reached small to medium effect size for some blinded primary outcomes in all studies. The smallest study[25] compared neurofeedback (tomographic SCP plus frequency neurofeedback) to EMG biofeedback with effective parent blinding. The advantage for tomographic neurofeedback was not significant but reached a medium effect size for all (blinded) parent ratings (ES = 0.57 for the total ADHD score). The larger study comparing individualized frequency training to sham control[45] included the data from Ref.[46] No significant advantage for the (blinded) primary outcomes was observed, but the effect for the decrease of hyperactivity/impulsivity symptoms reached a small to medium effect size (ES = 0.31, computed from their data). The largest recent study[47] used school-based neurofeedback. Although blinding of participants, parents, and teachers was not attempted in this study, blinded behavioral classroom observations indicated a significant reduction (ES = 0.43) of verbal-motor ADHD (off-task) behaviors corresponding to hyperactivity/impulsivity after the intervention,[47] as well as at follow-up when using a nonlinear model of change.[48] The advantage of neurofeedback was also maintained for blinded classroom observation when compared with an active computer training, including attention and working memory games of similar duration and intensity. However, when teacher ratings were used as the best blinded outcome for,[25,45] and when the classroom observations of inattention were included for,[49] following the protocol of,[11] these moderate effects were reduced substantially and no longer significant. This considerably less positive picture, and the lack of stability across properly blinded outcomes, may reflect reduced bias (due to an unknown mechanism given proper blinding), but could also suggest that teacher and classroom observations are less sensitive to neurofeedback effects on core ADHD symptoms than parent ratings. The results highlight the need for future studies to examine in more detail the reasons for the differences between outcomes.

Methodological issues

The most recent neurofeedback meta-analysis[11] has been criticized for underestimating neurofeedback efficacy because it included trials with training approaches with nonstandard protocols impeding learning and uncontrolled changes in medication dosage.[50] However, these criticisms reflect mainly problems inherent in the field rather than the meta-analysis per se. Controlling for medication changes (through sensitivity analysis) was indeed considered important and part of the authors' protocol,[11] but

Table 1
Characteristics of studies included in the meta-analysis of the European ADHD Guidelines Group

Study	Design	Duration of Treatment; Number of Sessions	Treatment	Control Condition	N Treatment	Control	Age Range in Years
Bakshayesh et al,[76] 2011	RCT; parallel groups	30 sessions; 10–15 wk	Theta-Beta	EMG	18	17	6–14
Beauregard & Levesque,[60] 2006	RCT; parallel groups	40 sessions; 13 wk	Theta-Beta	No treatment	15	5	8–12
Gevensleben et al,[44] 2009	RCT	36 sessions, 2 mo	18 sessions Theta-Beta + 18 sessions SCP in balanced order	Attention skills training	59	35	8–12
Heinrich et al,[35] 2004	RCT	25 sessions; 3 wk	SCP	Waiting list	13	9	7–13
Holtmann et al,[77] 2009	RCT; parallel groups	20 sessions in 2 wk	Theta-Beta	Attention skills training	20	14	7–12
Lansbergen et al,[46] 2011	Stratified, RCT	30 sessions, 3 mo	Individualized frequency band training	Placebo, neurofeedback	8	6	8–15
Linden et al,[34] 1996	RCT	40 sessions, 6 mo	Theta-Beta	Waiting list	9	9	5–15
Steiner et al,[49] 2011	RCT	Average 23.4 sessions, 4 mo	Theta-Beta	Waiting list	13	13	Not reported Mean 12.4 ± 0.9

Abbreviation: RCT, randomized controlled trial.
Adapted from Sonuga-Barke EJ, Brandeis D, Cortese S, et al. Nonpharmacological interventions for ADHD: systematic review and meta-analyses of randomized controlled trials of dietary and psychological treatments. Am J Psychiatry 2013;170(3):280.

Table 2
Characteristics of studies published following the meta-analysis of the European ADHD Guidelines Group meeting inclusion criteria or testing neurofeedback against medication

Study	Design	Duration of Treatment; Number of Sessions	Treatment	Control Condition	N Treatment Control		Age Range in Years
Van Dongen-Boomsma et al,[45] 2013	Stratified, RCT	30 sessions, 3 mo	Individualized frequency band training	Placebo, neurofeedback	22	19	8–15 Mean 10.62 ± 2.25
Maurizio et al,[25] 2014	RCT	36 units in 18 sessions, 6 mo	SCP and Theta-Beta (tomographic)	EMG biofeedback (matched)	13	12	8.5–12.9 Means 10.6 ± 1.3, 10.0 ± 1.2
Steiner et al,[47] 2014	RCT	40 sessions, 5 mo, at school	Theta-Beta	Community treatment/standard care	34	36	Not reported Mean 12.4 ± 0.9
Duric et al,[55] 2012	RCT, head-to-head, combination	30 sessions, 2.5 mo	Theta-Beta	Medication Medication + Theta-Beta			6–18
Meisel et al,[56] 2013	RCT, head-to-head	40 sessions, 5 mo	Theta-Beta	Medication management	12	11	7–14 Means 9.53 ± 1.8, 8.9± 1.53
Ogrim & Hestad,[54] 2013	RCT, head-to-head	30 sessions, 7–11 mo	Theta-Beta	Medication management			7–16

Abbreviation: RCT, randomized controlled trial.

Adapted from Sonuga-Barke EJ, Brandeis D, Cortese S, et al. Nonpharmacological interventions for ADHD: systematic review and meta-analyses of randomized controlled trials of dietary and psychological treatments. Am J Psychiatry 2013;170(3):280.

required a larger number of probably blinded studies.[51] The lack of standards regarding neurofeedback protocols is even more problematic for the field. Controlled studies on the optimal frequency bands, scalp sites, feedback timings, and thresholds are largely lacking, and clinical practice is still based on early animal studies and divergent clinical experience without control. This seems particularly problematic for QEEG (frequency band) training, whereby recent evidence no longer supports the presumption that increased theta and beta or SMR reduction are reliable ADHD markers (discussed above). These findings question the standard unidirectional "normalization" rationale of QEEG neurofeedback and suggest instead the adoption of bidirectional,[52] individualized,[46,53] or SCP-based regulation approaches. In addition, allowing "probably blinded" rather than strictly blinded measures in the largest studies may well have counterbalanced this bias in this meta-analysis.

A particularly relevant question from a clinical point of view is how neurofeedback compares to standard medication in the short term. Arns and coworkers[6] included a meta-analysis of 5 such head-to-head comparison studies of neurofeedback with stimulant medication and found no difference for impulsivity ratings. Although these studies were not randomized or blinded, the findings are difficult to explain through expectancy bias, which would be likely in favor of the "gold-standard" stimulant treatment in such a comparison. Several randomized controlled trial studies have since compared neurofeedback to medication alone or in combination (see **Table 2**). Although one of them[54] found neurofeedback effects inferior to medication effects, the other 2 studies[55,56] found no differences between medication and neurofeedback effects, and one study[55] reported that neurofeedback or medication alone was as effective as the combination.

Relation between training performance and clinical improvement

A key question regarding the specificity of the effects is whether treatment success is related to the degree of effective learning during neurofeedback (ie, the learning curve at the neural level). Some studies reported correlations between measures of improved cortical self-regulation and clinical gains. In one SCP study,[36] participants were divided into groups of successful or unsuccessful regulators, based on the ability to produce the required EEG activity in negativity trials without feedback. Children who showed good performance in cortical self-regulation demonstrated a better clinical outcome at the end of training than the unsuccessful regulators. Evidence from Ref.[57] points in a similar direction. Although only half the children in their neurofeedback condition learned to regulate cortical activation during a transfer condition (without direct feedback), the neurofeedback training performance of these good performers was closely related to clinical improvement in hyperactivity ($r = 0.81$) and impulsivity ($r = 0.75$). However, the poor regulators also showed comparable clinical improvement, indicating considerable nonspecific effects. Neurofeedback may also involve learning to reduce motor activity through artifact feedback and instructions to sit still, but this type of learning does not seem to directly account for clinical improvement.[52] Similarly, although learning was superior for EMG biofeedback (targeting motor control, the control condition) compared with neurofeedback (targeting cortical control) in one study,[25] the clinical effects did not reflect that advantage and even nonsignificantly favored neurofeedback. These results also illustrate that learning in the control condition may be required to match motivation and the experience of self-efficacy and suggest that sham control conditions that do not allow learning may not be suitable.

Together, these findings indicate that although learning can correlate with clinical improvement and thereby provide important evidence for the specificity of effects, the relation may not be trivial, may involve learning of other behavioral and physiologic states than the targeted ones, and may involve delays until evident in clinical improvement. Demographic, symptomatic, or other patient characteristics, which might predict successful neurofeedback learning and transfer performance, have not yet been identified.[6,57] In summary, the increased use of blinded ADHD measures and multiple control conditions in recent neurofeedback research is encouraging, but most recent results remain ambiguous without evidence for the learning of self-regulation[25,58] and leave open whether the neurofeedback protocols were compromised. Effect size considerations still tend to support some efficacy for neurofeedback, at least when considering some blinded outcomes, and may yield a slightly more positive picture than offered in the recent meta-analysis,[11] but evidence from larger studies using standard neurofeedback and examining learning under way[59] will be crucial to allow firmer conclusions. Also, most of these finding were obtained for groups including a considerable proportion of medicated ADHD patients, and most support the use of neurofeedback only in multimodal treatment schemes (but see Ref.[55]). However, the best blinded controlled effects were nonsignificant in the small group studies and remained considerably reduced when compared with more proximal ratings. These recent studies also raise the possibility that "good," partly active control conditions, may themselves bring about considerable improvement in ADHD symptoms, with 19% symptom reduction for EMG biofeedback[25] and 17.8% for sham neurofeedback,[45] compared with 9.4% reduction for the computer training control in the largest study.[44] Further research should clarify whether these sizable and clinically relevant effects are just nonspecific placebo effects mediated by expectancy, or whether active attempts to learn physiologic self-regulation through feedback and transfer, even though unsuccessful by design or targeting peripheral control, induce similar brain plasticity as implicated for neurofeedback.

Imaging studies
Neurofeedback appears to involve regulation of an extended cortical and subcortical network, with partly distinct regions for central negativity (activation) and positivity (deactivation) trials following successful SCP training. In a first controlled functional magnetic resonance imaging (fMRI) study on neurofeedback in ADHD,[60] it was reported that the enhancement of SMR, beta activity, and the suppression of theta activity led to a normalization of neural activity within brain regions key to selective attention and response inhibition (ie, the anterior cingulate cortex, caudate nucleus, and substantia nigra). As these studies lack an active control condition, the possibility that the effects may be explained by unspecific variables of the treatment setting cannot be excluded. An essential part of neurofeedback training is the reinforcement of desired "behavior," which will in itself induce the production of cortical (and, at least indirectly, subcortical) brain alterations in regions known to be involved in reinforcement processing. Via visual feedback, the trainee receives a high amount of rewarding stimuli throughout the training. It could, therefore, be hypothesized that part of the clinical outcome could be mediated by effects on the reward system. Simultaneous EEG-fMRI imaging findings during reward anticipation in fact demonstrated that negative SCPs (CNV activity) correlated with cortical and subcortical reward system activation.[61] Evidence to support this prediction in ADHD is still limited, but preliminary results of an ongoing study seem to point in this direction.[62] Although participants with ADHD showed a significant hypoactivation in the neural reward pathway before training compared with healthy controls,[20] sessions of SCP-neurofeedback led to a modification and partial functional normalization in pivotal reward-related structures.

Stability over time
A major advantage of neurofeedback and other neurotherapeutic approaches[63] over typical pharmacologic interventions (as for other behavioral, learning-based interventions) is the potential for sustained, long-term benefits after successful completion of treatment. Investigations[36] indeed found positive effects on ADHD symptoms being stable 6 months after training. Similarly, 2 studies[48,63] reported sustained advantages following neurofeedback at 6-month follow-ups, and one study[64] even reported stability after 2 years, following neurofeedback and a few booster sessions. However, interpretation of these findings is complicated by the fact that most ratings of long-term effects (except for the behavioral observation measure in Ref.[48]) were not blinded and thus subject to bias.

Despite evidence for beneficial effects of neurofeedback on ADHD symptoms, the National Institute for Health and Clinical Excellence (NICE) guidelines on ADHD do not recommend it as a treatment option,[65] but the most recently published studies were not yet part of the NICE review process.

CLINICAL DECISION-MAKING
Who Is Most Likely to Respond?

To guide the decision whether a training approach which is as intensive and time-consuming as neurofeedback is justified for a given patient, a better understanding is needed of how treatment effects are related to individual clinical and neurocognitive characteristics and electrophysiologic markers. Predictors and mediators of response in subgroups of ADHD patients and/or individual patients have only been studied in some of the most recent trials. Initial evidence for predictive and protocol-specific EEG or ERP markers is encouraging, as detailed in the following subsections.

Relation between pretreatment EEG characteristics and clinical improvement
Pretraining EEG measures seem to indicate later treatment response at least for SCP training (while similar findings have not yet been reported for EEG frequency band training). A larger pretraining CNV is associated with a larger reduction of ADHD symptoms for SCP training, accounting for about 20% of the variance in outcome.[66] Similarly, pretraining alpha resting activity is associated with behavioral improvements. Concerning the improvement of ADHD core symptoms induced by the SCP training, nearly 30% of the variance was explained by the combined predictor variables CNV and alpha activity.

Training intensity
Positive changes on the behavioral, neurophysiologic, and neuropsychological levels have been reported after as few as 20 and as many as 40 sessions of neurofeedback. Although no trial has systematically examined the number, frequency, and duration of sessions required to elicit a positive and enduring effect, a meta-analysis of 6 indicated a moderate positive correlation ($r = 0.55$) between the treatment effect on inattention and the number of training sessions across studies. Achievement of cortical self-regulation via neurofeedback was also related to the individual's ability for visual imagery.[67] This line of thought has not been further pursued in recent years, but the limited strength of the reported correlations ($r = 0.37$) and clinical experience suggests that imagery may only explain a small proportion of the interindividual variance in learning and treatment outcome and that other factors may play a substantial role in the mechanisms responsible for treatment response to neurofeedback.

Role of parents and parenting style on treatment success

Parenting style may moderate the effectiveness of neurofeedback. Patients whose parents were systematically using reinforcement principles in their normal practice were more likely to demonstrate a reduction in the frequency of core ADHD symptoms following neurofeedback training than children of parents with a nonsystematic parenting style.[68] When "systematic" parenting approaches were used, improvements were even maintained when the concomitant medication was discontinued. Similar results[57] indicated that parental support significantly mediates clinical improvement for both learners and nonlearners of self-regulation. Other less specific factors, such as effort, time (and attention!) invested, improved feedback and reward processing, and learning to reduce motor hyperactivity and to sit still to avoid artifacts,[52] may also contribute to the considerable effects common to neurofeedback and partly active control trainings.

What Outcomes Are Most Likely to Be Affected by Treatment?

Neurofeedback aims at the improvement of ADHD core symptoms and their underlying neuropsychological pathways. Regarding the 3 symptom domains of ADHD, current evidence suggests stronger effects of neurofeedback on attention and impulsivity than hyperactivity.[6]

What Are the Contraindications for Treatment?

There are no known contraindications for standard neurofeedback protocols. However, because epilepsy has been treated with SCP downregulation targeting positivity/deactivation,[69] epilepsy may represent a contraindication for the typical SCP upregulation protocol (ie, targeting negativity/activation in ADHD). Further research is required for this.

What Are Potential Adverse Effects of the Treatment?

To date, no severe or permanent side effects of neurofeedback have been reported, and adverse effects systematically decrease over training as for placebo control with blinded assessment.[45] Headaches and fatigue have been occasionally documented, which seem to be attributable to the intentional demands and associated muscular tension during training sessions.[33] Some patients with a simultaneous and well-tolerated regime of psychostimulants may experience typical medication side effects in the course of neurofeedback training that may require dose adjustment. This phenomenon might be related to the additional stimulating effect of the training.

How Should the Treatment Be Sequenced and/or Integrated with Drug Therapy and with Other Nondrug Treatments?

Although current evidence has not sufficiently addressed the differential efficacy of the existing neurofeedback protocols, evidence from one study suggests that the order of SCP and QEEG can affect results (favoring a start with the simpler QEEG training). Clinical practice may be based on established principles of learning; make use of clear instructions, the importance of regular, short, and repetitive sessions; and transfer into everyday life. Some of the high-quality studies with longer follow-up included "booster sessions" time-tabled after several weeks after treatment to refresh the ability of self-regulation and to maintain treatment effects.

FUTURE DIRECTIONS

The question whether one of the established training protocols (SCP training and training of EEG frequency bands) is more effective than the other is not yet fully resolved, but the initial evidence for distinct EEG and ERP outcome predictors suggests that the response may depend on the neurophysiologic subtype. Future research on neurofeedback should focus on such differential effects (which intervention works for whom?). Although EEG-based neurofeedback can build on a large evidence base of controlled studies and will continue to dominate for reasons of low cost and ease of use, new neurofeedback techniques based on hemodynamic measures are emerging. Both near infrared spectroscopy neurofeedback[70] and real-time fMRI neurofeedback may offer advantages in terms of targeting well-defined brain regions, and such studies are ongoing.[71] Notably, real-time fMRI additionally opens the possibility for more rapid learning to regulate deep structures, such as the dopaminergic midbrain regions[72] implicated in ADHD along with cortical regions.[73]

Additional Outcome Parameters

With regard to the multiple identified pathways to ADHD, initial steps have been undertaken to target deficits in executive dysfunction (eg, making use of inhibition or working memory trainings; see the article by Sonuga-Barke and colleagues elsewhere in this issue) and reward-related impairments. All neurofeedback protocols are characterized by reinforcement for the improvement of targeted "neural behavior," but the impact of training-induced neurobiological and neuropsychological changes on reward-related functions and structures has been rarely studied yet. In addition, temporal processing deficits as the third dissociable neuropsychological component of ADHD have not been explicitly addressed in many intervention studies. Neurofeedback studies aiming at the modulation of the CNV as an on-line marker of temporal coding and time-based decision-making may explicitly address impaired timing as an important treatment outcome.[74]

SUMMARY

Based on current knowledge, neurofeedback is likely to be used as an element in the broader set of nonpharmacologic treatments for ADHD in multimodal therapy. It has recently been claimed that neurofeedback is "efficacious and specific."[6,42] However, the authors think that in light of the most recent findings from sham-controlled studies[75] and the analysis of probably blinded measures,[11] there is a strong need for more evidence from well-blinded, methodologically sound and sensitive trials before neurofeedback can be assigned this highest level of evidence as a front-line treatment of ADHD. Firmer conclusions must await upcoming evidence from larger, well-controlled neurofeedback studies, which demonstrate learning of self-regulation in addition to using well-blinded and sensitive outcome measures.

DISCLOSURES

M. Holtmann served in an advisory or consultancy role for Lilly, Novartis, Shire, and Bristol-Myers Squibb and received conference attendance support or was paid for public speaking by AstraZeneca, Bristol-Myers Squibb, Janssen-Cilag, Lilly, Medice, Neuroconn, Novartis, and Shire. E. Sonuga-Barke has financial disclosures in relation to Shire Pharmaceuticals—speaker fees, consultancy, advisory board membership, research support, and conference attendance funds. Janssen Cilag has received speaker fees. Visiting chairs at Ghent University and Aarhus University. Grants awarded from MRC, Economic and Social Research Council, Wellcome Trust, Solent NHS Trust, European Union, Child Health Research Foundation New Zealand, National Institute on Handicapped Research, Nuffield Foundation, Fonds Wetenschappelijk Onderzoek–Vlaanderen (FWO). S. Cortese has no current relationships with drug companies. He receives royalties from Argon Healthcare Italy for educational activities on ADHD. Before 2010, he served as scientific consultant for Shire Pharmaceuticals and received support to attend meetings from Eli Lilly and from Shire. D. Brandeis has no disclosures to report.

REFERENCES

1. American Psychiatric Association. Diagnostic and statistical manual of mental disorders, 5th edition (DSM-5). Washington, DC: American Psychiatric Association Press; 2013.
2. Faraone SV, Biederman J, Mick E. The age-dependent decline of attention deficit hyperactivity disorder: a meta-analysis of follow-up studies. Psychol Med 2006;36(2):159–65.
3. Banaschewski T, Coghill D, Santosh P, et al. Long-acting medications for the hyperkinetic disorders. A systematic review and European treatment guideline. Eur Child Adolesc Psychiatry 2006;15(8):476–95.
4. Cortese S, Holtmann M, Banaschewski T, et al. Practitioner review: current best practice in the management of adverse events during treatment with ADHD medications in children and adolescents. J Child Psychol Psychiatry 2013;54(3):227–46.
5. Graham J, Banaschewski T, Buitelaar J, et al. European guidelines on managing adverse effects of medication for ADHD. Eur Child Adolesc Psychiatry 2011; 20(1):17–37.
6. Arns M, de Ridder S, Strehl U, et al. Efficacy of neurofeedback treatment in ADHD: the effects on inattention, impulsivity and hyperactivity: a meta-analysis. Clin EEG Neurosci 2009;40(3):180–9.
7. Fabiano GA, Pelham WE Jr, Coles EK, et al. A meta- analysis of behavioral treatments for attention-deficit/hyperactivity disorder. Clin Psychol Rev 2009;29(2): 129–40.
8. Nigg JT, Lewis K, Edinger T, et al. Meta-analysis of attention-deficit/hyperactivity disorder or attention-deficit/hyperactivity disorder symptoms, restriction diet, and synthetic food color additives. J Am Acad Child Adolesc Psychiatry 2012;51(1):86–97.e8.
9. Bloch MH, Qawasmi A. Omega-3 fatty acid supplementation for the treatment of children with attention-deficit/hyperactivity disorder symptomatology: systematic review and meta-analysis. J Am Acad Child Adolesc Psychiatry 2011; 50(10):991–1000.
10. Markomichali P, Donnelly N, Sonuga-Barke E. Cognitive training for attention, inhibition and working memory deficits: a potential treatment for ADHD? Advances in ADHD 2009;3:89–96.
11. Sonuga-Barke EJ, Brandeis D, Cortese S, et al. Nonpharmacological interventions for ADHD: systematic review and meta-analyses of randomized controlled trials of dietary and psychological treatments. Am J Psychiatry 2013;170(3):275–89.
12. Lubar JF, Shouse MN. EEG and behavioral changes in a hyperkinetic child concurrent with training of the sensorimotor rhythm (SMR): a preliminary report. Biofeedback Self Regul 1976;1:293–306.

13. Jasper H, Solomon P, Bradley C. Electroencephalographic analyses of behaviour problem children. Am J Psychiatry 1938;95:641–58.

14. Lindsley DB, Cutts K. Electroencephalograms of "constitutionally inferior" and behavior problem children: comparison with those of normal children and adults. Arch Neurol Psychiatr 1940;44(6):1199–212.

15. Lüchinger R, Michels L, Martin E, et al. Brain state regulation during normal development: intrinsic activity fluctuations in simultaneous EEG-fMRI. Neuroimage 2012;60(2):1426–39.

16. Gasser T, Verleger R, Bacher P, et al. Development of the EEG of school-age children and adolescents. I. Analysis of band power. Electroencephalogr Clin Neurophysiol 1988;69(2):91–9.

17. Becker K, Holtmann M. Role of electroencephalography in attention-deficit hyperactivity disorder. Expert Rev Neurother 2006;6(5):731–9.

18. Barry RJ, Clarke AR, Johnstone SJ. A review of electrophysiology in attention-deficit/hyperactivity disorder: I. Qualitative and quantitative electroencephalography. Clin Neurophysiol 2003;114(2):171–83.

19. Monastra VJ, Lubar JF, Linden M, et al. Assessing attention deficit hyperactivity disorder via quantitative electroencephalography: an initial validation study. Neuropsychology 1999;13(3):424–33.

20. Chabot RJ, Serfontein G. Quantitative electroencephalographic profiles of children with attention deficit disorder. Biol Psychiatry 1996;40:951–63.

21. Clarke AR, Barry RJ, McCarthy R, et al. EEG-defined subtypes of children with attention-deficit/hyperactivity disorder. Clin Neurophysiol 2001;112(11):2098–105.

22. Liechti M, Valko L, Müller UC, et al. Diagnostic value of resting electroencephalogram in attention deficit/hyperactivity disorder across the lifespan. Brain Topogr 2013;26(1):135–51.

23. Arns M, Conners CK, Kraemer HC. A decade of EEG theta/beta ratio research in ADHD: a meta-analysis. J Atten Disord 2013;17(5):374–83.

24. Barry RJ, Clarke AR, Johnstone SJ, et al. Electroencephalogram theta/beta ratio and arousal in attention-deficit/hyperactivity disorder: evidence of independent processes. Biol Psychiatry 2009;66(4):398–401.

25. Maurizio S, Liechti M, Heinrich H, et al. Comparing tomographic EEG neurofeedback and EMG biofeedback in children with attention-deficit/hyperactivity disorder. Biol Psychol 2014;95:31–44.

26. Clarke AR, Barry RJ, Dupuy FE, et al. Behavioural differences between EEG-defined subgroups of children with Attention-Deficit/Hyperactivity Disorder. Clin Neurophysiol 2011;22(7):1333–41.

27. Poil SS, Bollmann S, Ghisleni C, et al. Age-dependent electroencephalographic changes in Attention-Deficit/Hyperactivity Disorder (ADHD). Clin Neurophysiol 2014;125(8):1626–38.

28. Brandeis D, Banaschewski T, Baving L, et al. Multicenter P300 brain mapping of impaired attention to cues in hyperkinetic children. J Am Acad Child Adolesc Psychiatry 2002;41(8):990–8.

29. Birbaumer N, Elbert T, Canavan AG, et al. Slow potentials of the cerebral cortex and behavior. Physiol Rev 1990;70(1):1–41.

30. Macar F, Vidal F. Timing processes: an outline of behavioural and neural indices not systematically considered in timing models. Can J Exp Psychol 2009;63(3):227–39.

31. Doehnert M, Brandeis D, Schneider G, et al. A neurophysiological marker of impaired preparation in an 11-year follow-up study of attention-deficit/hyperactivity disorder (ADHD). J Child Psychol Psychiatry 2013;54(3):260–70.

32. Vernon D, Frick A, Gruzelier J. Neurofeedback as a treatment for ADHD: a methodological review with implications for future research. J Neurother 2004;8(2):53–82.
33. Nash JK. Treatment of attention deficit hyperactivity disorder with neurotherapy. Clin Electroencephalogr 2000;31(1):30–7.
34. Linden M, Habib T, Radojevic V. A controlled study of the effects of EEG biofeedback on cognition and behavior of children with attention deficit disorder and learning disabilities [Erratum appears in 1996;21(3):297]. Biofeedback Self Regul 1996;21(1):35–49.
35. Heinrich H, Gevensleben H, Freisleder FJ, et al. Training of slow cortical potentials in attention-deficit/hyperactivity disorder: evidence for positive behavioral and neurophysiological effects. Biol Psychiatry 2004;55:772–5.
36. Strehl U, Leins U, Goth G, et al. Self-regulation of slow cortical potentials: a new treatment for children with attention-deficit/hyperactivity disorder. Pediatrics 2006;118(5):1530–40.
37. Heinrich H, Gevensleben H, Strehl U. Annotation: neurofeedback - train your brain to train behaviour. J Child Psychol Psychiatry 2007;48(1):3–16.
38. Brandeis D. Neurofeedback training in ADHD: more news on specificity. Clin Neurophysiol 2011;122:856–7.
39. Gevensleben H, Kleemeyer M, Rothenberger L, et al. Neurofeedback in ADHD: further pieces of the puzzle. Brain Topogr 2014;27(1):20–32.
40. Holtmann M, Stadler C. Electroencephalographic biofeedback for the treatment of attention-deficit hyperactivity disorder in childhood and adolescence. Expert Rev Neurother 2006;6(4):533–40.
41. Holtmann M, Steiner S, Hohmann S, et al. Neurofeedback in autism spectrum disorders. Dev Med Child Neurol 2011;53(11):986–93.
42. Gevensleben H, Rothenberger A, Moll GH, et al. Neurofeedback in children with ADHD: validation and challenges. Expert Rev Neurother 2012;12(4):447–60.
43. Leins U, Goth G, Hinterberger T, et al. Neurofeedback for children with ADHD: a comparison of SCP and theta/beta protocols. Appl Psychophysiol Biofeedback 2007;32(2):73–88.
44. Gevensleben H, Holl B, Albrecht B, et al. Is neurofeedback an efficacious treatment for ADHD? A randomised controlled clinical trial. J Child Psychol Psychiatry 2009;50(7):780–9.
45. van Dongen-Boomsma M, Vollebregt MA, Slaats-Willemse D, et al. A randomized placebo-controlled trial of electroencephalographic (EEG) neurofeedback in children with attention-deficit/hyperactivity disorder. J Clin Psychiatry 2013;74(8):821–7.
46. Lansbergen MM, van Dongen-Boomsma M, Buitelaar JK, et al. ADHD and EEG-neurofeedback: a double-blind randomized placebo-controlled feasibility study. J Neural Transm 2011;118(2):275–84.
47. Steiner NJ, Frenette EC, Rene KM, et al. Neurofeedback and cognitive attention training for children with attention-deficit hyperactivity disorder in schools. J Dev Behav Pediatr 2014;35(1):18–27.
48. Steiner NJ, Frenette EC, Rene KM, et al. In-school neurofeedback training for ADHD: sustained improvements from a randomized control trial. Pediatrics 2014;133(3):483–92.
49. Steiner NJ, Sheldrick RC, Gotthelf D, et al. Computer-based attention training in the schools for children with attention deficit/hyperactivity disorder: a preliminary trial. Clin Pediatr (Phila) 2011;50(7):615–22.
50. Arns M, Strehl U. Evidence for efficacy of neurofeedback in ADHD? Am J Psychiatry 2013;170(7):799–800.

51. Sonuga-Barke EJ, Brandeis D, Cortese S, et al. Response to Chronis-Tuscano, et al. and Arns and Strehl. Am J Psychiatry 2013;170(7):800–2.
52. Liechti M, Maurizio S, Heinrich H, et al. First clinical trial of tomographic neuro-feedback in attention-deficit/hyperactivity disorder: evaluation of voluntary cortical control. Clin Neurophysiol 2012;123(10):1989–2005.
53. Arns M, Drinkenburg W, Leon Kenemans J. The effects of QEEG-informed neu-rofeedback in ADHD: an open-label pilot study. Appl Psychophysiol Biofeed-back 2012;7(3):171–80.
54. Ogrim G, Hestad KA. Effects of neurofeedback versus stimulant medication in attention-deficit/hyperactivity disorder: a randomized pilot study. J Child Ado-lesc Psychopharmacol 2013;23(7):448–57.
55. Duric N, Assmus J, Gundersen D, et al. Neurofeedback for the treatment of chil-dren and adolescents with ADHD: a randomized and controlled clinical trial us-ing parental reports. BMC Psychiatry 2012;12(1):107.
56. Meisel V, Servera M, Garcia-Banda G, et al. Neurofeedback and standard phar-macological intervention in ADHD: a randomized controlled trial with six-month follow-up. Biol Psychol 2013;94(1):12–21.
57. Drechsler R, Straub M, Döhnert M, et al. Controlled evaluation of a neurofeed-back training of slow cortical potentials in children with attention deficit/hyperac-tivity disorder (ADHD). Behav Brain Funct 2007;3(1):35.
58. Vollebregt MA, van Dongen-Boomsma M, Buitelaar JK, et al. Does EEG-neurofeedback improve neurocognitive functioning in children with attention-deficit/hyperactivity disorder? A systematic review and a double-blind placebo-controlled study. J Child Psychol Psychiatry 2013;55(5):460–72.
59. Holtmann M. Neurofeedback in children with attention deficit hyperactivity dis-order (ADHD): a single-blind randomised controlled trial. 2009. Available at: http://controlled-trials.com/ISRCTN76187185/neurofeedback. Accessed July 4, 2014.
60. Beauregard M, Levesque J. Functional magnetic resonance imaging investiga-tion of the effects of neurofeedback training on the neural bases of selective attention and response inhibition in children with attention-deficit/hyperactivity disorder. Appl Psychophysiol Biofeedback 2006;31(1):3–20.
61. Plichta MM, Wolf I, Hohmann S, et al. Simultaneous EEG and fMRI reveals a causally connected subcortical-cortical network during reward anticipation. J Neurosci 2013;33(36):14526–33.
62. Wolf I, Hohmann S, Baumeister S, et al. Effects of Biofeedback Training on the Brain Reward System of ADHD Patients. HBM 2013: 19th Annual Meeting of the Organization for Human Brain Mapping. Seattle, June 16-20, 2013.
63. Gevensleben H, Holl B, Albrecht B, et al. Neurofeedback training in children with ADHD: 6-month follow-up of a randomised controlled trial. Eur Child Adolesc Psychiatry 2010;19(9):715–24.
64. Gani C, Birbaumer N, Strehl U. Long term effects after feedback of slow cortical potentials and of theta-beta-amplitudes in children with attention-deficit/hyperactivity disorder (ADHD). Int J Bioelectromagn 2008;10(4):209–32.
65. NICE (National Institute for Health and Clinical Excellence). Attention deficit hy-peractivity disorder. Clinical guideline 72. 2008. Available at: http://www.nice.org.uk/nicemedia/live/12061/42060/42060.pdf. Accessed March 2, 2014.
66. Wangler S, Gevensleben H, Albrecht B, et al. Neurofeedback in children with ADHD: specific event-related potential findings of a randomized controlled trial. Clin Neurophysiol 2011;122(5):942–50.

67. Birbaumer N, Lang PJ, Cook E 3rd, et al. Slow brain potentials, imagery and hemispheric differences. Int J Neurosci 1988;39(1–2):101–16.
68. Monastra VJ, Lynn S, Linden M, et al. Electroencephalographic biofeedback in the treatment of attention-deficit/hyperactivity disorder. Appl Psychophysiol Biofeedback 2005;30(2):95–114.
69. Kotchoubey B, Strehl U, Uhlmann C, et al. Modification of slow cortical potentials in patients with refractory epilepsy: a controlled outcome study. Epilepsia 2001;42(3):406–16.
70. Mihara M, Miyai I, Hattori N, et al. Neurofeedback using real-time near-infrared spectroscopy enhances motor imagery related cortical activation. PLoS One 2012;7(3):e32234.
71. Rubia K. 2012. Available at: http://www.controlled-trials.com/ISRCTN12800253/rubia. Accessed July 4, 2014.
72. Sulzer J, Sitaram R, Blefari ML, et al. Neurofeedback-mediated self-regulation of the dopaminergic midbrain. Neuroimage 2013;75C:176–84.
73. Cortese S, Kelly C, Chabernaud C, et al. Toward systems neuroscience of ADHD: a meta-analysis of 55 fMRI studies. Am J Psychiatry 2012;169(10):1038–55.
74. Holtmann M. Commentary: persistent time estimation deficits in ADHD? from developmental trajectories to individual targets for intervention - reflections on Doehnert et al. (2013). J Child Psychol Psychiatry 2013;54(3):271–2.
75. Lofthouse N, Arnold LE, Hersch S, et al. A review of neurofeedback treatment for pediatric ADHD. J Atten Disord 2011;16(5):351–72.
76. Bakhshayesh A, Hänsch S, Wyschkon A, et al. Neurofeedback in ADHD: a single-blind randomized controlled trial. Eur Child Adolesc Psychiatry 2011; 20(9):481–91.
77. Holtmann M, Grasmann D, Cionek-Szpak E, et al. Spezifische Wirksamkeit von Neurofeedback auf die Impulsivität bei ADHS. [Specific effects of neurofeedback on impulsivity in ADHD]. Kindheit und Entwicklung 2009;18:95–104.

Computer-based Cognitive Training for ADHD
A Review of Current Evidence

Edmund Sonuga-Barke, PhD[a,b],*, Daniel Brandeis, PhD[c,d],
Martin Holtmann, MD[e], Samuele Cortese, MD, PhD[f,g]

KEYWORDS

- ADHD • Treatment • Cognitive training • Working memory • Inhibitory control
- Attentional control • Randomized controlled trial • Brain plasticity

KEY POINTS

- Cognitive training approaches, such as working memory training (WMT), are being increasingly used to target both the symptoms and the underlying neuropsychological deficits in patients with attention-deficit/hyperactivity disorder (ADHD). The rationale of these approaches is both biologically plausible and supported by basic cognitive neuroscience.
- There are now 14 randomized controlled trials (RCTs) with ADHD outcomes (8 published in the past 2 years or so).
- At present, given the inconsistency of extant findings, more evidence from well-blinded trials is required before cognitive training can be supported as a frontline treatment of ADHD.
- Evidence in relation to improved neuropsychological function maybe more positive, but additional research is required.
- Future research should focus on ways to improve the content and implementation, and increase the scope, of these potentially important therapeutic approaches.

Disclosures: See last page of article.
[a] Developmental Brain-Behaviour Laboratory, Psychology, Institute for Disorders of Impulse & Attention, University of Southampton, University Road, Southampton SO17 1BJ, UK; [b] Department of Experimental Clinical & Health Psychology, Ghent University, Henri Dunantlaan 2, Ghent B-9000, Belgium; [c] Department of Child and Adolescent Psychiatry, University of Zürich, Neumünsterallee 9/Fach, Zürich CH-8032, Switzerland; [d] Department of Child and Adolescent Psychiatry and Psychotherapy, Central Institute of Mental Health, Medical Faculty Mannheim, Heidelberg University, J5, Mannheim D-68159, Germany; [e] LWL-University Hospital for Child and Adolescent Psychiatry, Ruhr University Bochum, Heithofer Allee 64, Hamm D 59071, Germany; [f] Department of Child Psychiatry, Cambridge University Hospitals NHS Foundation Trust, Hills Road, Cambridge PE29 2BQ, UK; [g] Division of Psychiatry, Institute of Mental Health, University of Nottingham, Triumph Road, Nottingham NG7 2TU, UK
* Corresponding author. Developmental Brain-Behaviour Laboratory, Psychology, Institute for Disorders of Impulse & Attention, University of Southampton, University Road, Southampton SO17 1BJ, UK.
E-mail address: ejb3@soton.ac.uk

Child Adolesc Psychiatric Clin N Am 23 (2014) 807–824
http://dx.doi.org/10.1016/j.chc.2014.05.009
1056-4993/14/$ – see front matter © 2014 Elsevier Inc. All rights reserved.

Abbreviations	
ADHD	Attention-deficit/hyperactivity disorder
CI	Confidence interval
EF	Executive function
RCT	Randomized controlled trial
SMD	Standardized mean difference
TAU	Treatment as usual
WM	Working memory
WMT	Working memory training

INTRODUCTION
Target of Treatment: Distinguishing Clinical and Neuropsychological Elements

ADHD is a disorder of childhood onset marked by pervasive patterns of inattention, impulsivity, and/or hyperactivity, which often persist into later life.[1] ADHD is clinically complex and heterogeneous.[2] There are high rates of comorbid externalizing,[3,4] internalizing,[5,6] learning,[7] and pervasive developmental disorders.[8] Patients with ADHD are impaired across a range of domains in different settings (ie, at home, with peers, or at school and work), which leads to reduced quality of life.[9,10] ADHD affects the family and community more broadly, creating substantial burden for health, educational, and criminal justice systems.[11]

ADHD is associated with a broad range of neuropsychological impairments,[12] encompassing multiple brain networks known to underpin diverse cognitive and motivational processes.[13] In the cognitive domain these include frontostriatal inhibitory-based executive function networks,[12,14,15] frontoparietal working memory (WM),[16,17] thalamocorticocerebellar timing circuits,[18] as well as non-WM[19] and basic processing efficiency.[20] Motivational deficits seem multifarious and complex.[21,22] Task engagement is affected by altered patterns of intrinsic motivation[23] and altered sensitivity to punishment and reward[24] associated with specific brain circuits.[25,26] Deficits in response to delayed rewards are consistently observed.[27,28] The context-dependent nature of these deficits also points to the dysregulation of energetic processes (eg, effort, activation, and arousal[29]). More recently, there has been a focus on altered patterns of resting state connectivity in the default mode[30] and diminished suppression of resting state networks during active task performance,[31] which may explain periodic attention lapses and related increased intraindividual variability.[32] Crucially, the population of individuals with ADHD is heterogeneous in terms of their specific profile of neuropsychological deficits, with different individuals showing distinct neuropsychological and pathophysiological profiles, suggesting that there may be discrete ADHD subtypes with different cognitive, motivational, or energetic deficits.[30,33–38]

Neuropsychological deficits, and the impaired brain networks they reflect, are especially significant in guiding the development of neurotherapeutics for ADHD for 2 reasons. First, according to current causal models, they are conceptualized as pathophysiological mediators (ie, endophenotypes) of pathways between originating cases (genes, environments) and disorder manifestation.[39] Support for this comes from evidence of cosegregation of ADHD caseness with cognitive[40] and motivational deficits[41] in families. From a translational science perspective, they can be thought of as candidate ADHD treatment targets. The logic is that, for instance, as executive deficits, to some extent, are postulated to mediate the causal risk pathways to ADHD, remediating these deficits through training should alleviate ADHD symptoms and improve associated everyday functioning for that subgroup of patients marked by vulnerabilities in this neuropsychological domain. Second, neuropsychological deficits can be seen as targets for treatment in their own right, independent of any effects of executive training on ADHD symptoms. This fact is because such deficits are themselves (1) only partially overlapping with ADHD (being often found in individuals with other disorders or no disorders at all)[30,35] and (2) associated with deficits in daily functioning independent of ADHD.[42] In this sense over and above their role in causal pathways to ADHD, it may make sense to consider neuropsychological deficits as complicating factors or comorbid conditions.[43] Neuropsychological deficits themselves may even be considered as the primary treatment target for cognitive training interventions. In this sense, the use of cognitive training approaches to address neuropsychological deficits may be justified even if they are not effective treatments for ADHD symptoms.

Need for Treatment: Limitations of Pharmacologic and Behavioral Approaches in the Clinical and Neuropsychological Domains

Multimodal treatments, which combine pharmaceutical and psychological approaches, are currently recommended for the treatment of ADHD.[44] ADHD medications (ie, psychostimulant [eg, methylphenidate, D-amphetamine] and/or nonpsychostimulant [eg, atomoxetine, guanfacine]) demonstrate efficacy in short- and midterm RCTs[45] in terms of core symptoms, externalizing comorbidities, and improvements in daily functioning.[46] Neuropsychological impairments are also reduced by medication.[47] Coghill and colleagues[48] demonstrated significant effects of methylphenidate across 5 domains of executive functioning (executive memory, nonexecutive memory, reaction time, reaction time variability, and response inhibition). These effects were in general smaller than those seen for core symptoms. Medication also improves response to delayed reward[49] and increased intrinsic motivation.[23] Although recommended as a first-line treatment of ADHD (at least in more severe cases), some issues around medication use and response have motivated a search for effective nonpharmacologic alternatives.[50] These issues include (1) partial or no response,[45] (2) adverse effects[51] and long-term benefits/costs,[52,53] (3) poor adherence,[54] and (4) negative attitudes, from patients, parents, or clinicians, to medication.[55–57]

There are a range of nonpharmacologic treatment options (see this issue). Dietary exclusions can be valuable especially in individuals with food intolerances.[58] Polyunsaturated fatty acid supplementation seems to have small but generalized and robust effects.[58] Little is known about the effects of dietary treatments on either broader patterns of impairment or neuropsychological deficits. Psychosocial treatments based on social learning and behavior modification principles have been widely implemented often through parent-training-based approaches.[59] However, a recent meta-analysis has shown that positive reports by those closest to the therapeutic setting—typically unblinded and heavily treatment-invested parents—are not corroborated by more "blinded" measures (eg, direct observations).[50] In a second more recent meta-analysis, the investigators found some evidence that behavioral interventions reduced conduct disorder and improved social skills in children with ADHD.[60] There has been little or no study on the value of dietary or behavioral interventions for treating neuropsychological deficits in ADHD. A challenge for behavioral approaches has been to get effects to transfer from the specific focus on treatment and generalize from the intervention setting to other important settings. By attempting to target the core deficits rather than just ADHD behaviors, it is hoped that cognitive training and other neurotherapeutic approaches will lead to greater effect generalization and transfer.

In summary, limitations of existing treatments highlight the need for therapeutic innovation in ADHD to develop effective nonpharmacologic interventions that can improve short- and long-term outcomes on core symptoms, neuropsychological deficits, and more general patterns of impairment. Cognitive-based training approaches aim to both reduce ADHD core symptoms and improve neuropsychological functioning by targeting the underlying deficits thought to mediate ADHD causal pathways.

INTERVENTIONS
Theoretic Underpinnings: Why Should Cognitive Training Work?

Cognitive training has been defined as "the process of improving cognitive functioning by means of practice and/or intentional instructions."[61] Cognitive training needs to be differentiated from other neurotherapeutic approaches including neurofeedback, transcranial magnetic stimulation, transcranial electrical stimulation, meditation training, physical exercise, and music training. Two types of cognitive training have been described. The first are process-based approaches, which focus on *implicit* practice via repeated performance of cognitive tasks (eg, processing speed and inhibition); primary mental abilities (eg, inductive reasoning, spatial orientation, and episodic memory); higher-order cognitive constructs (eg, fluid intelligence and executive functioning); and global cognition, involving different cognitive domains such as attention and WM.[62] The second type involves strategy-based approaches, which use *explicit* task instructions aimed at promoting, for instance, the implementation of general metacognitive skills or specific strategies such as rehearsal, chunking, or mental imagery.[61] Recent studies in ADHD have focused on the former approaches, and this review does the same.

In a general sense, the theoretic rationale for cognitive training applied to ADHD builds on previous literature on both adult brain injury rehabilitation[63] and contemporary developmental neuroscience.[64] Both these approaches are grounded in the notion of neural plasticity and the reorganization of brain structure and function in response to structured environmental experience,[62] which drives learning and promotes the development of new cognitive skills even in patients experiencing lesion-based deficits and cognitive impairment.[65] From a developmental perspective Baltes[66] described 3 levels of cognitive performance. *Baseline performance* refers to the individual's initial level of performance without intervention. *Baseline plasticity* indicates the extended range of possible performances when additional resources are provided. *Developmental reserve capacity or developmental plasticity* refers to the additional performance improvement after intervention. Specific neurobiological models of the putative effects of particular cognitive training techniques used in patients with ADHD are lacking. Rather, they rest on both the assumption that particular neuropsychological deficits mediate ADHD pathogenesis (see above) and a generic "physical-energetic" model, according to which repeatedly loading a limited cognitive resource is expected to lead to its strengthening and improved function—similar to strengthening a muscle by repeated use.[8]

Although the precise mechanisms remain elusive, functional and structural correlates of cognitive training have been investigated. In terms of functional changes, 4 patterns have been reported[62,67]: (1) decreased activation in some brain regions after training,[68] which may reflect more efficient processing; (2) increased activation,[69] possibly linked to more extensive recruitment of cortical areas; indeed, some investigators have found an inverted U-shaped effect linking activation to training;[70] (3) a pattern of activation redistribution (second study),[69] characterized by a combination of activation and deactivation with the possibility that deactivation occurs in regions responsible for more general attention processes (eg, prefrontal cortex), while activation is in task-specific areas targeted by training; as well as (4) reorganization of networks,[71] which reflects a qualitative change in the process used to accomplish the trained task. Resting state networks also seem to show change, pointing to reduced interference among competing networks after training.[72] Structural brain changes in gray matter volume (in part overlapping with areas of functional changes) and white matter microstructure have been reported after training. Structural changes lend support to the brain plasticity hypothesis of cognitive training, because they may be considered as the most evident expression of lasting training effects. There is also evidence of neurochemical changes at the synapse after training—with effects found for WMT in dopamine function.[67] Two phases in the neurobiological effects of cognitive training have been described.[64] First, there are transient but large and widespread changes in task-specific cortical representations that do not persist outside of the training session. Second, there are more modest cognitive changes associated with reorganization of cortical task-specific representations as well as synaptogenesis. Finally, it should be noted that although the neuronal correlates of the training effects on proximal outcomes have begun to be elucidated, the neurobiological mechanisms underlying far transfer remain elusive.[73]

How Is the Treatment Delivered?

Cognitive training for ADHD is typically delivered using computers. The duration of each training session and the number of sessions and their frequency vary according to the specific protocol employed—although they typically involve a large number of sessions spread over several weeks. Training sessions may be implemented at school, at home, or in the clinic/research facility. Computerized approaches are especially appropriate given that they are suited to the implementation of adaptive training schedules—whereby the difficulty and intensity of the training is increased across the training regime to continually challenge the patient at the boundaries of their competence. For example, RoboMemo, one of the most popular WMT programs, is based on a total of 90 training sections (each day, lasting on an average for 40 minutes) spread over several weeks. The difficulty level is automatically adjusted by the software on a trial-by-trial basis, to match the improving WM span of the subject on each task to drive the learner to higher levels of performance as the training proceeds. Individualized adaptation of task difficulty also maintains a high trial-by-trial reward schedule, improving the brain's ability to engage. The underlying rationale derives from evidence from basic and neuroimaging studies suggesting that nonadaptive training does not bring persistent and sustained neuronal changes (for further discussion, please see Ref.[64]). **Table 1** presents descriptions of the most commonly used, commercially available, computerized cognitive training programs currently available.

Empirical Support

Effects on ADHD clinical symptoms
The first RCT evidence for the benefits of cognitive training as a treatment of ADHD was reported by Klingberg and colleagues[74] in 2005. This was a well-controlled trial comparing adaptive WMT against a placebo condition using low-demand nonadaptive training. There was a large effect on parent ratings of ADHD, but this did not generalize to teacher ratings. Subsequent RCTs focused on different training approaches targeting various cognitive functions and have used different designs.[50] There have been several qualitative and quantitative reviews of these studies related to ADHD.

| Table 1 |
| Most common computerized cognitive training programs | |
Name	Target
AIXTENT (CogniPlus)	Attention: selective, divided, focused, and constant
Captain's Log	Attention, working memory, visuomotor function, problem solving
Cogmed (RoboMemo)	Visuospatial and spatioverbal working memory
CogniPlus	Attention, working memory, visuomotor function, executive functions, long-term memory
Locu Tour	Acoustic, visual, and verbal attention; executive functions; acoustic and visual memory
Pay Attention!	Attention
RehaCom	Attention, memory, executive functions, visuomotor functions
REMINDER (partially computerized)	Memory storage and recall strategies

Adapted from Karch D, Albers L, Renner G, et al. The efficacy of cognitive training programs in children and adolescents: a meta-analysis. Dtsch Arztebl Int 2013;110(39):645.

Some of these meta-analyses have been difficult to interpret because they have sometimes combined clinical and typically developing samples,[75] have included both RCT and non-RCT studies,[76] or have included studies of both cognitive training and behavioral therapies.[77] One recent meta-analysis has focused solely on RCTs in ADHD populations,[50] employing stringent inclusion criteria and rigorous procedures. This meta-analysis also attempted to address the issue of blinding by comparing outcomes rated by individuals closest to the therapeutic setting (often heavily invested and either unblinded or probably not completely blinded) and a second analysis based on outcomes provided by reporters judged to be probably blinded. In trials in which an active or sham control was used to increase blinding of all raters, the best probably blinded rater was used. The results of this analysis must be viewed as preliminary because although many potential studies were reviewed, only 6 had sufficiently strong designs to be included (search in April 2012). Overall, the meta-analysis reported data from 126 subjects in active and 123 subjects in control conditions. There was considerable heterogeneity in the sorts of training used across the trials, but the effects of specific training approaches could not be compared given the small number of trials (Table 2). A range of different controls (active or waiting list) were also used. Overall, there was a moderate and highly significant effect in favor of intervention for most proximal ratings of ADHD (overall standard mean difference [SMD], 0.64; 95% confidence interval [CI], 0.33–0.95). However, when outcomes provided by probably blinded raters were considered, the effect dropped substantially and became not significant (overall SMD, 0.24; 95% CI, −0.24 to 0.72). This led the authors to argue that more evidence is needed from trials with well-blinded measures before cognitive training can be supported as an evidence-based treatment of ADHD.

By March 2014, 10 more reports of trials meeting the same inclusion criteria of Sonuga-Barke and colleagues[50] had been published, providing data from a total of 8 new RCTs (since Hovik and colleagues,[78] Egeland and colleagues,[79] as well as Steiner and colleagues[80,81] referred to the same data set). The characteristics of these additional studies are summarized in Table 3. These studies included a total of 244 subjects assigned to the active training conditions and 234 to the control conditions. Of these 8 RCTs, 5 focused on WMT, 1 implemented a combined WM and attention training, 1 was based on attention training, and 1 included a more general training

Table 2
Characteristics of studies included in the meta-analysis on cognitive training by the European ADHD Guidelines Group that included studies up to April 3, 2012

Trial (First Author and Year)	Design	Training Duration	Training Type	Control Condition	N[a] T C	Age Range in Months
Johnstone et al,[90] 2010	2 Parallel groups	5 wk	Adaptive inhibitory training and WMT	Nonadaptive low-difficulty WMT	20 20	95–149
Klingberg et al,[74] 2005	2 Parallel groups	5 wk	Adaptive WMT RoboMemo	Nonadaptive, low-difficulty WMT	26 27	116 (mean)
Rabiner[b] et al,[93] 2010	3 Parallel groups	14 wk	Adaptive attention training Captain's Log[c]	Waiting list	25 25[d]	NS
Shalev et al,[92] 2007	2 Parallel groups	8 wk	Adaptive attention training[e]	Matched computer games	20 16	72–156
Steiner[f] et al,[88] 2011	3 Parallel groups	Average 23.4 Sessions, 4 mo	Adaptive attention training/ WMT Brain Train[g]	Waiting list	13 15	No report; mean: 148.8 ± 10.8
Johnstone et al,[91] 2012	3 Parallel groups	5 wk	Adaptive inhibitory training and WMT	Waiting list	22 20	95–145

Note: the study by Klingberg et al[89] is not included in this table because it does not meet the inclusion criteria adopted in Sonuga-Barke et al.[50]
[a] N is the number of individuals in the treatment (T) and control (C) conditions.
[b] This study also included a treatment arm of computer-assisted instruction, not considered in the meta-analysis by Sonuga-Barke et al.[50]
[c] Braintrain http://www.braintrain.com/captainslogmentalgym/.
[d] 27 additional participants were allocated to computer-assisted instruction; 14 participants in the treatment group and 3 the control group received psychostimulants throughout the duration of the study. None were medicated during the training sessions or during the pretesting and posttesting sessions.
[e] (1) Computerized Continuous Performance Task, to improve sustained attention; (2) Conjunctive Search Task, to improve the function of Selective Attention; (3) Combined Orienting and Flanker Task to improve the function of Orienting Attention; as well as (4) Shift Stroop-like Task, designed to improve the function of Executive Attention.
[f] This trial also included an arm of neurofeedback considered against waiting list in neurofeedback analysis.
[g] http://www.braintrain.com.
Adapted from Sonuga-Barke EJ, Brandeis D, Cortese S, et al. Nonpharmacological interventions for ADHD: systematic review and meta-analyses of randomized controlled trials of dietary and psychological treatments. Am J Psychiatry 2013;170(3):275–89.

Table 3
Characteristics of cognitive/behavioral studies on cognitive training in ADHD published after April 3, 2012, meeting the same inclusion criteria as in Sonuga-Barke et al

Trial (First Author and Year)	Design	Training Duration	Training	Control Condition	N[a] T C	Age Range in Months
Gray et al,[86] 2012	2 Parallel groups	5 wk	Adaptive WMT *RoboMemo*	Adaptive math training *Academy of Math*	32 / 20	144–204
Green et al,[87] 2012	2 Parallel groups	25 d	Adaptive WMT *RoboMemo*	Nonadaptive, low-difficulty WMT	12 / 14	84–168
Tamm et al,[83] 2013	2 Parallel groups	8 wk	Adaptive attention training *Pay Attention!*	Waiting list	45 / 46	84–180
Chacko et al,[85] 2014	2 Parallel groups	5 wk	Adaptive WMT	Nonadaptive, low-difficulty WMT	44 / 41	84–132
Egeland[b] et al,[79] 2013	2 Parallel groups	25 d	Adaptive WMT *RoboMemo*	TAU	33 / 34	120–144
Hovik[b] et al,[78] 2013	2 Parallel groups	25 d	Adaptive WMT *RoboMemo*	TAU	33 / 34	120–144
Oord et al,[82] 2013	2 Parallel groups	5 wk	Adaptive EF training (inhibition, WM, cognitive flexibility)	Waiting list	18 / 22	96–144
Steiner et al,[81] 2014	3 Parallel groups (neurofeedback, cognitive training, control)	13 wk	Adaptive attention and WMT	TAU	34 / 36	No report; mean: 100.8 ± 14.8
Steiner[c] et al,[80] 2014	3 Parallel groups (neurofeedback, cognitive training, control)	13 wk	Adaptive attention and WMT	TAU	34 / 36	No report; mean: 100.8 ± 14.8
van Dongen-Boomsma et al,[84] 2014	2 Parallel groups	5 wk	Adaptive WMT	Nonadaptive, low-difficulty WMT	26 / 21	71.5–87.6

Studies are listed in chronologic order.

Abbreviations: EF, executive function; TAU, treatment as usual.

a N is the number of individuals in the Treatment (T) and Control (C) conditions.

b These 2 articles refer to the same study and present analyses on different outcomes.

c This article reports a follow-up of Steiner et al.[81]

Data from Sonuga-Barke EJ, Brandeis D, Cortese S, et al. Nonpharmacological interventions for ADHD: systematic review and meta-analyses of randomized controlled trials of dietary and psychological treatments. Am J Psychiatry 2013;170(3):275–89.

of executive functions. Considering ADHD core-symptom-related outcomes provided by raters closest to the training setting, 5 trials reported significant effects of training— 2 trials[82,83] reported effects of large (ie, >0.8) and 3 reported effects of moderate (>0.2 and <0.5) size.[78,81,84] Three trials found no effect.[85–87] Reports from probably blinded reporters were provided in 6 new RCTs. Three trials found significant effects: one[83] reported large, one[82] reported moderate, and one[85] reported a very small effect size (0.04). Three studies found no effect of training.[84,87,88] This inconsistent pattern of results for both most proximal and probably blinded ratings confirms the findings of the meta-analysis by Sonuga-Barke and colleagues[50] demonstrating markedly reduced effects with probably blinded raters.

Effects on neuropsychological deficits in individuals with ADHD

There has been no meta-analysis of cognitive training on ADHD-related neuropsychological deficits using the stringent inclusion criteria adopted in the above meta-analysis. However, many individual trials have assessed training effects on neuropsychological deficits alongside ADHD symptoms. **Table 4** summarizes the key results across the available studies for the 4 key neuropsychological outcomes. Although the results are mixed and indeed vary according to the specific domain and measure considered, a pattern seems to emerge supporting near transfer to untrained tasks tapping the same deficit as targeted by the intervention. For instance, 5 trials[74,78,85,86,89] of 12 including a component of WMT reported significant improvements on at least 1 non-trained measure of WM, whereas 1 trial[84] failed to replicate this finding and 6 did not report the assessment of near-transfer effects. Other examples of such near transfer relate to improvement of nontrained measures of sustained, selective, and alternating attention in the attention training trial by Tamm and colleagues[83] and significant improvements in Go/No-Go scores after response inhibition training in the trial by Johnstone and colleagues.[90] Further studies are required to examine how robust these effects are, given the modest nature of many of these effects and the fact that 5 trials[84–86,90,91] found no significant near-transfer effects in at least 1 measure of the targeted domain. Evidence for transfer to more distal processes is very patchy, but some evidence does exist. Improvement in reading performance after WMT were observed by Gray and colleagues,[86] reading comprehension and text copying after attention training,[92] reading performances after WMT by Egeland and colleagues,[79] and scores on the Raven's progressive matrices after WMT in Refs.[74,89]

Methodological issues

This evidence should be considered in the light of important methodological issues. First, the choice of the control group may significantly affect findings. The use of non-active control arms in some studies (eg, waiting list, treatment as usual) hinders blinding. At the same time, the choice of type of active control needs to be considered carefully because the use of low-demand, nonadaptive training adopted in many of trials recently can introduce differences between treatment and control arms in terms of extraneous factors such as motivation. Using adaptive training targeting neuropsychological domains other than those of interest may address this limitation (see Gray and colleagues[86]). Second, the range of outcome measures has been limited in trials and researchers should be cautious in generalizing the transfer effects of cognitive training based on one or few measures of the same domain/construct. Third, the length and intensity of training may affect the results of the program. In this respect, as shown in **Tables 2** and **3**, although available RCTs varied considerably with regard to these parameters, most lasted on an average for 4 to 5 weeks. However, there has been no study to establish optimal conditions. Fourth, there needs

Table 4
Significant improvement on nontrained neuropsychological tasks by domain

	Verbal WM	Visual WM	Inhibition	Attention
Klingberg et al,[89] 2002		*Span Board*	*Stroop*	2-choice RT task
Klingberg et al,[74] 2005	*Digit span*	*Span Board*	*Stroop*	
Johnstone et al,[90] 2010			Go/No-Go	
Johnstone et al,[91] 2012	Counting span		*Flanker* Go/No-Go	*Oddball task*
Green et al,[87] 2012	*WISC WM composite*			
Tamm et al,[83] 2013[a]	WJ-III (auditory WM) Digit Span		D-KEFS (Stroop)	*TEA-Ch*
Gray et al,[86] 2012	*Digit span*	*Spatial span* Spatial WM		D2 Attention Test: # *errors*, items process, total perform
Chacko et al,[85] 2014	*AWMA:* Digit recall Listening recall	*AWMA: Dot matrix* storage processing/ manipulation	CPT commissions	CPT omissions
Hovik et al,[78] 2013 & Egeland et al,[79] 2013	*Digit span*	*Visual span (Leiter)*	Stroop CPT: focus, sustained, vigilance	Trail making—B
van Dongen-Boomsma et al,[84] 2014	Digit span	Knox cubes LDT	Stroop "Shape school" (inhibition/ switching)	Sustained attention dots task

Only laboratory measures are reported. Rating scales and intelligence quotient tests are not included. Tests on which there was a significant effect of cognitive training are presented in bold and are italicized.

Abbreviations: AWMA, Automatic Working Memory Assessment; CPT, Continuous Performance Test; D-KEFS, Delis–Kaplan Executive Functioning System; LDT, Knox Cube Leidse Diagnostische Test; RT, Reaction Time; TEA-Ch, Test of Everyday Attention for Children; WISC, Wechsler Intelligence Scale for Children; WJ-III, Woodcock Johnson Tests of Achievement–III.

[a] This study also included the Quotient ADHD system, which is not shown in the table because its reliability and validity have not yet been established.

to be a focus on the longer-term persistence of any effects. A minority of RCTs have explored this (Johnstone and colleagues[90]: 6 weeks; Klingberg and colleagues[74]: 3 months; Rabiner and colleagues[93]: 6 months, Oord and colleagues[82]: 9 weeks; and Steiner and colleagues[80]: 6 months). Finally, despite being built on a rationale that ADHD arises because of deficits in specific neuropsychological processes, no trials have screened participants for these ADHD-related deficits before including them in trials. Given the heterogeneity of the condition, this is likely to reduce effect sizes.

CLINICAL DECISION MAKING

Given the current state of evidence and the lack of clinically useful data, it is premature to provide clinical guidance on the use of cognitive training technologies. It might be predicted that training regimes tailored to target the specific deficits experienced by individuals with ADHD may be more effective; however, there is currently no evidence to support this assertion. Evidence for corroborated core effects on ADHD remains inconsistent. Effects on targeted neuropsychological processes may be more robust, but more research is needed. There are currently no known contraindications. There is little evidence of adverse effects of cognitive training, although treatment can be expensive both in terms of time and money. The scheduling of treatment especially in relation to medication is yet to be explored in any depth.

FUTURE DIRECTIONS

Because of the inconsistency of evidence to date, more research is recommended to explore ways to improve treatment effects both on ADHD symptoms and underlying neuropsychological functions. Priority future questions are as follows.

Can Current Approaches Be Made More Effective?

Little is known about what training parameters and settings are optimal. Issues that require further study relate to (1) length, intensity, and scheduling/density; (2) varying treatment setting and context to promote generalization; (3) the development of more naturalistic everyday treatment setting (eg, the development of noncomputerized approaches); and (4) the appropriate use of incentives and instructions.

What Place Does Cognitive Training Have in Multimodal Treatment Approaches?

There is a particular need for studies examining the relative value of combined cognitive training and medication or dietary or other psychological approaches.[64]

Will Some Individuals with ADHD Be More Responsive to Cognitive Training?

Despite the strong theoretic belief that cognitive training targets underlying neuropsychological deficits and the obvious clinical and pathophysiological heterogeneity in the condition, there is almost no evidence about the sort of individuals with ADHD who respond best to different sorts of cognitive training. Trials in the future need to compare the response of clinical subtypes and neuropsychological subgroups to different forms of training.

What Are the Neuronal Correlates of Computerized, Adaptive Cognitive Training Programs?

Although there are 2 studies,[94,95] referring to the same data set, showing that a paper-and-pencil-based cognitive training program affected some of the neuroanatomical and functional abnormalities in ADHD, the neuronal correlates of computer-based programs are poorly understood. In relation to the previous point, baseline neuroanatomical and functional patterns as well as their changes after training could be used in studies aimed to infer prediction of response to treatment via multimodal neuroimaging support vector machine approaches.

Can Other Deficits Be Targeted?

As mentioned above, ADHD is a neuropsychologically heterogeneous condition implicating multiple cognitive, motivational, and state regulation deficits. Current approaches have focused on executive functions. Therapy developers need to think of ways to implement training approaches in the nonexecutive cognitive, motivational, and energetic domains.[96]

Will Value Be Increased Through Early Intervention?

Early intervention approaches for ADHD are increasingly supported in the field. Cognitive training approaches may play an important role in such approaches.[97] The challenge will be to introduce training regimes in ways that young children will find attractive and engaging. Noncomputerized play-based approaches are currently being investigated by several researchers.[98]

SUMMARY

Although biologically plausible and supported by basic neuroscience research, a stringent meta-analysis and overview of additional recent trials leads us to conclude that more consistent evidence from well-blinded studies is required before cognitive training can be supported as a frontline treatment of core ADHD. Effects on underlying ADHD-related neuropsychological deficits may be more consistent but seem to be limited to near-transfer effects. However, at the time of this writing, this has not been subjected to meta-analytic review. To date, there is a lack of sufficient evidence to know what role cognitive training may play in broader multimodal approaches or whether individuals with a particular type of ADHD or neuropsychological profile will benefit more.

DISCLOSURES

E. Sonuga-Barke has financial disclosures in relation to Shire pharmaceuticals—speaker fees, consultancy, advisory board membership, research support, and conference attendance funds; Janssen-Cilag—speaker fees; and visiting chairs at Ghent University and Aarhus University. Grants awarded from MRC, ESRC, Wellcome Trust, Solent NHS Trust, European Union, Child Health Research Foundation New Zealand, NIHR, Nuffield Foundation, and Fonds Wetenschappelijk Onderzoek, Vlaanderen (FWO). D. Brandeis has no disclosure to report. M. Holtmann served in an advisory or consultancy role for Lilly, Novartis, Shire, and Bristol-Myers Squibb and received conference attendance support or was paid for public speaking by AstraZeneca, Bristol-Myers Squibb, Janssen-Cilag, Lilly, Medice, Neuroconn, Novartis, and Shire. S. Cortese has no current relationships with drug companies. He receives royalties from Argon Healthcare, Italy, for educational activities on ADHD. Before 2010, he served as scientific consultant for Shire Pharmaceuticals and received support to attend meetings from Eli Lilly and from Shire.

REFERENCES

1. Ramos-Quiroga JA, Montoya A, Kutzelnigg A, et al. Attention deficit hyperactivity disorder in the European adult population: prevalence, disease awareness, and treatment guidelines. Curr Med Res Opin 2013;29(9):1093–104.
2. Willcutt EG, Nigg JT, Pennington BF, et al. Validity of DSM-IV attention deficit/hyperactivity disorder symptom dimensions and subtypes. J Abnorm Psychol 2012;121(4):991–1010.
3. Connor DF, Doerfler LA. ADHD with comorbid oppositional defiant disorder or conduct disorder: discrete or nondistinct disruptive behavior disorders? J Atten Disord 2008;12(2):126–34.
4. Williams ED, Reimherr FW, Marchant BK, et al. Personality disorder in ADHD Part 1: assessment of personality disorder in adult ADHD using data from a clinical trial of OROS methylphenidate. Ann Clin Psychiatry 2010;22(2):84–93.

5. Humphreys KL, Katz SJ, Lee SS, et al. The association of ADHD and depression: mediation by peer problems and parent-child difficulties in two complementary samples. J Abnorm Psychol 2013;122(3):854–67.
6. Lee SS, Falk AE, Aguirre VP. Association of comorbid anxiety with social functioning in school-age children with and without attention-deficit/hyperactivity disorder (ADHD). Psychiatry Res 2012;197(1–2):90–6.
7. Tannock R. Rethinking ADHD and LD in DSM-5: proposed changes in diagnostic criteria. J Learn Disabil 2013;46(1):5–25.
8. Antshel KM, Zhang-James Y, Faraone SV. The comorbidity of ADHD and autism spectrum disorder. Expert Rev Neurother 2013;13(10):1117–28.
9. Danckaerts M, Sonuga-Barke EJ, Banaschewski T, et al. The quality of life of children with attention deficit/hyperactivity disorder: a systematic review. Eur Child Adolesc Psychiatry 2010;19(2):83–105.
10. Garner AA, O'connor BC, Narad ME, et al. The relationship between ADHD symptom dimensions, clinical correlates, and functional impairments. J Dev Behav Pediatr 2013;34(7):469–77.
11. Schlander M, Trott GE, Schwarz O. The health economics of attention deficit hyperactivity disorder in Germany. Part 1: health care utilization and cost of illness. Nervenarzt 2010;81(3):289–300 [in German].
12. Willcutt EG, Sonuga-Barke EJS, Nigg JT, et al. Recent developments in neuropsychological models of childhood psychiatric disorders. In: Banaschewski T, Rohde LA, editors. Biological child psychiatry. Recent trends and developments. Advances in biological psychiatry, vol. 24. Basel (Switzerland): Karger; 2008. p. 195–226.
13. Cortese S, Kelly C, Chabernaud C, et al. Toward systems neuroscience of ADHD: a meta- analysis of 55 fMRI studies. Am J Psychiatry 2012;169(10): 1038–55.
14. Goos LM, Crosbie J, Payne S, et al. Validation and extension of the endophenotype model in ADHD patterns of inheritance in a family study of inhibitory control. Am J Psychiatry 2009;166(6):711–7.
15. Rubia K. "Cool" inferior frontostriatal dysfunction in attention-deficit/hyperactivity disorder versus "hot" ventromedial orbitofrontal-limbic dysfunction in conduct disorder: a review. Biol Psychiatry 2011;69(12):e69–87.
16. Kasper LJ, Alderson RM, Hudec KL. Moderators of working memory deficits in children with attention-deficit/hyperactivity disorder (ADHD): a meta-analytic review. Clin Psychol Rev 2012;32(7):605–17.
17. Silk TJ, Vance A, Rinehart N, et al. Dysfunction in the fronto-parietal network in attention deficit hyperactivity disorder (ADHD): an fMRI Study. Brain Imaging Behav 2008;2:123–31.
18. Noreika V, Falter CM, Rubia K. Timing deficits in attention-deficit/hyperactivity disorder (ADHD): evidence from neurocognitive and neuroimaging studies. Neuropsychologia 2013;51(2):235–66.
19. Rhodes SM, Park J, Seth S, et al. A comprehensive investigation of memory impairment in attention deficit hyperactivity disorder and oppositional defiant disorder. J Child Psychol Psychiatry 2012;53(2):128–37.
20. Metin B, Roeyers H, Wiersema JR, et al. ADHD performance reflects inefficient but not impulsive information processing: a diffusion model analysis. Neuropsychology 2013;27(2):193–200.
21. Sonuga-Barke EJ. Editorial: ADHD as a reinforcement disorder - moving from general effects to identifying (six) specific models to test. J Child Psychol Psychiatry 2011;52(9):917–8.

22. Sonuga-Barke EJ, Fairchild G. Neuroeconomics of attention-deficit/hyperactivity disorder: differential influences of medial, dorsal, and ventral prefrontal brain networks on suboptimal decision making? Biol Psychiatry 2012;72(2):126–33.

23. Volkow ND, Wang GJ, Newcorn JH, et al. Motivation deficit in ADHD is associated with dysfunction of the dopamine reward pathway. Mol Psychiatry 2011; 16(11):1147–54.

24. van Meel CS, Heslenfeld DJ, Oosterlaan J, et al. ERPs associated with monitoring and evaluation of monetary reward and punishment in children with ADHD. J Child Psychol Psychiatry 2011;52(9):942–53.

25. Lemiere J, Danckaerts M, Van HW, et al. Brain activation to cues predicting inescapable delay in adolescent attention deficit/hyperactivity disorder: an fMRI pilot study. Brain Res 2012;1450:57–66.

26. Scheres A, Dijkstra M, Ainslie E, et al. Temporal and probabilistic discounting of rewards in children and adolescents: effects of age and ADHD symptoms. Neuropsychologia 2006;44(11):2092–103.

27. Marco R, Miranda A, Schlotz W, et al. Delay and reward choice in ADHD: an experimental test of the role of delay aversion. Neuropsychology 2009;23(3): 367–80.

28. Wilbertz G, Trueg A, Sonuga-Barke EJ, et al. Neural and psychophysiological markers of delay aversion in attention-deficit hyperactivity disorder. J Abnorm Psychol 2013;122(2):566–72.

29. Sonuga-Barke EJ, Wiersema JR, van der Meere JJ, et al. Context-dependent dynamic processes in attention deficit/hyperactivity disorder: differentiating common and unique effects of state regulation deficits and delay aversion. Neuropsychol Rev 2010;20(1):86–102.

30. Fair DA, Bathula D, Nikolas MA, et al. Distinct neuropsychological subgroups in typically developing youth inform heterogeneity in children with ADHD. Proc Natl Acad Sci U S A 2012;109(17):6769–74.

31. Liddle EB, Hollis C, Batty MJ, et al. Task-related default mode network modulation and inhibitory control in ADHD: effects of motivation and methylphenidate. J Child Psychol Psychiatry 2011;52(7):761–71.

32. Sonuga-Barke EJ, Castellanos FX. Spontaneous attentional fluctuations in impaired states and pathological conditions: a neurobiological hypothesis. Neurosci Biobehav Rev 2007;31(7):977–86.

33. de ZP, Weusten J, van DS, et al. Deficits in cognitive control, timing and reward sensitivity appear to be dissociable in ADHD. PLoS One 2012;7(12): e51416.

34. Lambek R, Tannock R, Dalsgaard S, et al. Validating neuropsychological subtypes of ADHD: how do children with and without an executive function deficit differ? J Child Psychol Psychiatry 2010;51(8):895–904.

35. Nigg JT, Casey BJ. An integrative theory of attention-deficit/hyperactivity disorder based on the cognitive and affective neurosciences. Dev Psychopathol 2005;17(3):785–806.

36. Solanto MV, Abikoff H, Sonuga-Barke E, et al. The ecological validity of delay aversion and response inhibition as measures of impulsivity in AD/HD: a supplement to the NIMH multimodal treatment study of AD/HD. J Abnorm Child Psychol 2001;29(3):215–28.

37. Sonuga-Barke EJ. Psychological heterogeneity in AD/HD–a dual pathway model of behaviour and cognition. Behav Brain Res 2002;130(1–2):29–36.

38. Sonuga-Barke E, Bitsakou P, Thompson M. Beyond the dual pathway model: evidence for the dissociation of timing, inhibitory, and delay-related impairments

in attention- deficit/hyperactivity disorder. J Am Acad Child Adolesc Psychiatry 2010;49(4):345–55.

39. Coghill D, Nigg J, Rothenberger A, et al. Whither causal models in the neuroscience of ADHD? Dev Sci 2005;8(2):105–14.

40. Kuntsi J, Pinto R, Price TS, et al. The separation of ADHD inattention and hyperactivity-impulsivity symptoms: pathways from genetic effects to cognitive impairments and symptoms. J Abnorm Child Psychol 2014;42(1):127–36.

41. Bitsakou P, Psychogiou L, Thompson M, et al. Delay aversion in attention deficit/ hyperactivity disorder: an empirical investigation of the broader phenotype. Neuropsychologia 2009;47(2):446–56.

42. Holmes J, Gathercole SE, Dunning DL. Poor working memory: impact and interventions. In: Holmes J, editor. Advances in child development and behavior: developmental disorders and interventions, vol. 39. Burlington: Academic Press; 2010. p. 1–43.

43. Sonuga-Barke EJ, Sergeant JA, Nigg J, et al. Executive dysfunction and delay aversion in attention deficit hyperactivity disorder: nosologic and diagnostic implications. Child Adolesc Psychiatr Clin N Am 2008;17(2):367–84, ix.

44. Taylor E, Dopfner M, Sergeant J, et al. European clinical guidelines for hyperkinetic disorder – first upgrade. Eur Child Adolesc Psychiatry 2004;13(Suppl 1): I7–30.

45. Faraone SV, Buitelaar J. Comparing the efficacy of stimulants for ADHD in children and adolescents using meta-analysis. Eur Child Adolesc Psychiatry 2010; 19(4):353–64.

46. Banaschewski T, Soutullo C, Lecendreux M, et al. Health-related quality of life and functional outcomes from a randomized, controlled study of lisdexamfetamine dimesylate in children and adolescents with attention deficit hyperactivity disorder. CNS Drugs 2013;27(10):829–40.

47. Ni HC, Shang CY, Gau SS, et al. A head-to-head randomized clinical trial of methylphenidate and atomoxetine treatment for executive function in adults with attention-deficit hyperactivity disorder. Int J Neuropsychopharmacol 2013;16(9):1959–73.

48. Coghill DR, Seth S, Pedroso S, et al. Effects of methylphenidate on cognitive functions in children and adolescents with attention-deficit/hyperactivity disorder: evidence from a systematic review and a meta-analysis. Biol Psychiatry 2013. [Epub ahead of print].

49. Shiels K, Hawk LW Jr, Reynolds B, et al. Effects of methylphenidate on discounting of delayed rewards in attention deficit/hyperactivity disorder. Exp Clin Psychopharmacol 2009;17(5):291–301.

50. Sonuga-Barke EJ, Brandeis D, Cortese S, et al. Nonpharmacological interventions for ADHD: systematic review and meta-analyses of randomized controlled trials of dietary and psychological treatments. Am J Psychiatry 2013;170(3):275–89.

51. Cortese S, Holtmann M, Banaschewski T, et al. Practitioner review: current best practice in the management of adverse events during treatment with ADHD medications in children and adolescents. J Child Psychol Psychiatry 2013; 54(3):227–46.

52. Molina BS, Hinshaw SP, Swanson JM, et al. The MTA at 8 years: prospective follow-up of children treated for combined-type ADHD in a multisite study. J Am Acad Child Adolesc Psychiatry 2009;48(5):484–500.

53. van de Loo-Neus GH, Rommelse N, Buitelaar JK. To stop or not to stop? How long should medication treatment of attention-deficit hyperactivity disorder be extended? Eur Neuropsychopharmacol 2011;21(8):584–99.

54. Adler LD, Nierenberg AA. Review of medication adherence in children and adults with ADHD. Postgrad Med 2010;122(1):184–91.

55. Berger I, Dor T, Nevo Y, et al. Attitudes toward attention-deficit hyperactivity disorder (ADHD) treatment: parents' and children's perspectives. J Child Neurol 2008;23(9):1036–42.

56. Koerting J, Smith E, Knowles MM, et al. Barriers to, and facilitators of, parenting programmes for childhood behaviour problems: a qualitative synthesis of studies of parents' and professionals' perceptions. Eur Child Adolesc Psychiatry 2013;22(11):653–70.

57. Kovshoff H, Williams S, Vrijens M, et al. The decisions regarding ADHD management (DRAMa) study: uncertainties and complexities in assessment, diagnosis and treatment, from the clinician's point of view. Eur Child Adolesc Psychiatry 2012;21(2):87–99.

58. Stevenson J, Buitelaar J, Cortese S, et al. Research review: the role of diet in the treatment of attention-deficit/hyperactivity disorder - an appraisal of the evidence on efficacy and recommendations on the design of future studies. J Child Psychol Psychiatry 2014;55:416–27.

59. Fabiano GA, Pelham WE Jr, Coles EK, et al. A meta-analysis of behavioral treatments for attention-deficit/hyperactivity disorder. Clin Psychol Rev 2009;29(2): 129–40.

60. Daley D, Oord SV, Ferrin M, et al. The impact of behavioral interventions for children and adolescents with attention-deficit hyperactivity disorder: a meta-analysis of randomised controlled trials across multiple outcome domains. J Am Acad Child Adolesc Psychiatry 2014, in press.

61. Jolles DD, Crone EA. Training the developing brain: a neurocognitive perspective. Front Hum Neurosci 2012;6:76.

62. Willis SL, Schaie KW. Cognitive training and plasticity: theoretical perspective and methodological consequences. Restor Neurol Neurosci 2009;27(5): 375–89.

63. Bahar-Fuchs A, Clare L, Woods B. Cognitive training and cognitive rehabilitation for mild to moderate Alzheimer's disease and vascular dementia. Cochrane Database Syst Rev 2013;(6):CD003260.

64. Vinogradov S, Fisher M, de Villers-Sidani E. Cognitive training for impaired neural systems in neuropsychiatric illness. Neuropsychopharmacology 2012;37(1): 43–76.

65. Witte OW. Lesion-induced plasticity as a potential mechanism for recovery and rehabilitative training. Curr Opin Neurol 1998;11(6):655–62.

66. Baltes P. Theoretical propositions of life-span developmental psychology: on the dynamics between growth and decline. Dev Psychol 1987;23:611–26.

67. Buschkuehl M, Jaeggi SM, Jonides J. Neuronal effects following working memory training. Dev Cogn Neurosci 2012;2(Suppl 1):S167–79.

68. Haier RJ, Siegel BV Jr, MacLachlan A, et al. Regional glucose metabolic changes after learning a complex visuospatial/motor task: a positron emission tomographic study. Brain Res 1992;570(1–2):134–43.

69. Olesen PJ, Westerberg H, Klingberg T. Increased prefrontal and parietal activity after training of working memory. Nat Neurosci 2004;7(1):75–9.

70. Hempel A, Giesel FL, Garcia Caraballo NM, et al. Plasticity of cortical activation related to working memory during training. Am J Psychiatry 2004;161(4):745–7.

71. Poldrack RA, Gabrieli JD. Characterizing the neural mechanisms of skill learning and repetition priming: evidence from mirror reading. Brain 2001;124(Pt 1): 67–82.

72. Lewis CM, Baldassarre A, Committeri G, et al. Learning sculpts the spontaneous activity of the resting human brain. Proc Natl Acad Sci U S A 2009;106(41): 17558–63.

73. Dahlin E, Neely AS, Larsson A, et al. Transfer of learning after updating training mediated by the striatum. Science 2008;320(5882):1510–2.

74. Klingberg T, Fernell E, Olesen PJ, et al. Computerized training of working memory in children with ADHD–a randomized, controlled trial. J Am Acad Child Adolesc Psychiatry 2005;44(2):177–86.

75. Melby-Lervag M, Hulme C. Is working memory training effective? A meta-analytic review. Dev Psychol 2013;49(2):270–91.

76. Rapport MD, Orban SA, Kofler MJ, et al. Do programs designed to train working memory, other executive functions, and attention benefit children with ADHD? A meta- analytic review of cognitive, academic, and behavioral outcomes. Clin Psychol Rev 2013;33(8):1237–52.

77. Karch D, Albers L, Renner G, et al. The efficacy of cognitive training programs in children and adolescents: a meta-analysis. Dtsch Arztebl Int 2013;110(39):643–52.

78. Hovik KT, Saunes BK, Aarlien AK, et al. RCT of working memory training in ADHD: long-term near-transfer effects. PLoS One 2013;8(12):e80561.

79. Egeland J, Aarlien AK, Saunes BK. Few effects of far transfer of working memory training in ADHD: a randomized controlled trial. PLoS One 2013;8(10):e75660.

80. Steiner NJ, Frenette EC, Rene KM, et al. In-school neurofeedback training for ADHD: sustained improvements from a randomized control trial. Pediatrics 2014;133(3):483–92.

81. Steiner NJ, Frenette EC, Rene KM, et al. Neurofeedback and cognitive attention training for children with attention-deficit hyperactivity disorder in schools. J Dev Behav Pediatr 2014;35(1):18–27.

82. Oord SV, Ponsioen AJ, Geurts HM, et al. A Pilot Study of the efficacy of a computerized executive functioning remediation training with game elements for children with ADHD in an outpatient setting: outcome on parent- and teacher-rated executive functioning and ADHD behavior. J Atten Disord 2012. [Epub ahead of print].

83. Tamm L, Epstein JN, Peugh JL, et al. Preliminary data suggesting the efficacy of attention training for school-aged children with ADHD. Dev Cogn Neurosci 2013;4:16–28.

84. van Dongen-Boomsma M, Vollebregt MA, Buitelaar JK, et al. Working memory training in young children with ADHD: a randomized placebo-controlled trial. J Child Psychol Psychiatry 2014;55(5):460–72.

85. Chacko A, Bedard AC, Marks DJ, et al. A randomized clinical trial of Cogmed working memory training in school-age children with ADHD: a replication in a diverse sample using a control condition. J Child Psychol Psychiatry 2014; 55(3):247–55.

86. Gray SA, Chaban P, Martinussen R, et al. Effects of a computerized working memory training program on working memory, attention, and academics in adolescents with severe LD and comorbid ADHD: a randomized controlled trial. J Child Psychol Psychiatry 2012;53(12):1277–84.

87. Green CT, Long DL, Green D, et al. Will working memory training generalize to improve off-task behavior in children with attention-deficit/hyperactivity disorder? Neurotherapeutics 2012;9(3):639–48.

88. Steiner NJ, Sheldrick RC, Gotthelf D, et al. Computer-based attention training in the schools for children with attention deficit/hyperactivity disorder: a preliminary trial. Clin Pediatr (Phila) 2011;50(7):615–22.

89. Klingberg T, Forssberg H, Westerberg H. Training of working memory in children with ADHD. J Clin Exp Neuropsychol 2002;24(6):781–91.

90. Johnstone SJ, Roodenrys S, Phillips E, et al. A pilot study of combined working memory and inhibition training for children with AD/HD. Atten Defic Hyperact Disord 2010;2(1):31–42.

91. Johnstone SJ, Roodenrys S, Blackman R, et al. Neurocognitive training for children with and without AD/HD. Atten Defic Hyperact Disord 2012;4(1):11–23.

92. Shalev L, Tsal Y, Mevorach C. Computerized progressive Attentional (CPAT) Program: effective direct intervention for children with ADHD. Child Neuropsychol 2007;13:382–8.

93. Rabiner DL, Murray DW, Skinner AT, et al. A randomized trial of two promising computer-based interventions for students with attention difficulties. J Abnorm Child Psychol 2010;38(1):131–42.

94. Hoekzema E, Carmona S, Ramos-Quiroga J, et al. Training-induced neuroanatomical plasticity in ADHD: a tensor-based morphometric study. Hum Brain Mapp 2011;32(10):1741–9.

95. Hoekzema E, Carmona S, Tremols V. Enhanced neural activity in frontal and cerebellar circuits after cognitive training in children with attention-deficit/hyperactivity disorder. Hum Brain Mapp 2010;31(12):1942–50.

96. Sonuga-Barke EJ. On the reorganization of incentive structure to promote delay tolerance: a therapeutic possibility for AD/HD? Neural Plast 2004;11(1–2):23–8.

97. Sonuga-Barke EJ, Halperin JM. Developmental phenotypes and causal pathways in attention deficit/hyperactivity disorder: potential targets for early intervention? J Child Psychol Psychiatry 2010;51(4):368–89.

98. Halperin JM, Marks DJ, Bedard AC, et al. Training executive, attention, and motor skills: a proof-of-concept study in preschool children with ADHD. J Atten Disord 2013;17(8):711–21.

Cognitive Behavioral Therapy for Adolescents with ADHD

Kevin M. Antshel, PhD*, Amy K. Olszewski, MS

KEYWORDS

- ADHD • Cognitive behavioral therapy • CBT • Adolescence • Adolescent

KEY POINTS

- Attention deficit/hyperactivity disorder (ADHD) persists into adolescence quite often and although the medications are useful for managing ADHD symptoms, the medications are less effective for improving functioning.
- Existing adult cognitive behavioral therapy (CBT) interventions that may be used for adolescents with ADHD rely more on "behavioral" principles than "cognitive" principles. Any CBT intervention that is focused more on cognitive therapy (eg, modifying irrational thoughts, increasing self-monitoring) without concurrently incorporating contingency management principles, especially reinforcement, is not likely to be effective.
- Although including parents in the CBT therapy room may work against those adolescents with ADHD and comorbid oppositional defiant disorder, the inclusion of parents in the therapy room may be of benefit for adolescents with ADHD and a comorbid internalizing disorder.
- CBT interventions should be used in conjunction with medication management.

ADOLESCENT ATTENTION DEFICIT/HYPERACTIVITY DISORDER
Defining Features

As defined by the Diagnostic and Statistical Manual of Mental Disorders, 5th Edition (DSM-5),[1] attention deficit/hyperactivity disorder (ADHD) is characterized by developmentally inappropriate levels of inattention and/or hyperactivity-impulsivity that negatively affects functioning and cannot be better explained by another condition. The prevalence rate of ADHD is a much-debated statistic and ranges from approximately 3% to 9% of youth worldwide.[2–4] Although other psychiatric conditions such as anxiety, mood, and substance use disorders increase from childhood to adolescence, ADHD prevalence rates decrease with age.[5] However, longitudinal data report that

Neither author has any financial disclosures or conflicts of interest to report.
Department of Psychology, Syracuse University, 802 University Avenue, Syracuse, NY 13244, USA
* Corresponding author.
E-mail address: kmantshe@syr.edu

Child Adolesc Psychiatric Clin N Am 23 (2014) 825–842
http://dx.doi.org/10.1016/j.chc.2014.05.001
1056-4993/14/$ – see front matter © 2014 Elsevier Inc. All rights reserved.

Abbreviations	
ADHD	Attention deficit/hyperactivity disorder
BPT	Behavioral parent training
CBT	Cognitive behavioral therapy
CHP	Challenging Horizons Program
DSM	Diagnostic and Statistical Manual of Mental Disorders
OCEBM	Oxford Center for Evidence Based Medicine
SoP	Social phobia
STAND	Supporting Teens' Academic Needs Daily
STEER	Supporting a Teen's Effective Entry to the Roadway
TADS	Treatment of Adolescent Depression Study

50% to 70% of children with ADHD continue to show impairing symptoms into adolescence.[6] The decline in ADHD prevalence may be due to the finding that ADHD symptoms, especially hyperactivity, decline in typically developing populations as a function of age.[7,8] The loss of syndromal persistence in these populations may also be a function of DSM symptoms and symptom thresholds that have been described as developmentally inappropriate and too restrictive, respectively, to be applied to adolescents and adults.[9]

There are a variety of changes to ADHD as defined by DSM-5[1]; one of the more substantive changes was the addition of behavioral descriptors to Criterion 1 that were intended to be more representative of adolescents and adults. For example, the DSM-IV-TR[2] item, "often runs and climbs excessively" now has a qualifier listed about being limited to feeling restless in adolescents and adults.[1] The DSM-5 also reduced the symptom criterion threshold from 6 to 5 for ages 17 and over. Likewise, practice parameters of the American Academy of Child and Adolescent Psychiatry clearly outline practice guidelines for managing adolescents that are substantively different than child guidelines.[10] Twenty years ago, the prevailing notion was that ADHD was a disorder of childhood[11] and that children generally outgrew their impairing symptoms by adolescence. However, the zeitgeist about ADHD has shifted and the syndromal persistence of ADHD into adulthood is now well established.[9]

Predictors of the persistence of childhood ADHD into adolescence include severity of the childhood ADHD, family history of ADHD, comorbid psychiatric conditions, lower IQ, and parental psychopathology.[9,12,13] The most common comorbid psychiatric conditions in adolescent ADHD are (from most to least common): oppositional defiant disorder (30%–50%), anxiety disorders (20%–30%), conduct disorder (20%–30%), mood disorders (15%–25%), learning disorders (15%–25%), and substance use disorders (5%–15%).[13–15]

Although DSM defined hyperactivity decreases in adolescence,[6] adolescents with ADHD continue to have impairing symptoms of inattention, hyperactivity, and impulsivity[13] and experience the same domains of functional impairment as children with ADHD.[16] Academic,[17] social,[18] and family[19] domains are frequently impaired in adolescents with ADHD. Unlike children, however, several other domains of functioning that coalesce around risky behaviors (eg, motor vehicle operation, substance abuse, sexual risk taking) are also negatively affected by ADHD in adolescence.[9,20,21]

In sum, adolescents with ADHD remain symptomatic and have the same (and additional) functional impairments and psychiatric comorbidities as children with ADHD. Despite this extant descriptive research base, there have been far less research studies that have focused on treating adolescents with ADHD relative to children with ADHD[22] (and more recently, even adults with ADHD). Because of the syndromal persistence of ADHD and the continued associated functional impairments, there is a clear need for effective treatments for adolescents with ADHD.

Most Common Psychosocial Interventions for Adolescent ADHD

ADHD is a chronic disorder and both medication and psychosocial interventions are used to manage the disorder. Stimulant medications are effective for approximately 70% to 80% of youth with ADHD.[23] Oxford Center for Evidence Based Medicine (OCEBM) Level 1 meta-analyses have shown that the stimulants are more efficacious than nonstimulant medications.[23] There is less evidence that stimulants normalize functioning, although they do lessen ADHD symptoms.[24–27] Combining psychosocial treatments with stimulants can result in the need for lower doses of each form of treatment.[28] Parents are also more enthusiastic or interested in treatments that include psychosocial components.[27] For all of these reasons, treatments that include both medication and psychosocial interventions are typically recommended for adolescents.[10]

The 4 most common psychosocial interventions for managing adolescent ADHD are (1) behavioral parent training (BPT), (2) parent-adolescent training in problem-solving and communication skills, (3) training teachers in classroom applications of contingency management techniques, or (4) some combination of the above.[29] BPT programs are efficacious for children with ADHD,[30–36] yet are somewhat less effective for adolescents with ADHD.[37] Rather than ADHD symptom reductions, BPT generally results in decreases in adolescent oppositional behavior, suggesting that the treatment is most useful when parent-child conflict exists.[38] BPT most often consists of teaching parents operant conditioning techniques, such as applying consequences following behaviors. Despite the relatively common use of BPT for adolescent ADHD, less than 30% of adolescents with ADHD will respond positively to this intervention.[29]

Parent-adolescent training in problem-solving and communication skills is also used for adolescents with ADHD.[39] This intervention often involves training parents and adolescents in a 5-step problem-solving approach (eg, problem definition, brainstorming of possible solutions, negotiation, decision-making about a solution, implementation of the solution), helping parents and adolescents develop more effective communication skills while discussing family conflicts (eg, avoiding ultimatums, paraphrasing other concerns before speaking one's own) and cognitive restructuring (helping families to restructure irrational beliefs about their own or others' behaviors).[39] Similar to BPT, less than 30% of adolescents with ADHD will respond positively to this intervention.[29]

Contingency management procedures are the most effective teacher intervention for managing adolescents with ADHD in the classroom.[40] Applying reinforcers for reduced impulsivity and/or increased attention and incorporating more tangible rewards (eg, increased free time, privileges) is often required; simple praise may not be sufficient to increase or maintain on-task behavior in adolescents with ADHD in the classroom.[41,42] Once again, compared with the effect sizes for children with ADHD, effect sizes for teacher interventions for adolescents with ADHD are rather small,[29] possibly because of the larger number of teachers that interact with adolescents and difficulties maintaining consistency between the teachers.

Need for Novel Psychosocial Interventions for Adolescent ADHD

As noted above, several of the commonly used adolescent ADHD interventions (BPT, teacher training in contingency management) are similar to child ADHD interventions, yet are less effective for adolescents relative to children.[22] Adolescence is defined by increased autonomy striving,[43] which may lead to increased conflict with parents and subsequent discontinuation of BPT or parent-adolescent training in problem-solving and communication skills.[18] Likewise, in addition to the increased number of teachers that are involved in the education of an adolescent, there is some evidence that high school teachers may be less likely to implement contingency management strategies than elementary school teachers.[44]

Adolescence is a period marked by increased desire for independence and individuation from the family. Thus, rather than working primarily with parents (as exists in many child ADHD treatment paradigms), it makes clinical sense to more actively involve adolescents in treatment. For example, typically developing adolescents who have chronic medical conditions are more cognitively capable than children of taking an active role in their treatment decision-making and generally prefer to be involved.[45] Likewise, practice guidelines for the management of adult ADHD[46] highlight the need to get adolescents involved in their own care, helping to prepare them to manage their own treatment as adults.

Possibly as a function of their increased desire for independence, most adolescents with ADHD refuse to take their stimulant medications,[13] a decision that parents generally do not agree with.[47] Another way to not adhere to treatment is to misuse or divert the stimulant medication. Although more likely to happen in adolescents with ADHD and comorbid conduct disorder or substance abuse,[48,49] stimulant misuse/diversion is a possibility for many adolescents receiving stimulant therapy for ADHD.[50,51] Thus, although adolescents are more cognitively capable of participating in their treatment decision-making, adolescents with ADHD may be disinterested in adhering to the medical intervention. This finding similarly highlights the need for an effective psychosocial intervention.

The relative lack of psychosocial interventions for adolescents with ADHD is also puzzling given that parents of adolescents prefer psychosocial intervention to medication, yet are more likely to have access to medication.[52–54] Furthermore, parent satisfaction ratings are higher when parents received psychosocial treatment than when they received medication alone,[55] suggesting that despite the lack of research attention, psychosocial treatments may have a place in the treatment of adolescent ADHD.

One of the most common psychosocial interventions for adolescents with psychiatric disorders *other than ADHD* is cognitive behavioral therapy (CBT). The next section reviews what is known about CBT interventions in adolescence.

CBT OVERVIEW

CBT is a well-researched approach to managing a variety of disorders that includes both cognitive and behavioral intervention components. CBT is based on the premise that a combination of thoughts, feelings, and behaviors are all interrelated, and that addressing or changing one part of this triad will also modify the other elements. Most CBT interventions adopt the "mediational position" in that cognitive activity mediates an individual's response to the environment.[56]

The cognitive component is focused on identifying thinking patterns that negatively impact functioning and therefore therapeutic work is aimed at changing maladaptive thoughts and assumptions. Specific cognitive techniques used in CBT include psychoeducation and cognitive restructuring. Psychoeducation involves teaching the adolescent and family about the disorder and its symptoms as well as helping the adolescent and family to understand how CBT might help. The goal of cognitive restructuring is to help the adolescent think about him or herself and problems in a different way. Various cognitive restructuring methods are used in CBT, including recording automatic thoughts, helping the adolescent to identify cognitive errors, reframing problems, and examining the evidence for and against automatic thoughts.[57]

The behavioral component of CBT uses behavioral techniques to assist in modifying automatic thoughts. Behavioral techniques commonly used in CBT include role playing, contingent reinforcement, exposure, relaxation training, and activity scheduling.[57] Role playing allows the adolescent to practice the skills he or she has learned in session with the therapist, with the aim of helping the adolescent use the skills outside of session. Contingent reinforcement uses a reward system to help increase treatment adherence. For example, an adolescent may receive a special privilege for keeping a record of automatic thoughts for the week. Not all behavioral techniques are used in treating every psychiatric disorder. For example, exposure therapy is an essential component to CBT for anxiety disorders such as specific phobia and obsessive-compulsive disorder, whereas activity scheduling is a specific behavioral component of CBT for depression.[57] Relaxation training is also used in treatment of anxiety. In relaxation training, the adolescent learns how to manage the physiologic effects of anxiety by practicing deep breathing and progressive muscle relaxation. Activity scheduling or behavioral activation are used with the intention of helping the individual to engage in more activities he or she enjoys.

Finally, the CBT therapist will also assign tasks for the adolescent to complete before the next therapy session often referred to as homework. Homework is seen as an essential component in CBT, because it helps the adolescent to generalize the skills learned in session to other situations. Homework nonadherence can become an obstacle to effective treatment, particularly with adolescents, and therefore, the establishment of therapist-adolescent collaboration is central in CBT.[57] CBT can be provided to individual adolescents or in a group setting. Sessions usually take place weekly, with an average length of treatment lasting between 12 and 20 sessions.[57] In addition to the use of homework and the structured, time-limited nature of CBT, other defining CBT features include (1) the active direction of session activity by the therapist, (2) teaching of specific skills to manage symptoms, (3) an emphasis on the future and not the past, and (4) providing adolescents with information about their treatment and the disorder.[56]

ADOLESCENT CBT EVIDENCE BASE

Much of the research that has been conducted on the efficacy of CBT in adolescent populations has focused on anxiety disorders and depression. A brief overview of this literature is worthwhile given (1) both anxiety disorders and depression are common comorbid psychiatric conditions with ADHD in adolescence[13]; and (2) this literature demonstrates that adolescents respond well to CBT interventions.

Anxiety Disorders and Depression

There are a variety of studies examining the effectiveness of CBT for anxiety disorders that meet Level 1 OCEBM guidelines, as most are meta-analyses or systematic reviews. For example, Silverman and colleagues[58] used criteria from Chambless and Hollon[59] to study CBT effectiveness for a variety of anxiety disorders, including separation anxiety disorder, generalized anxiety disorder, and social phobia (SoP). Based on results of their review, it was concluded that individual CBT and group CBT for a variety of anxiety disorders and group CBT targeting SoP were all "probably efficacious" treatments. Similarly, Reynolds and colleagues[60] conducted a meta-analysis on the effects of psychotherapy for anxiety in children and adolescents. The authors reported that CBT for anxiety was "moderately effective," demonstrating that effect sizes were small to medium when compared with an active control in younger children. CBT studies for specific anxiety disorders in adolescents, particularly obsessive-compulsive disorder, had larger effect sizes.[60] Because of concerns about possible differences between older versus younger children and the received benefit from CBT, Bennett and colleagues[61] conducted an individual patient data meta-analysis examining age effects in CBT for child and adolescent anxiety. Although the authors predicted that children younger or older than the 8- to 11-year-old age group would respond differently to CBT, they found no statistically significant age by CBT interaction.[61]

CBT for depression has also been studied extensively with adolescents. However, whereas earlier meta-analyses (OCEBM Level 1) of CBT for adolescent depression demonstrated large effect sizes (average $d = 0.99$), more recent research has shown a decrease in the effect size.[62] Klein and colleagues[63] conducted a meta-analysis to better understand these changing effect sizes, suggesting that methodological differences have played a role in the effect size decrease. Klein and colleagues[63] found that CBT for depression involved 17.6 hours of therapy on average, with a medium mean posttreatment effect size for CBT ($d = 0.34$). They concluded that existing CBT for depression is not uniformly effective, and therefore, research needs to focus on which specific components of CBT are associated with improvement.[63]

Three recent adolescent depression studies meet OCEBM Level 2 criteria. A study currently underway[64] is a multisite randomized controlled trial examining the effectiveness of CBT among adolescents age 12 to 21. The authors compare CBT to treatment as usual, defined as interpersonal therapy, family therapy, parent counseling, medication, acceptance and commitment therapy, mindfulness training, or short-term psychodynamic therapy. The Treatment of Adolescent Depression Study (TADS)[65] is a multicenter, randomized effectiveness trial that examined short-term and long-term effects of fluoxetine, CBT, combination, and pill placebo. Individuals in the CBT group received 12 weeks of weekly individual CBT during stage 1. At stage 2, individuals who were still symptomatic received 6 more weeks of weekly CBT. Stage 3 lasted 18 weeks, wherein the CBT group received booster sessions every 6 weeks. Finally, stage 4 was completed at 1 year follow-up with no active treatment. Results showed that combination therapy was most effective, with a 71% response rate, followed by medication alone (60.6%), CBT alone (43.2%), and placebo (34.8%).[65]

In sum, there are a rather large number of OCEBM Level 1 and Level 2 studies that have demonstrated that CBT is an effective treatment of adolescent anxiety disorders and depression.

ADHD

Given the large extant literature suggesting that CBT is an effective treatment intervention for adolescent anxiety and depression, as well as the more modest sized OCEBM Level 1 literature suggesting that CBT can be effective for adolescent disruptive behavior disorders,[66] it is somewhat surprising that very few studies have even been conducted to assess the efficacy of CBT for managing ADHD in adolescents. The lack of empiric investigations of CBT for adolescent ADHD is especially remarkable in light of the emerging OCEBM Level 2 and 3 (nonrandomized controlled cohort study) literature suggesting that CBT can be effective for managing adult ADHD.[67–78]

Although behavioral therapy has been well researched for adolescents with ADHD,[79] far less empiric attention has been devoted to CBT in adolescents with ADHD, likely a function of previous findings that suggest that children and adolescents with ADHD have been deemed "treatment refractory" to any intervention deemed to be "cognitive."[80] Previous CBT interventions for child and adolescent ADHD focused on primarily changing self-talk and verbal mediation interventions,[80] yet were deemed to be ineffective.[81,82] Indeed, interventions for adolescents with ADHD have been grounded in behavioral principles far more than cognitive principles.[83]

Within the past 10 years, however, there have been data published on the efficacy of CBT for managing adult ADHD.[67–71,84] The CBT interventions in the adult ADHD population are focused on skill-building and teaching specific skills.[85] Although there is undoubtedly a cognitive component to the adult ADHD CBT interventions, all existing adult ADHD CBT interventions appear more heavily skewed toward teaching behavioral techniques. Given that the adult ADHD interventions appear to be effective and the adult interventions comprise more behavioral features than cognitive features, this raises the question of whether these adult CBT interventions can be effective for adolescents with ADHD. Anxiety and depression respond well to CBT and are common psychiatric comorbidities in adolescent ADHD; this is another reason that CBT interventions that adopt a skill-building emphasis may be worthwhile to consider for adolescents with ADHD. Presently, however, little data have been reported on using the adult ADHD interventions in adolescent ADHD samples.

Clinic-based Adolescent CBT Intervention

In one of the very few studies that assessed the efficacy of CBT for adolescent ADHD, Antshel and colleagues[86] used an open-label design (OCEBM Level 3) to investigate CBT outcomes in high school students (ages 14–18; mean age =16.4 years) with ADHD. In their clinically referred sample of 82 adolescents with ADHD that were recruited over a 4-year period, referrals were primarily from primary care physicians (34%), educational settings (33%), and parents (20%). There was roughly an even distribution between the Inattentive and Combined subtypes in the study. Seven adolescents with ADHD refused to participate in the CBT intervention and 4 failed to complete the CBT treatment protocol.

Most adolescents with ADHD had a comorbid condition; only 20% of adolescents had the single diagnosis of ADHD. Clinical rated Mean Global Assessment of Functioning[2] score was 52.2 (SD = 11.5), indicating moderate to serious symptoms and impairment.[2] Educationally, 61% of the adolescents with ADHD ($n = 41$) were served on some form of special education plan, generally an Americans with Disabilities Act 504 plan ($n = 27$) or an Individualized Education Plan ($n = 14$). All adolescents with ADHD who participated in the study also participated in concurrent pharmacotherapy. Fifty-nine of the adolescents were already prescribed stimulant ($n = 54$) or nonstimulant (atomoxetine) ($n = 5$) medication at the time of referral. In sum, this was a clinically referred sample of adolescents with ADHD that despite medication management continued to demonstrate rather significant functional impairments.

The Behavior Assessment System for Children–2nd edition,[87] the ADHD–Rating Scales[7] and the Impairment Rating Scale[88] served as outcome measures. In addition, several ecologically valid measures of real-world functioning were obtained. These measures included cumulative grade point average and number of school absences/tardies.

The intervention used in the study was a downward extension of the Safren and colleagues[71] CBT program for adults with ADHD. Safren's CBT program includes components of motivational interviewing, practice, review, and repetition of learned skills and comprises 3 core modules and 3 optional modules. In the Antshel and colleagues study, all adolescents received all 6 modules (core plus optional modules).

The first 4-session core module involved psychoeducation about ADHD as well as behavioral training in organization and planning skills. The second 3-session core module focused on the adolescent learning behavioral skills to reduce distractibility. The third core module used cognitive restructuring strategies. Unlike the other modules that were consistent in length, the cognitive restructuring module varied between 2 and 5 sessions (mean = 3.1 sessions; SD = 1.1 sessions) depending on the particular adolescent. The Safren and colleagues[71] optional modules were also completed by the adolescents with ADHD. These modules included 4 sessions focused on teaching behavioral skills aimed at reducing procrastination, improving communication skills (eg, reducing interruptions, improving active listening), and improving anger/frustration management.

At the conclusion of each session, a homework assignment was assigned and a handout describing the topics covered was provided to the parent/adolescent. Parents were included in the treatment and were in the therapy room during the first 7 sessions (core modules 1 and 2) as well as the one optional procrastination module. Parents were not in therapy room during core module 3 or the communication skills or anger management optional modules. When parents were present in the therapy room, parents were instructed explicitly that they were present only to "improve generalizability of the strategies to the real-world." The therapist directed most of the session toward the adolescent, with time for the parent to ask questions/seek clarification at the end of the 50-minute session. When parents were not included in the therapy room, parents were informed of the topics discussed and how to monitor homework, yet not the specific content of the topics.

Parents also explicitly used contingency management strategies with their adolescent in an attempt to improve homework adherence and generalization of the skills. For example, parents were instructed how to develop a reinforcement system specific to the CBT skills, how to monitor adherence, and how best to facilitate the adolescent engaging in the skill use outside of session. This a priori decision to (1) include parents heavily in the sessions and (2) train parents in the monitoring and application of contingency management strategies was based on the extant literature suggesting that purely cognitive-based interventions without the integration of behavioral principles and interventions lack an evidence-base for managing adolescents with ADHD.[89] Recent CBT suggestions for managing pediatric anxiety disorders that are comorbid with ADHD also highlight the need to actively involve parents in the therapy room.[90]

Results indicated that the Safren and colleagues[71] CBT intervention was modestly efficacious for high school students with ADHD. The largest effect sizes were observed for number of weekly missed classes, school tardies, stimulant medication doses, parent-reported externalizing behaviors, parent-reported inattention symptoms, and teacher-reported inattention symptoms. The adolescents reported less treatment changes than parents and teachers. No statistically significant interactions emerged between ADHD subtype or gender, time, and any of the dependent variables. Of interest, the group of adolescents with ADHD and comorbid oppositional defiant disorder was rated by parents and teachers as benefiting less from the CBT intervention, whereas the adolescents with ADHD and an anxiety disorder and the adolescents with ADHD and comorbid depression improved more than the ADHD-only group on several teacher report variables.[86] Antshel and colleagues[86] concluded that a downward extension of an empirically validated adult ADHD CBT protocol can benefit some adolescents with ADHD, especially with regard to functional parameters, yet less so for ADHD symptoms. Less optimistically, despite the improvements, most of the adolescents with ADHD did not normalize their functioning and remained both symptomatic and functionally impaired (as rated by teachers and parents) in at least one domain.[86]

Thus far, the study by Antshel and colleagues is the only clinic-based study that used CBT for managing ADHD in adolescents. Nonetheless, there have been other clinic-based studies that have analyzed ADHD and the impact on CBT in adolescents. For example, secondary analyses of abovementioned clinic-based TADS study[65] examined the role of comorbid ADHD as a moderator of treatment outcomes in adolescent depression. Data from these analyses suggested that comorbid ADHD did not negatively affect CBT response in adolescents with depression.[91] Likewise, in a clinic-based study of adolescent anxiety disorders, comorbid ADHD did not affect CBT treatment outcomes.[92] Thus, there is some reason to suggest that larger clinic-based OCEBM Level 2 trials for CBT in adolescent ADHD may be worthwhile to consider.

Although not referring to their intervention as CBT, Raggi and colleagues[93] studied a clinic-based homework intervention program for young adolescents (middle school students) that included multiple cognitive (eg, teaching methods for managing materials, teaching methods for time management) and behavioral interventions (eg, contingency contracting). Raggi and colleagues[93] demonstrated that the use of clinic-based cognitive behavioral *interventions* (not therapy) was beneficial for increasing homework adherence for 73% (or 8 of 11) middle school students in their study. In this OCEBM Level 4 study, positive change in grade point average was reported for 86% (or 7 of 8 participants).

Likewise, although not referring to their intervention as CBT, van de Weijer-Bergsma and colleagues[94] studied mindfulness training in adolescents with ADHD. Mindfulness interventions are commonly used within CBT treatments. In their clinic-based intervention, adolescents with ADHD met for 8 weekly 90-min sessions in groups of 4 to 6 adolescents. A reward system was implemented to assist in gaining adolescent engagement in treatment. In addition, parents concurrently participated in a mindful parenting intervention. The authors reported positive effects of the intervention on a variety of adolescent outcomes. Others have likewise reported that a mindfulness-based intervention delivered concurrently to parents and adolescents (ages 13–18) with ADHD can lead to positive outcomes, more so for parent-rated than adolescent-rated outcomes.[95] In both studies, however, it was not possible to determine which treatment component (adolescent intervention, parent intervention, combined) was responsible for the positive outcomes.

The Supporting Teens' Academic Needs Daily (STAND) program is a parent-adolescent collaborative behaviorally based intervention for adolescent ADHD that focuses exclusively on academic impairment.[96] A primary goal of the STAND program is to lessen the encumbrance on teachers by training parents to implement behaviorally based interventions that are typically administered at school. In the STAND intervention, relying on behavioral principles, parents are instructed on how to best increase adolescents' accountability for organization, time management, homework completion, studying, and note-taking via 8 weekly hour-long family sessions and 4 monthly group parent sessions.[96] A pilot investigation with 36 middle school students with ADHD suggested that the STAND program is a feasible and effective intervention for adolescents with ADHD.[96] In the pilot study, STAND was delivered in a clinic setting. Nonetheless, the STAND authors assert that clinicians in clinic, community, or school settings can deliver the intervention.[96]

Although the STAND program is specific to academics, another program with cognitive and behavioral elements has been developed to specifically target adolescent motor vehicle operation. The Supporting a Teen's Effective Entry to the Roadway (STEER) program is an 8-week 90-min intervention that integrates a motor vehicle targeted BPT program, communication training for the adolescent and parents, supervised practice in a driving simulator facilitated by clinician coaching, parental monitoring of objective driving behaviors using innovative technology, and contingency management aimed at promoting safe driving behaviors.[97] In the STEER program, parents and adolescents have concurrent 45-min sessions and a joint 45-min session following the concurrent session.

In the adolescent sessions, the focus of the clinician is on teaching self-monitoring behaviors, psychoeducation about safe driving practices, and discussion about how to resolve parent-adolescent conflict. In the parent sessions, contingency management strategies and reframing/restructuring unhelpful cognitions are covered. In the family sessions, the adolescent practiced on the driving simulator and reviewed objective driving data with parents. Behavioral contracts were also negotiated during the family sessions and linked to specific contingencies.[97] The STEER program has been investigated in a small pilot study of 7 adolescent drivers. Results indicate that the STEER program led to positive changes (especially from the perspective of fathers, less so from the adolescents) in driving-related impairments, yet less robust improvements in actual objectively measured driving behaviors.[97]

School-based Adolescent CBT Intervention

Although school-based interventions have several benefits, intervening with adolescents in the school often involves intervening with teachers. Evans and colleagues[98] described several challenges with working with teachers of adolescents with ADHD including teacher reluctance to implement suggested interventions as well as poor response to feedback from consultants.

Despite these challenges, and although not explicitly advertised as a CBT intervention, several previous studies have assessed school-based cognitive behavioral interventions (not therapy) for adolescents with ADHD. Most of these previous studies have occurred in the context of a larger school-based intervention package. For example, Evans and colleagues[99] studied an organizational intervention in young adolescents (middle school students) that was contained within a larger behaviorally based intervention. Their data suggest that combining a skill-based intervention with a behaviorally based reinforcement system can lead to improved organization in young adolescents.[99]

Evans and colleagues[100] have developed a comprehensive school-based program that integrates cognitive and behavioral interventions (not therapy). The Challenging Horizons Program (CHP) is a comprehensive afterschool psychosocial intervention that includes 2 meetings per week for 2 hours and 15 minutes per meeting for a portion of or an entire academic year. The activities included in the CHP include an education group (eg, teaching skills of note taking, teaching study skills), an interpersonal skills group (eg, teaching social problem-solving skills), recreation, and individual meeting times between students and counselors.[100] The CHP includes a behavioral management system that relies on rewards and privileges. Several family meetings focus on family problem-solving and communication are also conducted, yet not at the school. Most adolescents in the CHP trial were prescribed a stimulant medication.[100]

Evans and colleagues[100,101] have conducted several OCEBM Level 2 studies on the CHP. Results generally indicate a dose-response relationship; CHP delivered over the entire academic year is more effective than CHP delivered for only one semester and CHP delivered over 4 days per week is more effective than 2 days per week.[102] Teachers report being satisfied with the CHP program, and families in the program often do not pursue additional services besides the CHP.[100] CHP outcome data also generally suggest that the intervention is preventative; compared with control groups who decline in social and academic functioning over the course of the academic semester or year, CHP participants show less of a decline.[100] Evans and colleagues[100] stress that it is not possible to determine which CHP components are most central to the positive outcomes.

In sum, there are several reasons to be optimistic that CBT may be beneficial for adolescents with ADHD and is worthy of further investigation: (1) CBT is effective for many of the common comorbid conditions that coexist with adolescent ADHD; (2) several small pilot studies have demonstrated that CBT as well as cognitive behavioral interventions, delivered in the clinic as well as at school, can be beneficial for adolescents with ADHD.

CLINICAL DECISION-MAKING

The focus of this article is on assisting the clinic-based or school-based provider who would like to implement a CBT intervention (**Box 1**).

Who Is Most Likely to Respond to CBT?

The only CBT *therapy* study to date is the Antshel and colleagues[86] pilot study. Data from this investigation suggest that adolescents with ADHD who have comorbid depression and/or anxiety disorders are more likely to respond positively to CBT delivered in a clinic setting. Adolescents with oppositional defiant disorder were less likely to respond positively to the CBT intervention. In school-based studies, however, psychiatric comorbidity has not been a moderator of cognitive behavioral interventions for adolescents with ADHD.[103]

Although not assessed in the CBT study by Antshel and colleagues,[86] given the central role that parents maintained in the CBT intervention, it seems intuitive to suggest that parents who are able to attend treatment sessions regularly and consistently monitor the adolescent's use of the interventions at home may have a more positive treatment outcome. Nonetheless, this was not monitored in the study by Antshel and colleagues.[86] Finally, and although also not assessed by most of the extant studies, there is some evidence that having a strong therapeutic adolescent:provider alliance is associated with more positive outcomes.[103]

Box 1
Recommendations for clinicians

- Medications are more likely to positively affect ADHD symptoms than functioning. Thus, a psychosocial intervention may be important to consider for any adolescent that is continuing to demonstrate functional impairments despite medication management.

- Existing adult CBT interventions that may be used for adolescents with ADHD rely more on "behavioral" principles than "cognitive" principles. Any CBT intervention that is focused more on cognitive therapy components (eg, modifying irrational thoughts, increasing self-monitoring) without concurrently incorporating principles of contingency management, especially reinforcement, is not likely to be effective.

- Unlike CBT interventions for adult ADHD, parents are important to include in the treatment plan and ongoing treatment delivery. Although including parents in the therapy room may work against those adolescents with ADHD and a comorbid oppositional defiant disorder, the inclusion of parents in the therapy room may be of benefit for adolescents with ADHD and a comorbid internalizing disorder.

- CBT interventions should be used in conjunction with medication management. There are very little data suggesting that CBT can be used instead of medication management. CBT interventions may permit a lower dose of the medication and medication may permit a less intense CBT intervention to be effective.

- Although not CBT per se, there are multiple school-based interventions that rely on cognitive and behavioral principles and have demonstrated efficacy for adolescents with ADHD. Clinicians could work with school personnel to identify possible school-based interventions that may be available to supplement any clinic-based intervention.

What Outcomes Are Most Likely to Be Affected by Treatment?

Most of the CBT[86] and cognitive behavioral intervention[93,96,99,102] studies suggest that real-world functioning, not ADHD symptoms, is more likely to be positively affected by CBT or cognitive behavioral interventions.

What Are the Contraindications for Treatment?

All of the abovementioned CBT and cognitive behavioral intervention studies suggest that these interventions are feasible and relatively well received, especially by parents. Although there is some evidence that oppositional defiant disorder moderates treatment outcomes,[86] none of the reviewed studies suggest a contraindication for CBT or cognitive behavioral interventions.

What Are Potential Adverse Effects of the Treatment?

None of the reviewed studies suggests that CBT or cognitive behavioral interventions were associated with any adverse effects (eg, worsening of symptoms, iatrogenic effects).

How Should the Treatment Be Sequenced and/or Integrated with Drug Therapy and with Other Nondrug Treatments?

Most of the reviewed studies used CBT or cognitive behavioral interventions in conjunction with pre-existing pharmacologic interventions. Thus, at this point, the extant data suggest that CBT should be used as an adjunct to concurrent medication management, not in place of concurrent medication management. There are currently no data that have been reported on how CBT can be integrated with other psychosocial interventions (eg, biofeedback, nutritional therapies).

FUTURE DIRECTIONS

The efficacy of a specific adult ADHD CBT manualized intervention for managing adolescent ADHD has been studied in only one sample. An obvious need is to expand the research base on CBT interventions for adolescents with ADHD. The adult CBT models that exist are more behaviorally based than cognitive in nature. Many of the early attempts to use CBT for children (not adolescents) with ADHD were based on a more conventional model of CBT with heavy cognitive therapy components (eg, changing automatic thoughts). The adult ADHD CBT interventions, while including cognitive therapy components, are more skewed toward behaviorally based interventions. Future research should continue to assess the efficacy of these more contemporary and ADHD-specific CBT interventions for managing adolescent ADHD.

Future research should also continue to rely on multiple informants as well as ecologically valid functional outcome data points. For example, adolescents are more autonomous than children, yet deny impairments.[16] Thus, adolescents generally report less symptoms and impairments than parents, raising the question of which reporter is more accurate. Relying on ecologically valid functional outcome measures, such as academic output, driving simulator performance, and so on, may be beneficial to consider as outcome variables for CBT intervention studies. It is hoped that the primary focus on ADHD symptoms as the measure of treatment efficacy will be replaced by a primary focus on functional impairments.

Future adolescent ADHD CBT studies should continue to focus on better clarifying treatment moderators and mediators in an attempt to guide clinicians and families better in making treatment decisions. Finally, future studies should use longitudinal prospective designs to better evaluate treatment maintenance.

SUMMARY

In the past 10 years, there have been several CBT manuals that have been developed for adults with ADHD. These manuals are more behaviorally based than "cognitive" in nature. Thus far, only one study has assessed the efficacy of an adult CBT manual that was modified for work with adolescents with ADHD. Although this pilot study is suggestive of some promise for CBT for managing adolescent ADHD, far more studies need to be completed and the findings replicated before one can consider CBT an efficacious intervention for managing adolescent ADHD. Nonetheless, when viewed in light of the larger number of studies that have used cognitive behavioral *interventions* (not therapy) for adolescents with ADHD, there are reasons to suggest that this is a topic worthy of further investigation.

REFERENCES

1. APA. Diagnostic and statistical manual of mental disorders. 5th edition. Washington, DC: American Psychiatric Publishing; 2013.
2. APA. DSM-IV-TR. Washington, DC: American Psychiatric Association; 2000.
3. Froehlich TE, Lanphear BP, Epstein JN, et al. Prevalence, recognition, and treatment of attention-deficit/hyperactivity disorder in a national sample of US children. Arch Pediatr Adolesc Med 2007;161(9):857–64.
4. Faraone SV, Sergeant J, Gillberg C, et al. The worldwide prevalence of ADHD: is it an American condition? World Psychiatry 2003;2(2):104–13.
5. Costello EJ, Copeland W, Angold A. Trends in psychopathology across the adolescent years: what changes when children become adolescents, and when adolescents become adults? J Child Psychol Psychiatry 2011;52(10): 1015–25.
6. Faraone SV, Biederman J, Mick E. The age-dependent decline of attention deficit hyperactivity disorder: a meta-analysis of follow-up studies. Psychol Med 2006; 36(2):159–65.
7. Dupaul G, Power T, Anastopoulos A. ADHD rating scale-IV: checklists, norms, and clinical interpretation. New York: Guilford Press; 1998.
8. Hart EL, Lahey BB, Loeber R, et al. Developmental change in attention-deficit hyperactivity disorder in boys: a four-year longitudinal study. J Abnorm Child Psychol 1995;23(6):729–49.
9. Barkley RA, Murphy K, Fischer M. ADHD in adults: what the science says. New York: Guilford Press; 2008.
10. Pliszka S, AACAP Work Group on Quality Issues. Practice parameter for the assessment and treatment of children and adolescents with attention-deficit/ hyperactivity disorder. J Am Acad Child Adolesc Psychiatry 2007;46(7): 894–921.
11. Hill JC, Schoener EP. Age-dependent decline of attention deficit hyperactivity disorder. Am J Psychiatry 1996;153(9):1143–6.
12. Biederman J, Monuteaux MC, Mick E, et al. Young adult outcome of attention deficit hyperactivity disorder: a controlled 10-year follow-up study. Psychol Med 2006;36(2):167–79.
13. Molina BS, Hinshaw SP, Swanson JM, et al. The MTA at 8 years: prospective follow-up of children treated for combined-type ADHD in a multisite study. J Am Acad Child Adolesc Psychiatry 2009;48(5):484–500.
14. Biederman J, Faraone S, Milberger S, et al. Predictors of persistence and remission of ADHD into adolescence: results from a four-year prospective follow-up study. J Am Acad Child Adolesc Psychiatry 1996;35(3):343–51.

15. Barkley RA, Anastopoulos AD, Guevremont DC, et al. Adolescents with ADHD: patterns of behavioral adjustment, academic functioning, and treatment utilization. J Am Acad Child Adolesc Psychiatry 1991;30(5):752–61.

16. Sibley MH, Pelham WE Jr, Molina BS, et al. Diagnosing ADHD in adolescence. J Consult Clin Psychol 2012;80(1):139–50.

17. Kent KM, Pelham WE Jr, Molina BS, et al. The academic experience of male high school students with ADHD. J Abnorm Child Psychol 2011;39(3):451–62.

18. Edwards G, Barkley RA, Laneri M, et al. Parent-adolescent conflict in teenagers with ADHD and ODD. J Abnorm Child Psychol 2001;29(6):557–72.

19. Evans SW, Sibley M, Serpell ZN. Changes in caregiver strain over time in young adolescents with ADHD: the role of oppositional and delinquent behavior. J Atten Disord 2009;12(6):516–24.

20. Charach A, Yeung E, Climans T, et al. Childhood attention-deficit/hyperactivity disorder and future substance use disorders: comparative meta-analyses. J Am Acad Child Adolesc Psychiatry 2011;50(1):9–21.

21. Barkley RA, Cox D. A review of driving risks and impairments associated with attention-deficit/hyperactivity disorder and the effects of stimulant medication on driving performance. J Safety Res 2007;38(1):113–28.

22. Smith BH, Waschbusch DA, Willoughby MT, et al. The efficacy, safety, and practicality of treatments for adolescents with attention-deficit/hyperactivity disorder (ADHD). Clin Child Fam Psychol Rev 2000;3(4):243–67.

23. Faraone SV, Biederman J, Spencer TJ, et al. Comparing the efficacy of medications for ADHD using meta-analysis. MedGenMed 2006;8(4):4.

24. Hoza B, Gerdes AC, Mrug S, et al. Peer-assessed outcomes in the multimodal treatment study of children with attention deficit hyperactivity disorder. J Clin Child Adolesc Psychol 2005;34(1):74–86.

25. Johnston C, Mash EJ. Families of children with attention-deficit/hyperactivity disorder: review and recommendations for future research. Clin Child Fam Psychol Rev 2001;4(3):183–207.

26. Raggi VL, Chronis AM. Interventions to address the academic impairment of children and adolescents with ADHD. Clin Child Fam Psychol Rev 2006;9(2):85–111.

27. Pelham W, Fabiano GA, Gnagy EM, et al. ADHD. In: Hibbs ED, Jensen PS, editors. Psychosocial treatments for child and adolescent disorders: empirically based strategies for clinical practice. 2nd edition. Washington, DC: American Psychological Association; 2005.

28. Fabiano GA, Pelham WE Jr, Gnagy EM, et al. The single and combined effects of multiple intensities of behavior modification and methylphenidate for children with attention deficit hyperactivity disorder in a classroom setting. School Psychol Rev 2007;36:195–216.

29. Barkley RA. Adolescents with attention-deficit/hyperactivity disorder: an overview of empirically based treatments. J Psychiatr Pract 2004;10(1):39–56.

30. Chronis AM, Chacko A, Fabiano GA, et al. Enhancements to the behavioral parent training paradigm for families of children with ADHD: review and future directions. Clin Child Fam Psychol Rev 2004;7(1):1–27.

31. Chronis AM, Jones HA, Raggi VL. Evidence-based psychosocial treatments for children and adolescents with attention-deficit/hyperactivity disorder. Clin Psychol Rev 2006;26(4):486–502.

32. Chronis AM, Lahey BB, Pelham WE Jr, et al. Maternal depression and early positive parenting predict future conduct problems in young children with attention-deficit/hyperactivity disorder. Dev Psychol 2007;43(1):70–82.

33. Anastopoulos AD, DuPaul GJ, Barkley RA. Stimulant medication and parent training therapies for attention deficit-hyperactivity disorder. J Learn Disabil 1991;24(4):210–8.

34. Sonuga-Barke EJ, Daley D, Thompson M, et al. Parent-based therapies for pre-school attention-deficit/hyperactivity disorder: a randomized, controlled trial with a community sample. J Am Acad Child Adolesc Psychiatry 2001;40(4):402–8.

35. Sonuga-Barke EJ, Thompson M, Daley D, et al. Parent training for attention deficit/hyperactivity disorder: is it as effective when delivered as routine rather than as specialist care? Br J Clin Psychol 2004;43(Pt 4):449–57.

36. Strayhorn JM, Weidman CS. Reduction of attention deficit and internalizing symptoms in preschoolers through parent-child interaction training. J Am Acad Child Adolesc Psychiatry 1989;28(6):888–96.

37. Barkley RA, Guevremont DC, Anastopoulos AD, et al. A comparison of three family therapy programs for treating family conflicts in adolescents with attention-deficit hyperactivity disorder. J Consult Clin Psychol 1992;60(3):450–62.

38. Anastopoulos AD, Shelton TL, DuPaul GJ, et al. Parent training for attention-deficit hyperactivity disorder: its impact on parent functioning. J Abnorm Child Psychol 1993;21(5):581–96.

39. Barkley R, Edwards G, Robins AR. Defiant teens: a clinician's manual for family training. New York: Guiford; 1999.

40. DuPaul GJ, Eckert TL. The effects of school-based interventions for attention deficit hyperactivity disorder: a meta-analysis. Sch Psychol Dig 1997;26: 5–27.

41. Pfiffner LJ, Rosen LA, O'Leary SG. The efficacy of an all-positive approach to classroom management. J Appl Behav Anal 1985;18(3):257–61.

42. Pfiffner LJ, DuPaul GJ, Barkley R. Educational management. In: Barkley R, editor. Attention deficit hyperactivity disorder: a handbook for diagnosis and treatment, vol. 3. New York: Guilford Press; 2005. p. 547–89.

43. DiClemente RJ, Hansen WB, Ponton LE. Adolescents at risk. In: DiClemente R, Hansen W, Ponton L, editors. Handbook of adolescent health risk behavior. New York: Plenum Press; 1996. p. 1–4.

44. Weyandt LL, Dupaul GJ. Introduction to special series on college students with ADHD: psychosocial issues, comorbidity, and treatment. J Atten Disord 2012; 16(3):199–201.

45. Knopf JM, Hornung RW, Slap GB, et al. Views of treatment decision making from adolescents with chronic illnesses and their parents: a pilot study. Health Expect 2008;11(4):343–54.

46. Weiss M, Safren SA, Solanto MV, et al. Research forum on psychological treatment of adults with ADHD. J Atten Disord 2008;11(6):642–51.

47. Charach A, Ickowicz A, Schachar R. Stimulant treatment over five years: adherence, effectiveness, and adverse effects. J Am Acad Child Adolesc Psychiatry 2004;43(5):559–67.

48. Gordon SM, Tulak F, Troncale J. Prevalence and characteristics of adolescents patients with co-occurring ADHD and substance dependence. J Addict Dis 2004;23(4):31–40.

49. Thiruchelvam D, Charach A, Schachar RJ. Moderators and mediators of long-term adherence to stimulant treatment in children with ADHD. J Am Acad Child Adolesc Psychiatry 2001;40(8):922–8.

50. Wilens TE, Adler LA, Adams J, et al. Misuse and diversion of stimulants prescribed for ADHD: a systematic review of the literature. J Am Acad Child Adolesc Psychiatry 2008;47(1):21–31.

51. Faraone SV, Wilens TE. Effect of stimulant medications for attention-deficit/hyperactivity disorder on later substance use and the potential for stimulant misuse, abuse, and diversion. J Clin Psychiatry 2007;68(Suppl 11):15–22.
52. Bukstein OG. Satisfaction with treatment for attention-deficit/hyperactivity disorder. Am J Manag Care 2004;10(Suppl 4):S107–16.
53. Jensen PS, Kettle L, Roper MT, et al. Are stimulants overprescribed? Treatment of ADHD in four U.S. communities. J Am Acad Child Adolesc Psychiatry 1999; 38(7):797–804.
54. McLeod JD, Fettes DL, Jensen PS, et al. Public knowledge, beliefs, and treatment preferences concerning attention-deficit hyperactivity disorder. Psychiatr Serv 2007;58(5):626–31.
55. MTA Collaborative Group. Moderators and mediators of treatment response for children with attention-deficit/hyperactivity disorder: the multimodal treatment study of children with attention-deficit/hyperactivity disorder. Arch Gen Psychiatry 1999;56(12):1088–96.
56. Blagys MD, Hilsenroth MJ. Distinctive activities of cognitive-behavioral therapy. A review of the comparative psychotherapy process literature. Clin Psychol Rev 2002;22(5):671–706.
57. Weersing VR, Brent DA. Treating depression in adolescents using individual cognitive-behavioral therapy. In: Weisz JR, Kazdin AE, editors. Evidence-based psychotherapies for children and adolescents. 2nd edition. New York: Guilford Press; 2010. p. 126–39.
58. Silverman WK, Pina AA, Viswesvaran C. Evidence-based psychosocial treatments for phobic and anxiety disorders in children and adolescents. J Clin Child Adolesc Psychol 2008;37(1):105–30.
59. Chambless DL, Hollon SD. Defining empirically supported therapies. J Consult Clin Psychol 1998;66(1):7–18.
60. Reynolds S, Wilson C, Austin J, et al. Effects of psychotherapy for anxiety in children and adolescents: a meta-analytic review. Clin Psychol Rev 2012;32(4): 251–62.
61. Bennett K, Manassis K, Walter SD, et al. Cognitive behavioral therapy age effects in child and adolescent anxiety: an individual patient data metaanalysis. Depress Anxiety 2013;30(9):829–41.
62. Weisz JR, McCarty CA, Valeri SM. Effects of psychotherapy for depression in children and adolescents: a meta-analysis. Psychol Bull 2006;132(1): 132–49.
63. Klein JB, Jacobs RH, Reinecke MA. Cognitive-behavioral therapy for adolescent depression: a meta-analytic investigation of changes in effect-size estimates. J Am Acad Child Adolesc Psychiatry 2007;46(11):1403–13.
64. Stikkelbroek Y, Bodden DH, Dekovic M, et al. Effectiveness and cost effectiveness of cognitive behavioral therapy (CBT) in clinically depressed adolescents: individual CBT versus treatment as usual (TAU). BMC Psychiatry 2013; 13:314.
65. March J, Silva S, Curry J, et al. The treatment for adolescents with depression study (TADS): outcomes over 1 year of naturalistic follow-up. Am J Psychiatry 2009;166(10):1141–9.
66. Sukhodolsky DG, Kassinove H, Gorman BS. Cognitive-behavioral therapy for anger in children and adolescents: a meta-analysis. Aggress Violent Behav 2004;9(3):247–69.
67. Weiss M, Murray C, Wasdell M, et al. A randomized controlled trial of CBT therapy for adults with ADHD with and without medication. BMC Psychiatry 2012;12:30.

68. Emilsson B, Gudjonsson G, Sigurdsson JF, et al. Cognitive behaviour therapy in medication-treated adults with ADHD and persistent symptoms: a randomized controlled trial. BMC Psychiatry 2011;11:116.
69. Virta M, Salakari A, Antila M, et al. Short cognitive behavioral therapy and cognitive training for adults with ADHD - a randomized controlled pilot study. Neuropsychiatr Dis Treat 2010;6:443–53.
70. Bramham J, Young S, Bickerdike A, et al. Evaluation of group cognitive behavioral therapy for adults with ADHD. J Atten Disord 2009;12(5):434–41.
71. Safren SA, Otto MW, Sprich S, et al. Cognitive-behavioral therapy for ADHD in medication-treated adults with continued symptoms. Behav Res Ther 2005; 43(7):831–42.
72. Rostain AL, Ramsay JR. A combined treatment approach for adults with ADHD–results of an open study of 43 patients. J Atten Disord 2006;10(2):150–9.
73. Stevenson CS, Stevenson RJ, Whitmont S. A self-directed psychosocial intervention with minimal therapist contact for adults with attention deficit hyperactivity disorder. Clin Psychol Psychother 2003;10:93–101.
74. Stevenson CS, Whitmont S, Bornholt L, et al. A cognitive remediation programme for adults with attention deficit hyperactivity disorder. Aust N Z J Psychiatry 2002;36(5):610–6.
75. Safren SA, Sprich S, Mimiaga MJ, et al. Cognitive behavioral therapy vs relaxation with educational support for medication-treated adults with ADHD and persistent symptoms: a randomized controlled trial. JAMA 2010;304(8):875–80.
76. Solanto MV, Marks DJ, Wasserstein J, et al. Efficacy of meta-cognitive therapy for adult ADHD. Am J Psychiatry 2010;167(8):958–68.
77. Hesslinger B, Tebartz van Elst L, Nyberg E, et al. Psychotherapy of attention deficit hyperactivity disorder in adults–a pilot study using a structured skills training program. Eur Arch Psychiatry Clin Neurosci 2002;252(4):177–84.
78. Philipsen A, Richter H, Peters J, et al. Structured group psychotherapy in adults with attention deficit hyperactivity disorder: results of an open multicentre study. J Nerv Ment Dis 2007;195(12):1013–9.
79. Sibley MH, Kuriyan AB, Evans SW, et al. Pharmacological and psychosocial treatments for adolescents with ADHD: an updated systematic review of the literature. Clin Psychol Rev 2014;34(3):218–32.
80. Miller M, Hinshaw SP. Treatment for children and adolescents with ADHD. In: Kendall PC, editor. Child and adolescent therapy: cognitive-behavioral procedures. 4th edition. Guilford Press; 2012. p. 61–91.
81. Abikoff H. Tailored psychosocial treatments for ADHD: the search for a good fit. J Clin Child Psychol 2001;30(1):122–5.
82. Abikoff H. Cognitive training in ADHD children: less to it than meets the eye. J Learn Disabil 1991;24(4):205–9.
83. Fabiano GA, Pelham WE Jr, Coles EK, et al. A meta-analysis of behavioral treatments for attention-deficit/hyperactivity disorder. Clin Psychol Rev 2009;29(2): 129–40.
84. Mongia M, Hechtman L. Cognitive behavior therapy for adults with attention-deficit/hyperactivity disorder: a review of recent randomized controlled trials. Curr Psychiatry Rep 2012;14(5):561–7.
85. Knouse LE, Safren SA. Current status of cognitive behavioral therapy for adult attention-deficit hyperactivity disorder. Psychiatr Clin North Am 2010;33(3): 497–509.
86. Antshel KM, Faraone SV, Gordon M. Cognitive behavioral treatment outcomes in adolescent ADHD. J Atten Disord 2012. [Epub ahead of print].

87. Reynolds CR, Kamphaus RW. Behavior assessment scales for children. 2nd edition. Circle Pines (MN): American Guidance Services; 2006.
88. Fabiano GA, Pelham W, Waschbusch DA, et al. A practical measure of impairment: psychometric properties of the impairment rating scale in samples of children with attention deficit hyperactivity disorder and two school-based samples. J Clin Child Adolesc Psychol 2006;35:369–85.
89. Toplak ME, Connors L, Shuster J, et al. Review of cognitive, cognitive-behavioral, and neural-based interventions for Attention-Deficit/Hyperactivity Disorder (ADHD). Clin Psychol Rev 2008;28(5):801–23.
90. Haoodorsdottir T, Ollendick T. Comorbid ADHD: implications for the treatment of anxiety disorders in children and adolescents. Cognit Behav Pract 2014;21(3): 310–22.
91. Kratochvil CJ, May DE, Silva SG, et al. Treatment response in depressed adolescents with and without co-morbid attention-deficit/hyperactivity disorder in the treatment for adolescents with depression study. J Child Adolesc Psychopharmacol 2009;19(5):519–27.
92. Flannery-Schroeder E, Suveg C, Safford S, et al. Comorbid externalising disorders and child anxiety treatment outcomes. Behav Change 2004;21(1):14–25.
93. Raggi V, Chronis-Tuscano AM, Fishbein H, et al. Development of a brief, behavioral homework intervention for middle school students with attention-deficit/hyperactivity disorder. School Mental Health 2009;1:61–77.
94. van de Weijer-Bergsma E, Formsma AR, de Bruin EI, et al. The effectiveness of mindfulness training on behavioral problems and attentional functioning in adolescents with ADHD. J Child Fam Stud 2012;21(5):775–87.
95. Haydicky J, Shecter C, Wiener JM, et al. Evaluation of MBCT for adolescents with ADHD and their parents: impact on individual and family functioning. J Child Fam Stud 2013, in press.
96. Sibley MH, Pelham WE, Derefinko KJ, et al. A pilot trial of supporting teens' academic needs daily (STAND): a parent-adolescent collaborative intervention for ADHD. J Psychopathol Behav Assess 2013;35:436–49.
97. Fabiano GA, Hulme K, Linke S, et al. The supporting a teen's effective entry to the roadway (STEER) program: feasibility and preliminary support for a psychosocial intervention for teenage drivers with ADHD. Cognit Behav Pract 2011;18: 267–80.
98. Evans SW, Serpell ZN, Schultz BK, et al. Cumulative benefits of secondary school-based treatment of students with attention deficit hyperactivity disorder. School Psychol Rev 2007;36:256–73.
99. Evans SW, Schultz B, White L, et al. A school-based organization intervention for young adolescents with ADHD. School Mental Health 2009;1:78–88.
100. Evans SW, Schultz BK, Demars CE, et al. Effectiveness of the challenging horizons after-school program for young adolescents with ADHD. Behav Ther 2011; 42(3):462–74.
101. Evans SW, Langberg J, Raggi V, et al. Development of a school-based treatment program for middle school youth with ADHD. J Atten Disord 2005;9(1):343–53.
102. Langberg JM, Epstein JN, Urbanowicz CM, et al. Efficacy of an organization skills intervention to improve the academic functioning of students with attention-deficit/hyperactivity disorder. School Psychol Q 2008;23:407–17.
103. Langberg JM, Becker SP, Epstein JN, et al. Predictors of response and mechanisms of change in an organizational skills intervention for students with ADHD. J Child Fam Stud 2013;22(7):1000–12.

Neuropsychologically Informed Strategic Psychotherapy in Teenagers and Adults with ADHD

Larry J. Seidman, PhD

KEYWORDS

- ADHD • Neuropsychology • Psychotherapy • Mastery • Self-esteem
- Organization and control

KEY POINTS

- Psychotherapy, defined as a verbal, problem-solving ("strategic"), interpersonal interaction, may augment other treatments designed to increase self-regulation and self-control.
- Treatment may range from brief psychoeducational interventions of 1 to 5 sessions to longer term therapy of indefinite duration, depending on the needs and goals of the individual.
- This form of psychotherapy can adaptively weave cognitive–behavioral therapy, family therapy, and cognitive remediation into an integrated neuropsychologically informed treatment in which increasing mastery and competence of the individual forms the central core.
- Treatment could help to build a therapeutic alliance to improve adherence to medications, address other issues associated with attention deficit hyperactivity disorder, such as affective (eg, dysthymia, depression) or cognitive (eg, learning disabilities) comorbidities, and other life issues that require understanding and problem solving.

INTRODUCTION/BACKGROUND
Target of Treatment: Attention Deficit Hyperactivity Disorder Symptoms, Associated Features

Attention deficit hyperactivity disorder (ADHD) is a common neurobiological disorder estimated to affect up to 10% of children and 5% of adults worldwide.[1] Across the lifecycle it is associated with high levels of morbidity and disability, and exerts a significant toll in many areas of functioning, including academic, occupational, and

Disclosure: The author has nothing to disclose.
Commonwealth Research Center, Department of Psychiatry, Beth Israel Deaconess Medical Center, at the Massachusetts Mental Health Center, Room 542, 75 Fenwood Road, Boston, MA 02115, USA
E-mail address: lseidman@bidmc.harvard.edu

Child Adolesc Psychiatric Clin N Am 23 (2014) 843–852
http://dx.doi.org/10.1016/j.chc.2014.05.013
1056-4993/14/$ – see front matter © 2014 Elsevier Inc. All rights reserved.
childpsych.theclinics.com

Abbreviations	
ACC	Anterior cingulate cortex
ADHD	Attention deficit hyperactivity disorder
CBT	Cognitive–behavior therapy
PFC	Prefrontal cortex

interpersonal.[2] It is associated with underachievement in many aspects of life, including school, work, and interpersonal relations, and with additional psychiatric comorbidities, risk for addictions, accidents and injuries, and medical problems, among other adverse outcomes.[3]

Neurobiological evidence supports a brain basis for ADHD, with structural and functional brain alterations in widespread neural regions.[4–10] Although not all individuals with ADHD demonstrate neuropsychological dysfunctions on formal neuropsychological tests, approximately 40% to 50% can be considered to have neuropsychological deficits, at least of those who participate in research studies[11,12]; thus, neuropsychological dysfunctions, particularly executive dysfunction, must be considered to be part of the clinical picture requiring help, unless proven otherwise.[13–15]

Given the complexity of the disorder, individuals with ADHD should be treated from a comprehensive, biopsychosocial perspective.[16] Such a perspective embodies the notion that the clinical work must attend equally to subjective experience (the mind), the person in the social world, and the body, including brain and neurocognitive function, dysfunctions, and their consequences.[17,18]

Need for the Treatment

Considering the biopsychosocial perspective, the "symptoms" to be treated are wide ranging. Although stimulants remain the primary treatment for ADHD symptoms of inattention and hyperactivity–impulsivity, various forms of nonpharmacologic interventions may be helpful for a range of life issues. Psychotherapy, defined here as a verbal, problem-solving ("strategic"), interpersonal interaction, may augment other treatments designed to increase self-regulation, self-control, and increase competence.

In this article, we discuss a variety of strategies psychotherapists use in working with teenagers and young adults, although such approaches are relevant to adults throughout life. These include working with individuals who reject medications, or who take them suboptimally, and where a good therapeutic alliance may lead to better compliance. Moreover, individuals with ADHD often have other issues associated with ADHD such as affective (eg, dysthymia, depression) or cognitive (eg, learning disabilities) comorbidities that require understanding and problem solving. Individuals may want to deal with understanding what ADHD is and is not, the meaning of the disorder in their life, and how neuropsychological dysfunctions may play a role.[19,20] As ADHD has been increasingly accepted as a disorder continuing into adult life, more young adults grapple with the effect of its persistence in psychotherapy, for example, the pros and cons of revealing that they are taking medications and asking for accommodations for specialized examinations for school requirements. Frank education about these issues can help the individual to accept the disorder and cope more effectively. This includes addressing the neuropsychological strengths and weaknesses that they possess.[15,18,19]

Of course, having ADHD does not protect people from the vagaries of life that may in fact be more common in people with ADHD, such as head injuries and marital problems. Psychotherapy can help to disentangle "ADHD" from other issues and address them. All too often, the diagnosis of ADHD is a "phenocopy" of other executive disorders, and a good psychotherapist, who is knowledgeable about ADHD assessment, can help to improve diagnostic precision. For example, many people with a family history of schizophrenia manifest attention problems as part of their familial-genetic risk,[21–23] and yet attention difficulties associated with excess dopamine (eg, risk for schizophrenia) may be very important to treat differently than disorders of reduced dopamine (eg, ADHD). The risk for triggering a psychotic episode with stimulant treatment in ADHD-like persons with a positive family history of psychosis needs to be carefully considered in the assessment and treatment process.

This form of psychotherapy can adaptively weave in other treatments, including cognitive–behavioral therapy (CBT), family therapy, and cognitive remediation, into an integrated form of strategic treatment in which increasing mastery and competence of the individual forms the central core.[19] Treatment may range from short-term psychoeducational interventions of 1 to 5 sessions to longer term therapy of indefinite duration, depending on the needs and goals of the individual.[15,18,19]

INTERVENTIONS
Theoretic Overview: Why Does Theory Suggest the Treatment Should Work?

The empirical neurobiological data, including pharmacology of stimulants, genetics, structural and functional magnetic resonance imaging, and neuropsychological data, as well as behavioral data, form a coherent basis for postulating cortical–subcortical dysregulation, particularly prefrontal (PFC), anterior cingulate cortex (ACC), and parietal cortical cognitive networks, striatal motor and reward systems, and cerebellar cognitive, affective, and motor components.[6,8–10] This aggregation of dysfunctional structures forms a foundation for understanding ADHD core functional deficits as associated with cognitive control and working memory (cortex and cerebellum), and difficulties with reward (basal ganglia). In addition, intrinsic to the disorder, or owing to associated comorbidities of mood and other disorders, may be limbic (affective) dysfunctions.

The model suggests that treatments oriented toward self-regulation have the potential to improve the functioning of this suboptimal functional neuroanatomy. There are various theoretically sound methods for achieving this, at least in part, ranging from Tai Chi training, to cognitive remediation, to the verbal, interpersonal, problem-solving psychotherapy discussed herein.[24] Central to all of these techniques is a reliance on improving executive functions and, as needed, addressing other weaknesses such as excessive emotional arousal. Moreover, attention to reward and motivation is essential. This involves allying with the patient's goals and cognitive schemas, so the patient is an active collaborator in the therapeutic process. Perhaps central to the link to reward and motivation is the enhancement of experiences of mastery and competence, based on helping the patient become more of the driver and less out of control.[25]

The development of language, both phylogenetically and ontogentically, is clearly associated with the development of self-regulation and executive functions. Moreover, the literature on brain plasticity provides a strong foundation for understanding psychotherapy in terms of learning.[26–29] There are a number of examples in the literature demonstrating that an interpersonal, problem-solving therapy changes self-regulatory brain networks in ways that are similar to the changes induced by pharmacotherapy. Because there are few data thus far on psychotherapeutic treatment for ADHD and subsequent changes in the brain, a few studies on brain changes after psychotherapy for anxiety disorders, depression, and borderline personality disorders are discussed briefly.

More than 20 years ago, the first study was published indicating that both fluoxetine and CBT induced similar brain changes, particularly in the caudate nucleus.[30] Many other studies have been performed over the last 2 decades.[31] Taken together, there is growing evidence that CBT, dialectic behavior therapy, psychodynamic psychotherapy, and interpersonal psychotherapy alter brain function in patients with a variety of disorders. These disorders include obsessive–compulsive disorder, panic, anxiety and phobic disorders, major depressive disorder, borderline personality disorder, and posttraumatic stress disorder. Most of these studies have reported similar brain changes after psychotherapy and medication, although there are differences.

The therapies invoked in these studies, similar to the approach described herein is oriented toward enhancing problem-solving (executive) capacities, self-representation (self-esteem, sense of self), and regulation of emotional states. The brain areas that play a role in these functions include the dorsolateral and ventrolateral PFC, ACC, medial PFC, precuneus, insular cortex, and amygdala. It seems plausible to suggest that cognitive control, involving emotional regulation, planning, and impulse control, can be improved by a better functional balance of cortical, especially PFC, and subcortical structures, including the limbic structures involved in emotional processing. Thus, verbal psychotherapy has a good theoretic basis for working with motivated teenagers or adults who choose this approach.

Description: How Is Treatment Delivered?

Treatment is typically delivered in an office, in a conventional way in which clinician and patient are usually sitting across from one another. However, in principle, there is no reason that this could not take place in other settings that help to motivate the patient and make him or her more comfortable and motivated.

The first phase of treatment involves careful assessment. An effective, neuropsychologically oriented evaluation emphasizes a patient's adaptive strengths and weaknesses while also clarifying diagnostic issues. Neuropsychologists emphasize the importance of addressing cognitive, medical (including pharmacologic), developmental, social, personality, and environmental factors that could be affecting an individual's cognitive functioning, as well as his or her psychosocial adjustment. Such an evaluation often includes dynamically and neuropsychologically informed interviewing in addition to the possible use of clinical psychological and neuropsychological instruments.[32] These techniques are designed to produce a description of adaptive strengths and weaknesses, as well as an understanding of the patient's experience of his or her illness or disability, the meaning of the disorder, its impact on self-esteem, the cognitive deficits that limit adaptation (eg, impaired verbal mediation leading to aggressive or impulsive behaviors), and the direct effects of the disorder on such realms as affective experience, sexuality, mood, and autonomic reactivity. As Silver points out,[33] developmental cognitive disorders are "life disabilities" that affect cognition, emotion, social life, and family life.

The neuropsychologist ought to play a substantial role in integrating the assessment of such features. Based on a careful evaluation of neurocognitive and personality factors, the neuropsychologist can offer an objective view of the patient's experience and adaptive resources or limitations. I would emphasize that, although formal neuropsychological testing is often helpful in framing the psychotherapy, it is not a requirement. However, a neuropsychologically informed perspective is essential, because it is highly relevant to the experience of the patient. Many patients and their family members have misconceptions regarding their "cognitive deficits" and a realistic appraisal in teenage years or young adulthood can go a long way in effective life planning. Such a perspective may indeed be objective without sacrificing empathy and is crucial for development of a therapeutic alliance, the foundation of any treatment.

The next phase of treatment depends on the goals defined as a result of the assessment. Many paths flow out of that initial framing. These are discussed at some length by Seidman.[19] In this article, I briefly describe 1 central theme that often defines the next phase of treatment. Although the course of treatment varies with the individual patient, a common theme from the perspective of the individual with ADHD that emerges during the assessment is the experience of disappointing adults, especially parents, and the experience of parents who seemed to demand too much, especially in relation to school. Such themes are frequent and intense for many teenagers and young adults with ADHD and are amplified when they have comorbid learning disabilities. When these themes are pursued in psychotherapy, it sometimes is evident that the patient's parents are often neither as harsh nor as demanding as the patient's conscious perception of them. Rather, the patients are carrying around an old, sometimes archaic experience of their parents' expectations and their own disappointments. Accurate understanding of these issues helps the patient and his or her family to work together more realistically. In the case of teens or young adults in their 20s, often a very important communication is a testing feedback session, with both patient and parents, in which the actual test performance is shown (with the patient's permission) to all. Such a demonstration allows parents to distinguish their child's failures from a willful lack of effort. A new realization of longstanding developmental cognitive difficulty often breaks a logjam between parent and child, who may have misunderstood one another for years. It also may allow them to plan more effectively for work or school.

Empirical Support

The treatment described herein does not exist as a formal, manualized treatment that has been tested and demonstrated to be evidence based. Rather, it is an amalgam of other treatment approaches melded together with a neuropsychological and neurobiological perspective that frames the treatment techniques within a cognitive neuroscience perspective. Nevertheless, it incorporates techniques supported by some research, particularly CBT and metacognitive training. A review of the empirical psychotherapy literature about ADHD is succinctly summarized by Philipsen,[34] is relevant to the application of this treatment, and some of those results are reported herein.

Philipsen's review, focusing on adults, acknowledges the same set of issues that have been discussed already in this article (eg, low self-esteem, depression and anxiety, in addition to inattention and hyperactivity–impulsivity). This treatment is thought to be applicable to teenagers from high school age or older. Philipsen notes that formal clinical trials of standardized treatment programs began in the 1990s and that the last decade has shown an increasing focus, with CBT receiving the lion's share of the attention. In general, these manualized treatments begin with a psychoeducational introduction, followed by a number of modules including "self-monitoring, mindfulness, emotion regulation, dysfunctional cognitions, time management and organization" (p. 1217). It has been more typical to do these modules in a group therapy rather than individual therapy format, and the CBT results have been positive.[34–36]

Individual CBT approaches that are more structured than the treatment described herein but cover many of the same topic areas have been generally successful. An open-label study demonstrated improvement on measures of ADHD, functioning, and comorbid symptoms.[37] Randomized, controlled trials of individual CBT have found positive results, including ADHD symptoms, clinical global impression, depression, and anxiety.[38,39] Overall, the results in these and other adult CBT studies are promising. Although these indicate that elements of the treatment described herein have received support, one cannot be sure that the "package" delivered in the more eclectic form of individual therapy is as effective as the manualized treatments until formally tested. At this point, using Oxford Center for Evidence Based Medicine guidelines, the use of a neuropsychologically informed strategic psychotherapy in teenagers and adults with ADHD has Level 5 support.

CLINICAL DECISION MAKING
Who Is Most Likely to Respond?

There is no research on who is most likely to respond to the treatment described herein (eg, patient characteristics, family variables) and there are limited data on patient characteristics observed in the manualized treatments. In a study of group therapy of metacognitive therapy compared with supportive therapy, female patients and those of the inattentive subtype were more likely to finish the treatment program than others. This sample may be somewhat atypical because of the high IQ and composition of the sample (mainly women).[40] No formal studies of demographics and comorbid characteristics as moderators of psychotherapeutic treatment have yet been carried out.

What Outcomes Are Most Likely to Be Affected by Treatment?

The review by Philipsen[34] indicated that the CBT treatments have all had effectiveness with ADHD symptoms, and some of the interventions were successful in improving comorbid symptoms including social functioning, anxiety, and depression. Anecdotally, the treatment described herein has been effective in self-esteem and social and role functioning improvements, perhaps secondary to better coping strategies for neuropsychological deficits.

What Are the Contraindications for Treatment?

No specific contraindications have been described. In general, psychosocial treatments have lower side effects than pharmacologic treatments. Nevertheless, harm could be caused by a provider who uses psychosocial treatments exclusively and does not appropriately discuss the potential benefits of pharmacologic treatments or is ideologically biased against such treatments. A good therapeutic alliance depends in part on a frank discussion of various options, the state of knowledge in the field, and respect for the wishes of the patient. Violations of those principles can be harmful to the patient, and also inhibit their capacity to obtain other empirically validated treatments.

What Are Potential Adverse Effects of the Treatment?

As noted, because this is not an empirically validated treatment per se (although it contains many elements of CBT and other structured treatments), it may not be generally effective. There are no known adverse effects of the treatment.

How Should the Treatment Be Sequenced and/or Integrated with Other Therapies?

Because drug therapy is the best-validated treatment for ADHD,[41] stand alone or combination therapy would optimally be combined with it, and may enhance the outcomes.[34] The treatment begins with a careful assessment described earlier, which may include neuropsychological testing, not for diagnostic purposes, but to provide a detailed understanding of the cognitive strengths and weaknesses of the individual. If the patient has not yet received drug treatment, an assessment before medications is valuable for documenting the "natural" state of cognition in the context of ADHD. Moreover, such an assessment helps to identify or rule out learning disabilities, and in general to provide an accurate understanding of the patient's cognitive capacities, because this is often not updated since childhood examinations.[15,18,19] This may also give clues to the most effective "windows" into the patient's concerns. Meetings with parents may also be included in this early phase of the first five sessions. A clear set of goals and their probable sequence of attention should emerge from the assessment and this initial "psychoeducational" phase of treatment.

The typical sequence of subsequent interventions involves discussion of medications and their effects and side effects on a regular basis, and then depending on the patient, a focus on self-monitoring, mindfulness, emotional regulation, and dysfunctional cognitions, followed by strategic cognitive guidance regarding organization, decision making, planning, aids to memory, and so on. Because some patients dislike taking medications or because they may have unpleasant side effects, an empathic approach to this challenge may help adherence or at least lead to rational choices.

FUTURE DIRECTIONS

This treatment could be manualized and then formally tested. Alternatively, the neuropsychological capacity evaluation could be integrated into existing CBT treatments, followed by psychoeducation about the cognitive strengths and weaknesses. This domain could then be used as a predictor of treatment outcome. Finally, the neurocognitive deficits found in many adults with ADHD[7,12,22] could be a target for cognitive remediation programs.[24]

SUMMARY

Nonpharmacologic interventions have developed rapidly over the past 20 to 30 years, and their empirical testing has grown substantially in the past 10 to 15 years. The treatment described herein does not yet have empirical support, but combines elements of empirically supported treatments. It is recommended that the role of neurocognition be enlarged for both assessment and potential treatment and be integrated within structured treatments like CBT.

CLINICIAN RECOMMENDATIONS

Sequence	Brief Summary
Assessment	Careful assessment of neurocognitive strengths and weaknesses, with or without formal neurocognitive testing, along with a detailed history, and full range of coverage of all aspects of life, including feelings the patient has about himself or herself.
Feedback	Discuss the results of your assessment with the patient and possibly with his or her parents. A frank discussion may clarify long-held distortions and elicit key issues for treatment.
Psychoeducation	This involves a more extensive discussion of what is ADHD, how it plays out in the patients life, cognitive strengths and weaknesses, the neurobiological basis of ADHD, the implications for everyday life with specific examples, and further elucidation of the patient's goals.
Goal setting	Development of a shared treatment plan based on a consensual view of the disorder's impact on the patient, what they can do about it, and the patient's plans for their life.
Treatment	A sequence of strategies should be implemented, including self-monitoring and mindfulness (to correct cognitive distortions), emotion regulation, time management, organizational skills, memory aids, and other neurocognitive skills-building exercises. Attention to medication status and side effects and relationship issues should be ongoing.

REFERENCES

1. Kessler RC, Adler L, Barkley R, et al. The prevalence and correlates of adult ADHD in the United States: results from the National Comorbidity Survey Replication. Am J Psychiatry 2006;163:716–23.
2. Biederman J. Attention deficit hyperactivity disorder: a selective overview. Biol Psychiatry 2005;57:1215–20.
3. Faraone SV, Biederman J, Spencer T, et al. Attention deficit disorder in adults: a review. Biol Psychiatry 2000;48:9–20.
4. Krain AL, Castellanos FX. Brain development and ADHD. Clin Psychol Rev 2006; 26(4):433–44.
5. Dickstein SG, Bannon K, Xavier Castellanos F, et al. The neural correlates of attention deficit hyperactivity disorder: an ALE meta-analysis. J Child Psychol Psychiatry 2006;47:1051–62.
6. Seidman LJ, Valera E, Bush G. Brain function and structure in adults with attention-deficit hyperactivity disorder. Psychiatr Clin North Am 2004;27: 323–47.
7. Seidman LJ, Doyle A, Fried R, et al. Neuropsychological function in adults with attention-deficit hyperactivity disorder. Psychiatr Clin North Am 2004;27:261–82.
8. Seidman LJ, Valera EM, Makris NM. Structural brain imaging of attention-deficit/ hyperactivity disorder. Biol Psychiatry 2005;57:1263–72.
9. Bush G, Valera EM, Seidman LJ. Functional neuroimaging of attention-deficit/ hyperactivity disorder: a review and suggested future directions. Biol Psychiatry 2005;57:1273–84.
10. Makris N, Biederman J, Monuteaux MC, et al. Towards conceptualizing a neural systems-based anatomy of attention-deficit/hyperactivity disorder. Dev Neurosci 2009;21:36–49.
11. Doyle AE, Biederman J, Seidman LJ, et al. Diagnostic efficiency of neuropsychological test scores for discriminating boys with and without ADHD. J Consult Clin Psychol 2000;68:477–88.
12. Seidman LJ. Neuropsychological function in people with ADHD across the lifespan. Clin Psychol Rev 2006;26:466–85.
13. Allen JG, Lewis L, Peebles MJ, et al. Neuropsychological assessment in a psychoanalytic setting: the mind· body problem in clinical practice. Bull Menninger Clin 1986;50:5–21.
14. Lewis L. Individual psychotherapy with patients having combined psychological and neurological disorders. Bull Menninger Clin 1986;50:75–87.
15. Seidman LJ, Bruder G, Giuliano AJ. Neuropsychological testing and neurophysiological assessment. In: Tasman A, Kay J, Lieberman JA, et al, editors. Psychiatry. 3rd edition. London: John Wiley & Sons, Ltd; 2008. p. 556–69.
16. Engel GL. The need for a new medical model: a challenge for biomedicine. Science 1977;196:129–36.
17. Kandel ER. A new intellectual framework for psychiatry. Am J Psychiatry 1998; 155:457–69.
18. Weinstein CS, Seidman LJ. The role of neuropsychological assessment in adult psychiatry. In: Ellison J, Weinstein CS, Hodel–Malinofsky T, editors. Psychotherapist's guide to neuropsychiatric patients: diagnostic and treatment issues. Washington, DC: American Psychiatric Press, Inc; 1994. p. 53–106.
19. Seidman LJ. Listening, meaning and empathy in neuropsychological disorders: case examples of assessment and treatment. In: Ellison J, Weinstein CS, Hodel–Malinofsky T, editors. Psychotherapist's guide to neuropsychiatric

patients: diagnostic and treatment issues. Washington, DC: American Psychiatric Press, Inc; 1994. p. 1–22.

20. Rosenberger J. Self psychology as a theoretical base for understanding the impact of learning disabilities. Child Adolesc Social Work J 1988;5:269–80.

21. Nuechterlein KH. Signal detection in vigilance tasks and behavioral attributes among offspring of schizophrenic mothers and among hyperactive children. J Abnorm Psychol 1983;92:4–28.

22. Seidman LJ, Van-Manen KJ, Gamser DM, et al. Effects of increasing processing load on vigilance in schizophrenia and in adults with attentional and learning disorders. Schizophr Res 1998;34:101–12.

23. Seidman LJ, Meyer EC, Giuliano AJ, et al. Auditory working memory impairments in individuals at familial high risk for schizophrenia. Neuropsychology 2012;26: 288–303.

24. Diamond A, Lee K. Interventions shown to improve executive function development in children 4-12 years old. Science 2011;333:959–64.

25. White RW. Motivation reconsidered: the concept of competence. Psychol Rev 1959;66:297–333.

26. May A. Experience-dependent structural plasticity in the adult human brain. Trends Cogn Sci 2011;15:475–82.

27. Zatorre RJ, Fields RD, Johansen-Berg H. Plasticity in gray and white: neuroimaging changes in brain structure during learning. Nat Neurosci 2012;15: 528–36.

28. Lövdén M, Wenger E, Mårtensson J, et al. Structural brain plasticity in adult learning and development. Neurosci Biobehav Rev 2013;37:2296–310.

29. Cibu T, Baker CI. Teaching an adult brain new tricks: a critical review of evidence for training-dependent structural plasticity in humans. Neuroimage 2013;73: 225–36.

30. Baxter LR Jr, Schwartz JM, Bergman KS, et al. Caudate glucose metabolic rate changes with both drug and behavior therapy for obsessive-compulsive disorder. Arch Gen Psychiatry 1992;49:681–9.

31. Frewen PA, Dozois DJ, Lanius RA. Neuroimaging studies of psychological interventions for mood and anxiety disorders: empirical and methodological review. Clin Psychol Rev 2008;28:228–46.

32. Seidman LJ, Toomey R. The clinical use of psychological and neuropsychological tests. In: Nicholi A, editor. The Harvard guide to psychiatry. 3rd edition. Cambridge (MA): Harvard University Press; 1999. p. 40–65.

33. Silver LB. Psychological and family problems associated with learning disabilities: assessment and intervention. J Am Acad Child Adolesc Psychiatry 1989; 28:319–25.

34. Philipsen A. Psychotherapy in adult attention deficit hyperactivity disorder. Expert Rev Neurother 2012;12:1217–25.

35. Bramham J, Young S, Bickerdike A, et al. Evaluation of group cognitive behavioral therapy for adults with ADHD. J Atten Disord 2009;12:434–41.

36. Philipsen A, Richter H, Peters J, et al. Structured group psychotherapy in adults with attention deficit hyperactivity disorder: results of an open multicentre study. J Nerv Ment Dis 2007;195:1013–9.

37. Rostain AL, Ramsay JR. A combined treatment approach for adults with ADHD – results of an open study of 43 patients. J Atten Disord 2006;10:150–9.

38. Safren SA, Otto MW, Sprich S, et al. Cognitive-behavioral therapy for ADHD in medication-treated adults with continued symptoms. Behav Res Ther 2005;43: 831–42.

39. Safren SA, Sprich S, Mimiaga MJ, et al. Cognitive behavioral therapy vs. relaxation with educational support for medication-treated adults with ADHD and persistent symptoms: a randomized controlled trial. JAMA 2010;304:875–80.
40. Solanto MV, Marks DJ, Wasserstein J, et al. Efficacy of meta-cognitive therapy for adult ADHD. Am J Psychiatry 2010;167:958–68.
41. Seixas M, Weiss M, Muller U. Systematic review of national and international guidelines on attention-deficit hyperactivity disorder. J Psychopharmacol 2011; 26:753–65.

Traditional Chinese Medicine in the Treatment of ADHD: A Review

Xinqiang Ni, MD, PhD[a], Yanli Zhang-James, PhD[b],
Xinmin Han, MD, PhD[a,*], Shuang Lei, MD, PhD[a], Jichao Sun, MD[a],
Rongyi Zhou, MD[a]

KEYWORDS

- Traditional Chinese medicine • Chinese herb medicine • Acupuncture • Tui na
- Tai chi chuan • Diet • Attention-deficit/hyperactivity disorder

KEY POINTS

- This is the first systematic review of traditional Chinese medicine (TCM) used in the treatment of attention-deficit/hyperactivity disorder (ADHD) in the English language.
- TCM is a natural therapy that has a rich cultural influence and is characterized by holism and individualized treatments based on traditional medicine theories and syndrome differentiation.
- TCM therapies, characterized by the combination and individualized use of herbal medicine, acupuncture, tui na, tai chi chuan, and diet, have been proven to be effective in improving ADHD symptoms in conjunction with Western pharmacologic therapy or alone.
- TCM is safe and has less side effects than pharmacologic therapy.
- TCM is commonly accepted and practiced in Asian countries. However, it is not well known or commonly used in Western countries.

INTRODUCTION/BACKGROUND

Target of Treatment: Attention-Deficit/Hyperactivity Disorder Symptoms, Associated Features

Attention-deficit/hyperactivity disorder (ADHD) is a prevalent childhood-onset neuro-psychiatric disorder that occurs in approximately 5.29% of school-aged children worldwide, with an estimated 66% of these children retaining ADHD symptoms into adulthood.[1–3] ADHD is characterized by age-inappropriate inattention and/or

Disclosure: This study was supported by the National Natural Science Foundation Project of China (No. 81273801) and the Specialized Research Fund for the Doctoral Program of Higher Education of China (No. 20123237110002). The authors do not have any conflict of interest.
[a] Department of Pediatrics of Chinese Medicine, Nanjing University of Traditional Chinese Medicine, 138 Xian Lin Avenue, Nanjing, China, 210046; [b] Department of Psychiatry, SUNY Upstate Medical University, 766 Irving Avenue, Syracuse, NY 13210, USA
* Corresponding author.
E-mail address: hxm1nj@163.com

Child Adolesc Psychiatric Clin N Am 23 (2014) 853–881
http://dx.doi.org/10.1016/j.chc.2014.05.011
1056-4993/14/$ – see front matter © 2014 Elsevier Inc. All rights reserved.

Abbreviations	
ADHD	Attention-deficit/hyperactivity disorder
CHM	Chinese herbal medicine
MPH	Methylphenidate
TCM	Traditional Chinese medicine

hyperactivity-impulsivity and can be comorbid with oppositional defiant, conduct, anxiety, mood, substance use, and learning disorders.[4–6] It impairs academic achievement, social functioning, relationships with family and peers, self-esteem, and quality of life.[7–10]

Traditional Chinese medicine (TCM) has been a comprehensive system of medical practice for more than 2000 years. There was no specialized term for ADHD as a diagnostic syndrome in ancient TCM literatures. However, ADHD and comorbid symptoms were described with many terms such as forgetfulness, dysphoria, injudicious, and so forth. ADHD-like symptom description and management methods can be found in many ancient Chinese medical documents. *Plain Questions* (*Huangdi Neijing, Suwen*), written 2500 years ago, states "Powerful Yang strengthens legs, thus climbing easily to the highest; Excess Yang leads to raving speech, chiding and cursing regardless of who is present." *Essays on the Pathogenesis and Manifestations of Various Diseases* (*Zhubingyuanhoulun*; 610 AD) states, "Children who were characterized by bowel and visceral sthenia, exuberance of blood and Qi, would be restless and fidgety." Sun Si-miao's *Thousand Golden Prescriptions* (*Qian Jin Fang*; 652 AD) states, "Silence, talkativeness for no reason, or disorderly excessive activities with short concentration of mind." *Achieving Longevity by Guarding the Source* (*Shoushibaoyuan*; 1616 AD) adopted the Cleverness Pill for school-aged absent-minded children who always started well but not ended well and talked but always forgot what they were talking about. A Western medicine practitioner first reviewed ADHD, known as *minimal brain dysfunction syndrome* at the time, in a Chinese journal in 1975.[11] Subsequently, the first Chinese workshop on ADHD in children, held by the China Association of Chinese Medicine in 1986, proposed ADHD diagnostic criteria and recommended Chinese herbal medicine (CHM) to treat ADHD. Since then, TCM theoretic and clinical systems for treating ADHD have been developed.

In TCM theories, ADHD is a condition affecting the mind, thought, and emotion. The main affected systems are the heart, liver, spleen, and kidney; the pathogenesis is caused by the imbalance of yin-yang and dysfunction of the Zang-fu (viscera) organs. *Plain Questions* (*Huangdi Neijing, Suwen*) states, "Only when Yin is at peace and Yang is compact, can essence-spirit be normal." Yin-yang theory holds that yin and yang are opposing and constraining, interdependent and mutually promoting each other. Yin and yang within our body are in dynamic balance, and diseases arise if the balance is damaged. Yin masters calmness, and yang masters movement; equilibrium between yin and yang produces coordination. The common physiologic functions of the 5 Zang (ie, 5 organs [heart, liver, spleen, lung, kidney]) are to produce and store essence, such as blood, qi, and body fluid. Vital essence in the 5 Zang is the physical basis of the human mind and spirit: (1) The heart is the master of the Zang-fu, which governs the blood, harbors the spirit, and controls mental and emotional activities. Sufficient heart-yin and heart-blood moisten and nourish the spirit and make it at peace. (2) The liver is an unyielding viscus, storing blood and governing tendons. The liver controls activities and stores the ethereal soul and corresponds to anger in emotion and shouting in sound. (3) The spleen stores intention, attention, and intelligence and corresponds to thinking in cognition. The nature of the spleen is quiet.

(4) The kidney stores mind and essence, dominates bone, produces marrow, and then passes it on to brain. Kidney deficiency may result in insufficiency of brain marrow and, thus, affects mental activities. Children have delicate organs, their physique and qi are not fully developed. The physiologic functions of the yin-yang and 5 Zang in children are marked by characteristics of 3 abundances and 4 insufficiencies: constant abundances of liver, heart, and yang and constant insufficiencies of the lung, spleen, kidney, and yin. When children have a congenital insufficiency, improper postnatal nursing, improper education, environmental impact, trauma, or emotional disturbance, there will be an imbalance of yin-yang (insufficient yin and excessive yang) combined with the pathogenesis of the 5 Zang organs.

TCM's diagnosis and treatment of ADHD are based on the holistic and unique syndrome differentiation in TCM theories.[12,13] TCM syndromes refer to the generalization of pathologic causes, organs, and the nature and the evolution of the symptoms and signs. Syndrome differentiation in TCM mainly relies on the comprehensive analysis of clinical information (symptoms, signs, pulse conditions, and tongue pictures) gathered by the 4 main diagnostic procedures: observation, auscultation and olfaction, questioning, and pulse analysis. Syndrome differentiation analysis is then used to establish therapies, such as the choice of herbs and formulae. Overall TCM symptoms are often divided into main and secondary symptoms according to their contribution to the diagnosis. The main symptoms reflect the basic attributes of the syndrome and determine the disease essence.[14]

The Chinese medical diagnosis and treatment of ADHD Project (Trial version)[15] divides ADHD into 5 main syndromes:

1. Heat in heart and liver
2. Internal disturbance of pyrophlegm
3. Deficiency of liver-yin and kidney-yin
4. Heartspleen deficiency
5. Liver depression and spleen deficiency

Clinical manifestations of each syndrome are further described by the main symptoms, secondary symptoms, and typical tongue and pulse presentations. The establishment of each syndrome must meet the following 3 criteria:

1. All or most of the main symptoms
2. Any secondary symptoms
3. Typical tongue and pulse presentations

The correlation between the 5 TCM syndromes and 3 *Diagnostic and Statistical Manual of Mental Disorders* (Fourth Edition) subtypes (predominantly inattentive, predominantly hyperactive/impulsive, or combined) of ADHD[16,17] are listed in **Table 1**. The differentiation of Zang-fu, deficiency-excess, and yin-yang are determined by trained TCM practitioners. However, it may be difficult for nonprofessionals. It is described in **Box 1**.

Need for the Treatment

In the last 2 decades, the authors have witnessed an increased use of the diagnosis of ADHD. The escalating and long-term use of psychostimulants in children has been controversial.[18] In addition, about 30% of children and adolescents with ADHD fail to respond to stimulants or cannot tolerate the adverse drug effects, such as the reduced appetite, insomnia, gastrointestinal pain, headache, and anxiety.[19–21] Many nonstimulants, such as atomoxetine, bupropion, guanfacine, and clonidine, also have side effects.[22–25] From the lifespan persistence point of view, ADHD is a chronic

Table 1
The correlation between TCM syndromes and subgroups of ADHD

TCM Syndrome	Clinical Manifestations	Therapeutic Principles	ADHD Subtypes
Heat in heart and liver	Main symptoms 1. Overactivity and talkativeness, impulsiveness and willfulness, interrupts others, quarrels and fights noisily; irritability and explosiveness, recklessness, talks back to authority, loses temper 2. Inattention Secondary symptoms 1. Reddish complexion, irritable feverish sensation in chest, sore in tongue and mouth 2. Ocular redness, headache and bitter taste in mouth, constipation, deep-colored urine Typical tongue and pulses: red tongue or tongue tip, thin yellow tongue coating, wiry and rapid pulse	Clearing the heart fire and soothing the liver, quieting spirit and stabilizing mind	Predominantly hyperactive-impulsive
Internal disturbance of pyrophlegm	Main symptoms 1. Extremely arrogant and restless, talkative and noisy, crying and screaming, howling and cursing angrily, talking nonsense, beating people and smashing objects 2. Inattention, reddish complexion and yellow sputum Secondary symptoms 1. Irritable feverish sensation in chest, vexation and dreaminess, fickle interest, woolly headed 2. Deep-colored urine, dry stool Typical tongue and pulses: red tongue, yellow greasy tongue coating, slippery and rapid pulse	Clearing heat-fire, resolving phlegm and quieting heart	Predominantly hyperactive-impulsive
Deficiency of liver-yin and kidney-yin	Main symptoms 1. Restlessness and unsettled, impatience and tantrums, impulsiveness and willfulness 2. Inattention, poor memory, poor academic achievement Secondary symptoms 1. Dysphoria in chest and palms-soles, night sweating, aching limbs and lack of strength 2. Lusterless nails and hair 3. Insomnia and dreaminess, sleep talking, or enuresis 4. Dry mouth and pharynx, likes cool drinks Typical tongue and pulses: red or dark red tongue, thin or little tongue coating, fine wiry pulse or fine rapid pulse	Nourishing the kidney and liver, calming the liver, and suppressing yang	Combined type

(continued on next page)

Table 1 (continued)			
TCM Syndrome	**Clinical Manifestations**	**Therapeutic Principles**	**ADHD Subtypes**
Heart-spleen deficiency	**Main symptoms** 1. Absentmindedness, inattention, fickle interests, dilatoriness 2. Hyperactivity with especially excessive little trick, no bad temper, reckless speech, impulsiveness 3. Fatigued spirit and lack of strength, lusterless facial complexion **Secondary symptoms** 1. Poor memory, slowness of thinking, poor sleep 2. Monophagia and reduced food intake, abdominal distention, loose stool 3. Spontaneous sweating, heart palpitations, shortness of breath 4. Emaciation or puffiness Typical tongue and pulses: pale tongue, little tongue coating, or thin white coating, fine weak pulse	Nourishing heart and soothing the nerves, invigorating spleen and supplementing qi	Inattentive type
Liver depression and spleen deficiency	**Main symptoms** 1. Absentmindedness, inattention, excessive little trick, impulsiveness and willfulness, irritability 2. Fatigued spirit and lack of strength, abdominal fullness and distention, reduced appetite and slow intake **Secondary symptoms** 1. Pessimism, depression, frequent sighing 2. Lusterless facial complexion, emaciation, cold extremities, irregular stools, constipation or sloppy stool Typical tongue and pulses: white greasy tongue coating, wiry slow pulse	Soothing liver and strengthening spleen, tonifying qi and resolving depression	Combined type

Data from Ma R, Han XM. Pediatrics of Chinese medicine. Beijing (China): People's Medical Publishing House; 2012. p. 123–4 [in Chinese]; and National Administration of Traditional Chinese Medicine. Chinese medical diagnosis and treatment project for 105 diseases in 24 majors. Beijing (China): National Administration of Traditional Chinese Medicine; 2012. p. 490–4 [in Chinese].

condition requiring long-term medication. Poor adherence and subsequent treatment failure are prevalent in childhood/adolescent ADHD because of the side effects or lack of effect.[26,27] As a safer approach with fewer side effects, complementary and alternative medicine, including TCM, has gained popularity.[28]

In TCM, the treatment goal for ADHD in children is full remission, which is defined as "A loss of diagnostic status, minimal or no symptoms, and optimal functioning when individuals are being treated with or without medication."[29,30] More specifically, a successful TCM treatment (1) eliminates ADHD core symptoms, improves comorbid conditions, and maximally improves children's behavior, emotion, social functioning, and quality of life; (2) strengthens the body's resistance, eliminates endogenous and

Box 1
Syndrome differentiation for ADHD

1. Zang-fu differentiation

   If the disease is located in the heart, the symptoms include inattention, emotional lability, dreaminess, and dysphoria. If the disease is located in the liver, the symptoms include impulsiveness, hyperkinesia, irritability, and lack of in self-control. If the disease is located in the spleen, the symptoms include inattentiveness and poor memory. If the disease is located in the kidney, the symptoms include poor academic achievement and memory, enuresis, soreness, and weakness of the waist and knees.

2. Deficiency-excess differentiation

   Excess syndromes are always found in the early stage of ADHD, dominated by heat in the heart and liver, internal disturbance of pyrophlegm, liver depression, and spleen deficiency. Deficiency syndromes are always found in the late stage of ADHD, dominated by a deficiency of liver-yin and kidney-yin and heart-spleen deficiency. ADHD has a complicated cause and a long course, which can result in a deficiency in origin, yet an excess in superficiality or a complex deficiency-excess syndrome representation.

3. Yin-yang differentiation

   If there is a yin deficiency, the symptoms include inattention, poor self-control, emotional lability, and absent-mindedness. If there is a yang excess, the symptoms include hyperactivity, hyperactivity and talkativeness, impulsiveness and willfulness, and irritability.

exogenous pathogenic factors, and eliminates the underlying cause of ADHD; (3) strengthens and consolidates the effects of conventional medication, then safely and gradually reduces the dose of conventional medication or discontinues them, and reduces the course of treatment and the recurrence rate; (4) reduces the side effects of conventional medication and TCM; and (5) markedly reduces health care costs and the use of limited medical resources.

INTERVENTIONS
Theoretic Overview: Does TCM Work?

Historically, TCM has been the mainstream medicine in East Asia, including China, Japan, and Korea. The theoretic framework of TCM, such as the theories of yin-yang and the 5 elements, derives from Chinese explanations of phenomena in the universe, which embodies rich dialectical thought and materialism. *Yellow Emperor's Inner Canon* (*Huangdi Neijing*) states, "The existence of human beings depends on the interaction between the celestial qi and terrestrial qi." "The human body is a small universe." Therefore, the main tenet of TCM theory is holism. TCM assumes that the human being is an organic whole of the body, energy, and the mind, which are interconnected by Zang-fu organs and meridians. TCM states that human diseases, including ADHD, are the results of disharmony within the body and between the body and environment. Therefore, TCM adopts a holistic approach to cure disease by reestablishing equilibrium in the human body, mind, and emotion as well as between the individual and the environment.

TCM treatment is tailored to each individual based on their syndrome differentiation and the disease progression. The general therapeutic principle of TCM for disease includes searching for and treating of the primary cause of the disease, strengthening the body's resistance to pathogenic factors, regulating yin-yang and the function of the Zang-fu organs, and regulating qi-blood. The treatment design for each individual also considers the variability of climate and geographic locality. TCM treatments are based on 3 basic principles: reinforcing deficiency and reducing excess, regulating the function of Zang-fu organs, and balancing yin-yang with individualized treatment adjustments aimed at each unique symptom (see **Table 1**). TCM values the importance of monitoring dynamic changes of syndromes during the course of treatment. Adjustments to treatments are tailored to respond to the individual's condition. These adjustments often assist in maintaining the effectiveness of the main treatments and balancing the Zang-Fu and yin-yang.

The focus of TCM treatment is on the individual patient rather than the disease. Although the pathophysiologic mechanism underlying ADHD is still not clear, it is well recognized that gene and environment interactions play a significant role in ADHD.[31–33] Such interactions are well recognized in the TCM theory of Unity of Man and Universe. TCM theories and treatments consider 5 interconnected dimensions, time-space-social-psychological-biological, which are more complex than the modern Western medical model of biological-psychological-social.[34] Western medicine is often based on laboratory findings and uses drugs targeting specific symptoms and biological mechanisms. TCM practice is patient-oriented with an emphasis on the overall improvement in all dimensions. It has been recognized in Asian cultures that chronic diseases with an unclear cause, multi-pathogenic factors, and complex pathophysiology have always been the preponderant illnesses for TCM therapy. ADHD was officially recognized as one of the preponderant illnesses in pediatric TCM in 2011 in China.[35,36]

Description: How Is the Treatment Delivered?

According to the above-mentioned principles, TCM clinicians prescribe individually designed therapies for each patient, composed mainly of CHM, with adjuvant acupuncture, tui na, tai chi chuan, and diet (**Fig 1**).[37] Based on the clinical and theoretic research of the past 3 decades, Chinese TCM society has established a set of basic treatment guidelines for the 5 subtypes of ADHD TCM diagnosis, with the recommendation of appropriate combination of CHM, acupuncture, tui na, and diet therapy (**Table 2**).[37] However, these guidelines are always subjected to appropriate adjustments for each individual and can be adjusted during the course of treatment. In the following section, the authors describe each of the treatment methods and provide the empirical evidence that supports their use for treating ADHD.

Chinese herbal medicine

There are many effective CHM formulae (prescriptions with several types of herbs, animal drugs, or minerals) used by TCM physicians to treat different syndromes of ADHD. Generally, the compatibility of Chinese medicine is the basis of CHM formulae, which includes the theory of seven features of compatibility[38] and the monarch-minister-assistant-guide (Jun-Chen-Zuo-Shi). Under the compatibility guideline, medical herbs are prescribed as a well-balanced formula that aims to bring yin-yang and Zang-fu into equilibrium based on the different effects of the herbs. Traditional medicine evaluates the function of the medicinal herbs according to their known 4 properties (cold, hot, warm, and cool), 5 tastes (sweet, sour, bitter, pungent, and salty), channel tropism, and lifting, lowering, floating, and sinking properties. There are often multiple ingredients in each herb; the aims of compatibility are to remove the undesired effects of certain ingredients, to enhance the effectiveness of the main ingredient, and to reduce toxicity. CHM promotes multi-targeted effects and produces synergistic results that can be achieved with low doses.

Adherent to this same principle, different physicians often design and prescribe different variations of formulae for treating ADHD. For example, Duodongning granule

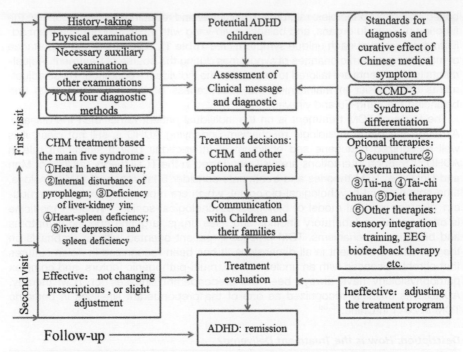

Fig. 1. Clinical pathway of TCM treating ADHD. EEG, electroencephalogram; CCMD-3, Chinese Classification of Mental Disorders Version 3. (*Adapted from* National Administration of Traditional Chinese Medicine. Chinese medical diagnosis and treatment project for 105 diseases in 24 majors. Beijing (China): National Administration of Traditional Chinese Medicine; 2012. p. 490–4 [in Chinese]; with permission.)

used for ADHD consists of Gouqizi (Fructus lycii), Shudihuang (*Rehmanniae radix preparata*), Wuweizi (*Schisandra chinensis*), Renshen (*Ginseng radix et rhizome*), Fuling (*Poriacocos*), and Gancao (*Glycyrrhizae radix et rhizoma*). It invigorates the heart and kidney, calms the nerves, and reinforces intelligence. In a randomized and double-blind clinical trial,[39] children with ADHD (N = 37) treated with Duodongning granule achieved the similar total effective rate (89.2%) as the methylphenidate (MPH) (10 mg/d)-treated group (N = 33, 87.9%) after 4 weeks of treatment. The Duodongning granule group was not different from the MPH group in the improvements of Conners hyperactivity index, social functioning, and academic achievements. Fewer cases developed side effects, such as loss of appetite or insomnia (3 in the Duodongning group and 8 in MPH group). The Yizhi mixture is composed of 10 herbs, including Lujiaoshuang (*Cervi cornu degelatinatum*), Guiban (*Testudinis carapacis et plastri*), Shudihuang (*Rehmanniae radix preparata*), and Gouteng (*Uncariaeramulus cum uncis*), synergistically supplementing the liver-kidney yin to tranquilize the liver yang. In a randomized trial of 12 weeks treatment,[40] combined treatment with the Yizhi mixture and MPH group was significantly more effective than the Yizhi mixture or MPH (10–30 mg/d) treatment alone (N = 70 each); both the Yizhi-mixture-alone group and the combined group had significantly fewer side effects than the MPH-treatment-alone group.

Jingling oral liquid was used in combination with MPH in treating ADHD children with transient tic disorder (N = 50) and was significantly more effective in improving ADHD and tic symptoms than MPH (10–40 mg/d) alone (N = 44) in a randomized trial.[41] Jingling oral liquid is composed of 12 herbs also including some commonly used in other formulae, such as Shudihuang (*Rehmanniae radix preparata*), Shanyao (*Rhizome Dioscoreae*), Yuanzhi (*Polygalae radix*), Longgu (*Os Draconis*), and Shichangpu (*Rhizoma Acori Tatarinowii*). The overall design of the Jingling oral liquid is to synergistically nourish yin for suppressing hyperactive Yang, to calm spirit and to promote intelligence. Another formula Ningdong granule, comprising 8 herbs, such as Tianma (*Gastrodiae rhizoma*), Dangshen (*Codonopsis radix*), Maidong (*Ophiopogonis radix*), and Baishao (*Paeoniae alba radix*), synergistically nourishes the heart and liver, calms endogenous wind and relieves convulsion. Eight weeks of treatment in a randomized and double-blind trial showed that Ningdong granule is more effective and safer than MPH (1 mg/kg/d) treatment (N = 36 each) and could increase serum homovanillic concentration, suggesting that Ningdong granule treatment could regulate dopamine metabolism.[42] Several other studies[43–47] showed that CHM treatment increases the serum concentration of calcium and zinc in children with ADHD, with inconsistent findings in reducing the higher levels of serum lead in some children with ADHD.

In the authors' recent meta-analysis, they summarized that there were 39 different CHM formulae containing a total of 94 herbs used for treating ADHD in the studies that they included in the meta-analysis. Despite many variations of the CHM formulae used, TCM clinicians follow the principle of compatibility and theories of syndrome differentiation. In **Table 1**, the authors list examples of CHMs and their recommended uses for ADHD subtypes. The overall efficacy of the various CHM formulae in the treatment of ADHD is further reviewed in the empirical support section.

Acupuncture

Acupuncture procedure is performed by inserting sterilized fine needles at specific surface acupoints on the body, followed by applying lifting-thrusting and twisting-rotating manipulations to induce the psychophysical responses known as *De-qi*, a sensory experience related to clinical efficacy. De-qi can be perceived as tingling, numbness, heaviness, and other sensations that occur after an acupuncture needle has properly been placed in the acupoints. The needles are retained for a period of time and then removed. The acupoints are linked through 14 meridians throughout the human body, which connect to the Zang-fu. Acupuncture treats ADHD by dredging the meridian, regulating yin-yang and Zang-fu with reinforcing and reducing methods, which refers to puncture along and against the direction of the meridians, respectively. Acupuncture can be performed on the body, scalp, or ear acupoints.

Acupuncture is often applied in combination with CHM for treating ADHD. Similar to the herbal components, the choice of the main and adjunct acupoints is based on syndrome differentiation. In an article by Chai,[48] 155 children with ADHD received acupuncture with Four-Shen point, Brain-Three–needles, and Jin-Three–needles in comparison with 58 children treated with MPH (5 mg/d). Head acupoints were horizontally inserted 1 cun in depth with 1.5-cun sterilized needles; limb acupoints were perpendicularly inserted in regular depth recommended by the recognized textbook *Acupuncture*.[49] Cun, or Chinese inch, equal to 3.33 cm, is often measured by the width of the individual's thumb at the knuckle, a traditional charting method for acupuncture. Needles were retained for 30 minutes after De-qi and twirled once every 10 minutes with an even reinforcing-reducing method. Acupuncture was performed 5 days a week for 2 weeks for 6 courses of treatment. After 6 courses, the acupuncture group and MPH group had similar rates of efficacy response (82.5% and 87.93%, respectively; P>.05). However, the long-term efficacy rates for the acupuncture group

Table 2
TCM recommended therapies and their clinical evidence grading

	Heat in Heart and Liver	Internal Disturbance of Pyrophlegm	Deficiency of Liver-Yin and Kidney-Yin	Heart-Spleen Deficiency	Liver Depression and Spleen Deficiency
Recommended TCM formula	Modified Anshen Dingzhi decoction[88,89] (II)	Modified Huanglian Wendan decoction[90] (II)	Modified Qiju Dihuang wan[91] (II)	Modified Guipi decoction combined with Ganmai Dazao decoction[15] (IV)	Modified Xiaoyao powder[15] (IV)
Alternative TCM formula	1. Modified Lingjiao Gouteng decoction[92] (II) 2. Modified Daochi San combined with Longdan Xiegan decoction[93] (II)	Ditan decoction[94] (IV)	Modified Zuogui yin[94] (IV) yin	Modified Liushen powder combined with Guizhi Gancao Longgu Muli decoction[94] (IV)	Modified Sini decoction[94] (IV)
Alternative Chinese patent medicine	1. Xiegan Anshen Pill[94] (IV) 2. Zhusha Anshen Pill[95] (IV)	1. Mengshi Guntan pill[94] (IV) 2. Zhuli Datan pill[94] (IV)	1. Jingling oral liquid[96,97] (II)[98-101] 2. Xiaoer Zhili syrup[46,47,102-104] (II)	1. Guipi mixture[94] (IV) 2. Bozi Yangxin pill[94] (IV)	1. Xiaoyao pill[94] (IV) 2. Chihu Shugan pill[94] (IV)
Recommended acupoints in body acupuncture[94] (IV)	Shenmen (HT 7), Taichong (LR 3), Fengchi (GB 20), Xinshu (BL 15), Ganshu (BL 18), Shenshu (BL 23), Sishencong (EX-HN 1)	Dazhui (GV 14), Neiguan (PC 6), Fenglong (ST 40)	Neiguan (PC 6), Taichong (LR 3), Dazhui (GV 14), Quchi (LI 11)	Fengfu (GV 16), Fengchi (GB 20), Shangxing (GV 23), Jianshi (PC 5), Zusanli (ST 36), Taichong (LR 3), Qihai (CV 6), Geshu (BL 17)	Shenmen (HT 7), Shenting (GV 24), Baihui (DU 20), Houxi (SI 3), Zusanli (ST 36), Pishu (BL 20), Ganshu (BL 18), Taichong (LR 3)

Recommended tui-namanipulation[94] (IV)	Clear Ganjing, clear Xinjing, knead Xiaotianxin, clear Tianheshui	Clear Ganjing, clear Xinjing, clear Tianheshui, push Pijing	Reinforce Shenjing, clear Ganjing, clear Xinjing, separate-push yin-yang, knead Xiaotianxin, knead Yong-quan (KI 1)	Tonify Pijing, separate-push yin-yang, push-knead Pi-shu (BL 20) and Wei-shu (BL 21), push and knead Zusanli (ST 36), pinch spine	Tonify Pijing, clear Ganjing, transport Neibagua, pinch spine
Recommended diet therapies[94] (IV)	1. Suanzaoren (Semen Ziziphi Spinosae) dearing heart gruel 2. White chrysanthemum and Juemingzi (Cassiae semen) tea	1. Chuanbeimu (Fritillariae Cirrhosae Bulbus) gruel 2. Zhuru (Caulis bambusae in taenia) and Chixiaodou (Vignae semen) gruel	Mulberry and Baihe (Bulbus Lilii) honey cream	1. Renshen (Ginseng radix et rhizome) egg soup 2. Lianzi (Nelumbinis semen) soup	1. Foshou (Fructus citri sarcodactylis) and Yujin (Curcumae Radix) gruel 2. Taizishen (Radix Pseudostellariae) and Qingpi (Pericarpium Citri Reticulatae Viride) stewed crucian

Abbreviations: BL, Bladder Meridian of Foot-Taiyang; CV, Conception Vessel; DU, Du Meridian; EX-HN, Extra Point in Head and Neck; GB, Gallbaldder Meridian of Foot-Shaoyang; GV, Governor Vessel; HT, Heart Meridian of Hand-Shaoyin; KI, Kidney Meridian of Foot-Shaoyin; LI, Large Intestine Meridian of Hand-Yangming; LR, Liver Meridian of Foot-Jueyin; PC, Pericardium Meridian of Hand-Jueyin; SI, Small Intestine Meridian of Hand-Taiyang; ST, Stomach Meridian of Foot-Yangming.

Data from Ma R, Han XM. Pediatrics of Chinese medicine [M]. Beijing (China): People's Medical Publishing House; 2012. p. 123–4 [in Chinese]; and Leng FN, Ling YX, Peng GC, et al. Clinical therapeutics of children with attention deficit hyperactivity disorder [M]. Beijing (China): People's Military Medical Publisher; 2010 [in Chinese].

(82.58%) 1 month after stopping the treatment were significantly higher than for the MPH-treated group (32.76%, *P*<.01). These results suggest that acupuncture therapy has long-term effects for ADHD. In addition, the efficacy of acupuncture was highly correlated with the treatment duration and the age of patients. A younger age and a longer treatment course produce better treatment outcomes.[48] When acupuncture was used in combination with Jingling oral liquid in a randomized, double-blind trial,[50] the combined TCM treatment group had a similar total response rate as MPH (15 mg/d) treatment alone (91.4% vs 90.0%, *P*>.05; N = 50 each). However, the TCM group had no side effects; the MPH group had nausea and loss of appetite (N = 10), dizziness (N = 2), and insomnia (N = 1). In this study, acupuncture used the following acupoints: Nei-guan (Pericardium Meridian of Hand-Jueyin [PC 6]), Tai-chong (Large Intestine Meridian of Hand-Yangming [LI 3]), Tai-xi (Kidney Meridian of Foot-shaoyin [KI 3]), Qu-chi (Large Intestine Meridian of Hand-Yangming [LI 11]) as main points; Bai-hui (Governor Vessel [GV 20]), Shen-men (Heart Meridian of Hand-shaoyin [HT 7]), and Si-shen-cong (EX-HN 1), which are 4 points around Bai-hui (GV 20) for inattention; Lie-que (Lung Meridian of Hand-Taiyin [LU 7]), Xin-shu (Bladder Meridian of Foot-Taiyang [BL15]), and Ding-shen (an extra point at the junction of the lower one-third and upper two-thirds of the philtrum) for restlessness; Shen-ting (GV 24), Zhao-hai (KI 6), and Dan-zhong (Conception Vessel [CV 17]) for emotional irritability and instability; Xin-shu (BL 15), Zu-san-li (Stomach Meridian of Foot-Yangming, [ST 36]), and San-Yin-jiao (Spleen Meridian of Foot-Taiyin [SP 6]) for yin deficiency of the heart-spleen. Altogether, the acupoints synergistically dredge channels, nourish yin for suppressing hyperactive yang, regulate the liver-kidney-heart-spleen, boost brain function, calm the spirit, enlighten, and reinforce intelligence. Needles were retained for 30 minutes after De-qi, with 4 acupoints alternately used in each session. Treatment sessions were performed once every other day, with 7 sessions in one course. A total of 3 courses were performed in the study.

Tui na (Chinese medical massage)

Tui na for children is a nondrug and noninvasive naturopathy in which special manipulations (pressing, rubbing, nipping, kneading, pushing, transporting, foulage, and rotating) are gently and dexterously applied to the special meridians and acupoints on the skin surface of children. Tui na dredges meridians, promotes the flow of qi and circulates blood, strengthens the body resistance to pathogenic factors, and harmonizes yin-yang. Children are sensitive to the stimulation of tui na manipulation because their skin and muscle are so thin that the meridians and points are relatively shallow. In children, tui na manipulation requires moderate, gentle, stable, and penetrative techniques because of their special physiologic character, including tender Zang-fu, vulnerable striae and interstitial space, timid spirit-qi, and weak skin and bones. Professionally performed tui na should be noninvasive, painless, and easily accepted by children.

Tui na is often used as an ADHD treatment in conjunction with other therapies, such as CHM and/or acupuncture. The recommended tui na manipulation for ADHD is listed in **Table 3**. There are a few clinical trials that have evaluated the clinical efficacy of tui na therapy for ADHD. Wang and Shi[51] applied tui na to 33 Swiss children with ADHD using routine manipulation on the head, chest, abdomen, and back. After an average of 18 treatments, 10 cases were no longer meeting the diagnosis of ADHD (cured), 18 cases showed remarkable improvement, and 5 had no effect. In a randomized trial comparing tui na with MPH treatment (N = 20 each), Zhuo[52] found that after 1 month of treatment (**Box 2**), tui na and MPH (5 mg, twice a day) had a similar total response rate (85% vs 90%, P>.05); However, after 6 months posttreatment, the tui na group showed a significantly lower recurrence rate than the MPH-treated group (20% vs 55%, P<.05). These results suggest that tui na may be a safe and effective therapy for ADHD with long-term effects.

Tai chi chuan

Tai chi chuan (commonly known as tai chi, Taiji, and so forth) is a 300-year-old Chinese martial art form that is gaining popularity in Western culture. The basic principle of tai chi chuan is yin-yang balance and deficiency-excess change, which share the same principles as TCM theories. Only when one follows the ideas of yin-yang and deficiency-excess in TCM can one attain the acme of perfection in tai chi chuan.[53] Tai chi chuan features slow movements of both dynamic and static forms. By exercising breathing and body movements, tai chi chuan activates and harmonizes qi-blood. Every form and motion of tai chi chuan is guided by thought (Yi-nian) and combined with slowly regulated breathing to synchronize both the inner and outer universe and to improve mental concentration. An integration of diaphragmatic breathing (deep, full, and shallow) and body movements (slow, gentle, graceful) can quell inner restlessness, quiet the mind, and slowly transfer the underlying distracting thoughts into the tai chi chuan postures that concentrate attention. Long-term practicing of tai chi chuan improves attention, reduces hot temper, anxiety, and irritability and thereby alleviates ADHD symptoms.[54,55]

There have been few clinical trials using tai chi chuan for the treatment of ADHD. Wen[56] randomized ADHD children into a tai chi chuan group (16 cases) and a control group (14 cases). In a 12-week training program, tai chi chuan was practiced 3 times per week for 45 minutes. The forms practiced were modified from the Chen-tai-chi old style. The tai chi chuan group was superior to the control group in reducing hyperactivity and aggressiveness and improving vestibular function, proprioception, and learning abilities. Hernandez-Reif and colleagues[57] observed 13 adolescents with ADHD practicing tai chi chuan twice a week for 5 weeks. The adolescents displayed improvement in anxiety, daydreaming, inappropriate emotions, hyperactivity, and conduct disorder, which persisted at the 2-week posttreatment follow-up.

TCM diet therapy (Yaoshan)

TCM diet therapy is typically part of a treatment program for ADHD. In TCM theories, food has 4 properties (cold, hot, cool, and warm), 5 flavors (sweet, sour, bitter, pungent, and salty), tendency of drug effect (ascending and descending, floating and sinking), and channel tropism. TCM diet therapy follows the principles of TCM treatment, such as reinforcing deficiency and reducing excess, treating cold with hot drugs, and treating heat with cold drugs, then establishing the 8 treatment methods including diaphoresis, harmonizing, purgation, dispersion, emesis, clearing, warming, and toning. Foods alone or combined with Chinese medicine are used to mutually promote their respective advantages via cooking methods, such as stewing, braising, steaming, boiling, and frying. For example, Suanzaoren (Semen Ziziphi Spinosae) clearing heart gruel is recommended for heat in heart and liver syndrome of ADHD. To prepare it, 30 g of smashed Suanzaoren (Semen Ziziphi Spinosae), 6 g of Dengxincao (Junci Medulla), and 3 g of Danzhuye (Lophatheri Herba) are boiled down to concentrate the juice. After removing the drug sediment, 100 g of rice is added to the juice concentrate and cooked into gruel. The gruel is administered in the mornings and evenings with no defined treatment course. There are many empirical studies on TCM diet therapy for ADHD; all of them are considered to benefit patients with ADHD,[50] but no clinical trials have been conducted to confirm the efficacy of TCM diet therapy.

Table 3
Recommended tui na manipulation and their action

Tui Na Manipulation	Location of Acupoints	Manipulation Procedure	Action
Tonifying Pijing	The thumb ball or the line from the tip to root on the radial border of thumb	Bend child's thumb; push along the radial border of thumb to finger root for 300 times, respectively	Invigorate spleen and stomach, tonify qi and blood
Clearing Ganjing	The index fingertip	Push from the distal interphalangeal joint crease of the index finger to the fingertip for 300 times	Clear the liver, drain fire, extinguish wind, sedate fright, relieve depression and dysphoria
Clearing Xinjing	The fingertip of the middle finger	Push straight from the distal interphalangeal joint crease to fingertip for 300 times	Clear heart and purge fire
Reinforcing Shenjing	The fingertip of the little finger	Push fingertip of little finger in circles for 300 times	Nourish kidney, tonify brain, warm and strengthen kidney qi
Kneading Xiaotianxin	In the depression of the junction between greater and hypothenar eminences	Knead the point with middle finger tip for 300 times	Clear heat, sedate convulsion, diuresis, and improve vision
Transporting Neibagua	Taking palm center as the center, draw a circle with the radius from the center to the point at inner two-thirds of distance between palm center and transverse crease of middle finger toot; Neibagua indicates area within the circle	Apply transporting manipulation on the area with thumb belly for 300 times	Enlarge chest and benefit diaphragm, regulate qi and resolve phlegm, remove food retention and promote digestion

Clearing the Heavenly River	Midline of the forearm from wrist to elbow	Push from transverse crease of wrist to transverse crease of elbow with the pads of the index and middle fingers for 300 times	Clear heat, relieve the exterior, purge heart fire, resolve restlessness and moisten dryness
Pinching Spine	The straight line between Dazhui (DU14) and Changqiang (DU 1)	Pinching along the spine from the lower side to the upper side is called pinching along the spine; lifting the skin on the spine once after every 3 times of pinching is called the method of one lifting after 3 pinching	Harmonize yin-yang, regulate qi and blood, normalize Zang-fu organs, dredge channels and collaterals, strengthen original qi
Kneading Yong-quan	On the sole, in the depression when foot is in plantar flexion	Knead the point with thumb tip for 100 times	Guide fire to origin, fade deficiency fire, treat vomiting and diarrhea
Kneading Pi-shu (BL 20) and Wei-shu (BL 21)	BL 20: 1.5 cun lateral to lower border of spinous process of the 11th thoracic vertebra; BL 21: 1.5 cun lateral to lower border of spinous process of the 12th thoracic vertebra	Knead the points with thumb tip for 200 times	Strengthen the function of spleen and nourish qi, reconcile the function of stomach and descend adverse qi
Pressing-kneading Zusanli (ST 36)	3 cun below Dubi (ST 35), one fingerbreadth from the anterior border of tibia	Press-knead the point with thumb tip for 200 times	Invigorate spleen and supplement qi
Separating-pushing Dahengwen also known as separating yin and yang	On the palmar transverse crease of the wrist, the radial end close to the thumb is known as Yangchi (SJ 4), and the ulnar end close to the little finger is called Yinchi	Push from the midpoint of the palmar transverse crease of wrist is toward the sides of wrist with the 2 thumbs, respectively	Balance yin-yang and harmonize qi-blood, resolve food retention, promote digestion, resolve phlegm, and eliminate masses

Abbreviations: BL, Bladder Meridian of Foot-Taiyang; DU, Du Meridian; SJ, Sanjiao Meridian of Hand-shaoyang; ST, Stomach Meridian of Foot-Yangming.

Adapted from Leng FN, Ling YX, Peng GC, et al. Clinical therapeutics of children with attention deficit hyperactivity disorder [M]. Beijing (China): People's Military Medical Publisher; 2010 [in Chinese]; with permission.

Box 2
Tui na therapy

Children began treatment in a supine position; Bai-hui (GV 20) and Si-shen-cong (EX-HN 1) were pressed and kneaded by the forefinger and middle finger for 1 minute, pushing yin-tang (EX-HN3, midpoint between the medial ends of the supraciliary arches) to shen-ting (GV 24) and were conducted with single-finger meditation pushing therapy 3 times. Bilateral Tai-yang (EX-HN 5) were pressed and kneaded with the fingertip of middle finger for 1 to 2 minutes; wiping manipulation with both thumbs was applied from Cuan-zhu (BL 2) to Tai-yang (EX-HN 5) through the superciliary arch 5 to 7 times. Qi-hai (CV 6) and Guan-yuan (CV 4) were pressed and kneaded with the fingertip of the middle finger for 1 to 2 minutes each and followed by rubbing the abdomen for 1 to 2 minutes. Children were then treated in a prone position and treated with chiropractic for 5 to 7 times back and forth, grasping the neck and Jian-jing (GB 21) for 1 to 2 minutes. Ear point application therapy was be applied according to TCM syndrome classification.

Summary and Conclusions: Empirical Support for the TCM Treatment of ADHD

TCM for the treatment of ADHD has not been acknowledged and accepted by most Westerners for 2 main reasons: (1) TCM theories are complex and difficult to understand. (2) There is a lack of data addressing the efficacy and safety of TCM treatments. TCM has evolved as a traditional medicine by constantly summarizing clinical medical data from TCM practitioners since ancient times. These data have been validated repeatedly on large human samples in clinical settings. These centuries of clinical practice have been an important part of developing the TCM academic system. Modern TCM researchers have conducted a series of clinical studies of ADHD using the research methodology of Western medicine, such as multicenter, large-sample, and randomized case-controlled studies. These studies have provided some evidences to support the efficacy of TCM for ADHD. It is, however, difficult to study the advantages of individualized treatments that are based on syndrome differentiation and the holism concepts of TCM. As a result, most TCM studies are still individual case reports or consensus reports, which Western scientists would view as a low level of supporting evidence.

TCM's approach to evaluate efficacy and safety differs from the standards of Western medicine.[59-61] The grading criteria proposed by the Oxford Center for Evidence-Based Medicine[62] emphasizes the importance of external research evidence, randomized trials, and systematic reviews (including meta-analyses); but expert experience is not taken into consideration. TCM researchers consider that unique cultural characteristics and consensus historical experiences should be of importance when grading the clinical evidence as well as the consensus professional opinions shared by contemporary experts in the field. The recommended TCM evidence classification system focuses on treatment effectiveness (**Table 4**).[63] Using this system, the authors ranked CHM, acupuncture, tui na, and diet therapy accordingly in **Table 2**.

Nevertheless, the authors highly value and recommend large TCM clinical trials of ADHD with rigorous design and appropriate methodology. This point may be a breakthrough point for international acceptance. Indeed, very few TCM clinical trials have been accepted and published in the international journals. "The Guideline for Prevention and Treatment of ADHD (2007)" issued by the Chinese Medical Association states that there was a scarcity of large-sample, double-blind, randomized controlled trials to support the efficacy of TCM formulae in the treatment of ADHD.[64] A meta-analyses and a systematic review on TCM used in treating ADHD also support the aforementioned findings.[65,66] One Cochrane review found that there was no evidence of

Table 4	
TCM criteria for grading evidence	
Level of Evidence	Criteria
I	Large-sample randomized studies with clear results, low risk of false-positive error or false-negative error
II	Small-sample randomized studies with uncertain results, moderate to high risk of false-positive error and/or false-negative error
III	Nonrandomized, concurrent controlled studies, and TCM expert consensus based on the ancient and modern literature[a]
IV	Nonrandomized, historical controlled trials, and the modern TCM experts' consensus[b]
V	Case reports, noncontrolled studies, and expert opinions[c]

[a] Refers to those that were recorded in the ancient medical writings, are still used today, and have reached consensus based on a scientific opinion survey of modern experts.
[b] Refers to those that were defined through questionnaire survey of modern experts.
[c] Refers to some individual expert opinions.
Adapted from Wang SC, Chen ZG, Xu S, et al. Study on evidence grading system in evidence-based clinical practice guidelines of traditional Chinese medicine. World Sci Technol Mod Tradit Chin Med 2013;15(7):1488–92 [in Chinese]; with permission.

randomized or quasi-randomized controlled trials to support acupuncture as an effective treatment of ADHD in children and adolescents.[67]

The authors' group performed a more recent and thorough meta-analysis and systematic review (Xinqiang Ni, MD, PhD, unpublished data, 2014) using the inclusion and exclusion criteria based on a combination of TCM characteristics and international standards that included 48 randomized controlled trials and 6 clinical controlled trials (CHM formula or CHM combined with MPH vs MPH alone) ranging from 1999 to 2013. In these studies, 39 different CHM formulae containing a total of 94 herbs were used, with each formula consisting of 5 to 17 different herbs. Fifteen herbs that were used most often (frequency ≥ 8) are listed in **Table 5**. Shichangpu (*Rhizoma acori tatarinowii*) and Yuanzhi (*Polygala tenuifolia*) are the 2 most frequently used herbs and have long been used to treat psychotic illnesses for hundreds of years in TCM. The extracts from both herbs can easily pass through the blood-brain barrier, improve memory, and reduce the hyperactivity.[68–70] The authors' meta-analysis results showed that CHM therapies were similarly effective as the MPH treatment in reducing ADHD symptoms; however, the combined CHM and MPH therapy was superior to MPH alone with fewer side effects (unpublished).

The authors' meta-analysis also revealed many methodological issues and heterogeneity of the TCM trials. For example, many studies used various criteria for diagnosis and outcome measures. TCM individualized therapy (various doses and herbal components according to different syndrome differentiation and symptom evolution) poses a major challenge to Western scientists who wish to evaluate TCM in a controlled manner.

CLINICAL DECISION MAKING
Who Is Most Likely to Respond? (eg, Patient Characteristics, Family Variables, and So Forth)

TCM clinical efficacy depends on correct syndrome differentiation, appropriate treatment principles and therapies, and acceptance and compliance of children

Table 5
Most frequently used Chinese herbs for ADHD and their hypothesized function

Chinese Herbs	Frequency (n ≥8)	Dosage (g)	Meridian Distribution	Effect
Shichangpu (Rhizoma Acori Tatarinowii)	25	3–10	Heart, stomach	Induce resuscitation and restore consciousness, tranquilize the mind and promote intelligence, remove dampness to regulate stomach
Yuanzhi (Polygalae radix)	20	3–10	Heart, kidney, lung	Calm the mind and reinforce intelligence, induce resuscitation by dispelling phlegm, eliminate carbuncle
Fuling (Poriacocos)	18	10–15	Heart, spleen, kidney	Remove dampness and promote diuresis, invigorate the spleen and tranquilize the mind
Shudihuang (Rehmanniae radix preparata)	18	9–15	Liver, kidney	Nourish yin and blood, replenish vital essence, and benefit marrow
Guiban (Testudinis carapacis et plastri)	17	9–24	Liver, kidney, heart	Nourish yin and suppress yang, tonify the kidney, strengthen the bones, nourish blood, and tonify the heart
Gancao (Glycyrrhizae radix et rhizome)	15	2–10	Heart, lung, spleen, stomach	Invigorate the spleen, replenish qi, expel phlegm to arrest cough, relieve spasm and pain, clear heat and detoxicate, and coordinate the drug actions of a prescription
Longgu (Os Draconis)	14	15	Heart, liver, kidney	Overcome the fears and tranquilize the mind, calm the liver and check exuberance of yang, induce astringency

Shanzhuyu (Cornifructus)	12	Liver, kidney	Invigorate the kidney and liver, relieve and restore depletion
Wuweizi (Schisandraefructuschinensis)	12	Lung, heart, kidney	Constrain perspiration, nourish qi and generate body fluid, tonify kidney, and calm the heart
Baishao (Paeoniae Radix Alba)	10	Liver, spleen	Nourish blood and retain yin, smooth the liver to stop pain, subdue the hyperactivity liver-yang
Shanyao (Dioscoreae Rhizoma)	10	Spleen, lung, kidney	Tonify spleen, lung, and kidney; promote the production of body fluid; tonify kidney to secure genital essence
Gouteng (Uncariae Ramulus cum Uncis)	9	Liver, pericardium	Calm the liver by clearing away the heat, relieve spasm by calming endogenous wind
Muli (Concha ostreae)	9	Liver, gallbladder, kidney	Tranquilize, calm the liver yang and check exuberance of yang, soften and resolve the hard lumps, induce astringency
Yizhiren (Alpiniaeoxyphyllae Fructus)	9	Spleen, kidney	Tonify kidney to control nocturnal emission and decrease urination, warm spleen to promote appetite and control saliva
Zhenzhumu (Concha margaritiferausta)	8	Liver, heart	Calm the mind and tranquilize, improve acuity of vision and remove nebula, detoxicate and promote tissue regeneration

Adapted from Gao XM. Chinese medicine [M]. Beijing (China): Chinese Press of Traditional Chinese Medicine; 2007 [in Chinese]; with permission.

and their families. TCM features holism, and treatment is based on the individual's syndrome differentiation. Patients will usually respond to the therapies prescribed by experienced traditional medicine physicians. TCM theory originates from the ancient Chinese culture and philosophy that have been deeply ingrained and rooted within the entire Chinese population. Cultural acceptance leads to belief and good compliance, resulting in the expected treatment effect.[71] Recently, TCM theory and practice have been being increasingly adopted and explored by the Western community. However, acceptance and compliance are still far less than in Asian countries.

The efficacy of TCM practice for Western patients with ADHD should also take into account the following factors: recognition and evaluation of the impact of the cultural differences in the symptoms/syndrome differentiation of ADHD, genetic polymorphisms, influence of geographic environment, diet, lifestyle, and other factors. The main types of syndrome differentiation, response to TCM therapies, and treatment courses may be different than those of East Asians. Two preliminary studies have suggested that TCM syndrome differentiation can also be conducted in patients of other races, but the main types of TCM syndrome differentiation are not always consistent with those used for Chinese patients.[72,73] Additional studies are still needed to evaluate the syndrome differentiations of ADHD in none-Asian populations. In addition, the response and tolerability of TCM treatment methods (CHM, acupuncture, tui na, cupping, and moxibustion) may be different among different races.[74,75] For example, as for the response sensitivity to the same CHM dose, the Black race has the most sensitivity, followed by Caucasians; Asians are the least sensitive. The tolerance to the therapies ranging from weak to strong also follows the order of Black, Caucasian, and Asian as well as the length of the sustained effective period of CHM treatment from long to short.

What Outcomes Are Most Likely to be Affected by Treatment? (eg, ADHD Symptoms, Academic Impairment, Parental Stress, and So Forth)

TCM treatment of ADHD focuses on the restoration of the functional balance of the body in a holistic manner and attempts to bring the body, mind, and spirit into harmony. It has been recognized that TCM treatment can improve the core symptoms of ADHD as well as the overall quality of life, such as appetite, sleep quality, memory, and academic performance. By doing so, it also relieves parental and family stress, reduces classroom disturbances, improves children's self-esteem, and restores personal relationships.

What Are the Contraindications for Treatment?

Contraindications for the TCM treatment of ADHD are a complicated issue. TCM, if used inappropriately, can cause harmful effects to human beings. The TCM practitioner must assess patients' comprehensive conditions to determine the appropriate therapies. TCM therapy for ADHD should consider contraindications related to the disease diagnostic, syndrome differentiation, constitution, food taboo, acupuncture, herbal incompatibility (eg, 18 incompatible medicaments and 19 medicaments of mutual antagonisms), as well as patients' daily life. Children's Zang-fu is tender and delicate. In CHM formula treatment of ADHD, yin should be nourished without the impairment of the spleen. The pathogenic fire should be removed without causing excessive bitterness-coldness. Pathogens should be eliminated without impairment of the body resistance. Tonic herbs should be used without causing an obstruction in the middle burner (portion of the body housing the stomach and spleen). The full extent of contraindications for CHM can be found elsewhere.[76]

Acupuncture and tui na are considered relatively safe if appropriately used by well-trained practitioners. However, they are not free of risk; various guidelines govern the employment of specific acupoints, safe depth, the directions of needling, and many other details. Commonly recognized contraindications and precautions for acupuncture and tui na are outlined in **Table 6**.

Contraindications for TCM diet therapy for ADHD consider the food taboo, drug-food interaction, seasonal influences of food intake, the changing course of disease, pregnancy, and parturition. Some foods and drugs, when paired together inappropriately, may reduce the original efficacy of each component and even produce side effects, such as Renshen (*Ginseng radix et rhizome*) and radish or tea, carp and Houpo (*Cortex Magnoliae officinalis*), Haizao (*Sagrassum*), and Gancao (*Glycyrrhizae radix et rhizome*). Certain foods, when ingested together, may also produce an undesired effect, for example, soft-shell turtle and 3-colored amaranth, honey and raw onions, egg and soybean milk, and so forth.

Table 6
Contraindications and precautions for use of acupuncture and tui na in ADHD

Therapies	Contraindications
Acupuncture[49]	Acupuncture is contraindicated 1. In patients who are hungry, overeating, drunken, in rage, frightened, or show over fatigue or mental tension 2. On body areas that have infections, ulcers and scars 3. In patients with acute infectious disease, coagulation disorders, serious heart disease, severe diabetes mellitus, severe anemia, acute inflammation, heart failure, tendency to bleed spontaneously or blood-clotting problem Precautions 1. Strong needle manipulations should be avoided for patients with weak constitutions or with severe or chronic illness and deficiencies of qi and blood and who should be treated in the supine position. 2. Large vessels should be avoided. 3. Care should be taken to the depths, angles, and direction of needling for acupoints in the chests, ribs, lumbar region, upper back, around the eyes, and along the spine. 4. Acupoints around the fontanelle should not be acupunctured for children whose fontanelle are unclosed. 5. Needle retaining is not recommended for infants or for children who do not cooperate or move restlessly.
Tui na[105]	Tui na cannot be performed when the children have the following complications: 1. Some acute infectious diseases, such as scarlet fever, chickenpox, hepatitis, and pulmonary tuberculosis 2. Local places of various kinds of malignant tumor 3. Hemorrhagic disease, local places in bleeding, and internal bleeding 4. Bone and joint tuberculosis, septic arthritis 5. Local places of burns, scald and any skin breaks, injured skin places of all kinds of dermatoses 6. Early phase of fractures and paraplegia 7. Extremely feeble patients with critical illness, serious heart and kidney disease, diseases with unexplained diagnoses

Data from Shi XM. Acupuncture. Beijing (China): Chinese Press of Traditional Chinese Medicine; 2002. p. 154–5 [in Chinese]; and China Association of Chinese Medicine (ZYYXH/T171-2010). Technical specification of health preservation and prevention of traditional Chinese medicine-massage for children. Beijing (China): Chinese Medicine Press; First version 2010. p. 14–5.

What Are Potential Adverse Effects of the Treatment?

Adverse effects of TCM therapies when used appropriately are usually limited, such as a loss of appetite, insomnia, and mild abdomen pain.[65,66] These symptoms usually go away by themselves and have no impact on continued treatment. Because many of the medicinal herbs contain different levels of noxiousness, which are usually diminished through proper processing and compatible design of the medicine formulae, it is usually thought that "The adverse effects of Chinese medicine were from the doctors, not from the Chinese medicine itself."[77] When used improperly, some adverse effects and complications can be painful and life threatening. There were a total of 20 potential side effects summarized in the authors' meta-analysis, which include anorexia/decreased appetite, insomnia, nausea/vomiting, dry mouth, headache, constipation, dizziness, weight loss, sweating, blurred vision, akathisia, tachycardia, dermatologic changes, increased appetite, anxiety/nervousness, abdominal pain, diarrhea, hypersomnia, hallucination, and slow growth (unpublished).

Fewer side effects were reported in the clinical trials of acupuncture for the treatment of ADHD. Those side effects included loss of appetite, dry mouth, nausea, and constipation. However, because only one study was reported,[78] the authors cannot fully evaluate the side effects of acupuncture yet. There can be accidents during the acupuncture procedure, including fainting; a needle stuck, bent, or broken; hematomas; and traumatic pneumothorax. These accidents are often the results of carelessness, violation or neglect of the rules, inappropriately strong manipulations, or inadequate knowledge of human acupoints and anatomy.

Chinese herbal medicines are always obtained from hospitals or pharmacies where raw herbs are purchased from different growers/manufacturers, some of which may not have rigorous quality control in the cultivation, collection, and processing. Some herbs may occasionally be contaminated with bacteria, microbe, heavy metal, pesticides, and chemicals. Using contaminated herbs can cause damage to human health and reduce the efficacy of the therapies.

How Should Treatment Be Sequenced and/or Integrated with Drug Therapy and with Other Nondrug Treatments (eg, Stand Alone, Combination Therapy, and So Forth)

Single-modal TCM therapy or multimodal therapies can be prescribed by TCM doctors according to patients' conditions and the wishes of the children and their families. CHM formulae and acupuncture are the most often used therapies for ADHD. Each or both are often combined with other auxiliary TCM therapies, such as tui na, tai chi chuan, diet therapy, and sometimes with Western ADHD medicines.

FUTURE DIRECTIONS

The theoretic system and clinical practice of TCM in treating ADHD remain to be questioned and evaluated by the international society. Admittedly, because of the special theory and unique clinical system, a lack of large high-quality clinical trials, unknown modern scientific interpretation of the mechanisms of action, despite the long history of safe clinical practice and efficacy of treatment in China and other Asian countries, it is still a challenge to introduce TCM as an alternative medicine for treating ADHD in non-Asian cultures. In addition, more efforts are needed to address cultural and racial differences in both the diagnostic and treatment systems.

The current Chinese medical diagnosis and treatment guideline for ADHD should be amended and revised through more experts communication and evaluation as well as verification from larger multicentered, double-blind, randomized controlled clinical trials. Physicians should continue to explore and refine more effective CHM formulae and their active constituent, acupuncture, tui na, tai chi chuan, and diet, as well as the more effective combination of these therapies.

Finally, more laboratory studies are needed to help understand the neurobiological basis of the TCM treatment. Although it is difficult to study the TCM theories and holistic approaches in laboratory animals, a few animal studies have shown that the CHM formulae or herbal extracts can reduce ADHD phenotypes in animal models. This finding may be caused by targeting the catecholamine neurotransmitter systems in the brain,[79–82] which are the same neurobiological targets of Western pharmacologic treatments.[83–87] Obviously, complex CHM formulae are likely to target many organs and systems and, most importantly, target the individual as a whole. Modern scientific methods using model systems or modern techniques, such as functional magnetic resonance imaging, may help us to finally understand the scientific basis of this ancient medicine.

SUMMARY

ADHD treatment is individualized when using TCM guidelines of holism and treatment principles derived from syndrome differentiation. The special theoretic and clinical systems of TCM possess a profound cultural origin. Since the 1980s, a series of clinical documents including clinical trials, case reports, and expert experiences have been conducted by TCM researchers to diagnose and treat ADHD, leading to the current understanding and summarized guidelines that are used by TCM physicians. Because ADHD is a lifelong disorder for some patients and has a complex multifactorial cause that includes gene and environmental interactions, ADHD is considered one of the preponderant illnesses for TCM therapy by the State Administration of Traditional Chinese Medicine in China. The existing published studies, although limited, have demonstrated the safety and potential beneficial effects of TCM in treating ADHD. However, larger studies are still needed and collaborations are encouraged. For Western society, although we still know very little about the cultural and racial differences in the response and tolerance to the TCM therapies, some of the most important TCM practicing principles, such as holism and individualized medicine, should also be valuable for modern psychiatric practice in managing and treating ADHD.

ACKNOWLEDGMENTS

The authors thank Gail Depalma for help revising the article.

REFERENCES

1. Polanczyk G, de Lima MS, Horta BL, et al. The worldwide prevalence of ADHD: a systematic review and metaregression analysis. Am J Psychiatry 2007;164(6): 942–8.
2. Faraone S, Biederman J, Mick E. The age dependent decline of attention-deficit/ hyperactivity disorder: a meta-analysis of follow-up studies. Psychol Med 2006; 36(2):159–65.
3. Faraone SV, Sergeant J, Gillberg C, et al. The worldwide prevalence of ADHD: is it an American condition? World Psychiatry 2003;2(2):104–13.
4. American Psychiatric Association. Diagnostic and statistical manual of mental disorders. 4th edition. Washington, DC: American Psychiatric Association; 2000.
5. Pliszka SR. Comorbidity of attention-deficit/hyperactivity disorder with psychiatric disorder: an overview. J Clin Psychiatry 1998;59(Suppl 7):50–8.

6. Van de Glind G, Konstenius M, Koeter MW, et al. Variability in the prevalence of adult ADHD in treatment seeking substance use disorder patients: results from an international multi-center study exploring DSM-IV and DSM-5 criteria. Drug Alcohol Depend 2014;134(134):158–66.

7. DuPaul GJ, McGoey KE, Eckert TL, et al. Preschool children with attention-deficit/hyperactivity disorder: impairments in behavioral, social, and school functioning. J Am Acad Child Adolesc Psychiatry 2001;40(5):508–15.

8. Harpin VA. The effect of ADHD on the life of an individual, their family, and community from preschool to adult life. Arch Dis Child 2005;90(Suppl 1):i2–7.

9. Barkley RA. Global issues related to the impact of untreated attention-deficit/hyperactivity disorder from childhood to young adulthood. Postgrad Med 2008;120(3):48–59.

10. Pliszka S, AACAP Work Group on Quality Issues. Practice parameter for the assessment and treatment of children and adolescents with attention-deficit/hyperactivity disorder. J Am Acad Child Adolesc Psychiatry 2007;46(7):894–921.

11. Li XR. Minimal brain dysfunction syndrome in children. Journal International Psychiatry 1975;(2):55–9 [in Chinese].

12. Jiang J. Limitations of treatment based on syndrome differentiation and necessity of combining syndrome differentiation with disease differentiation. Journal Chinese Integrative Medicine 2005;3(2):85–7 [in Chinese].

13. Lu A, Jiang M, Zhang C, et al. An integrative approach of linking traditional Chinese medicine pattern classification and biomedicine diagnosis. J Ethnopharmacol 2012;141(2):549–56.

14. Zheng XY. Clinical guideline of new drugs for traditional Chinese medicine. Beijing (China): Medicine Science and Technology Press of China; 2002. p. 29–30 [in Chinese].

15. State Administration of Traditional Chinese Medicine. Chinese medical diagnosis and treatment project of ADHD. 2012. [in Chinese].

16. Mo S, Deng LS, Li WY, et al. Research of correlation between the three ADHD subtypes and TCM syndromes. Journal Liaoning University TCM 2011;13(9):102–4 [in Chinese].

17. Guo YJ, Gao JF. Research of efficacy difference of TCM treatment based on syndrome differentiation and correlation between the TCM syndromes and Western medicine subtypes. Journal Inner Mongolia Chinese Medicine 2013;(17):5–6 [in Chinese].

18. Breggin PR. Questioning the treatment for ADHD. Science 2001;291(5504):595.

19. Spencer T, Biederman J, Wilens T, et al. Pharmacotherapy of attention-deficit hyperactivity disorder across the life cycle. J Am Acad Child Adolesc Psychiatry 1996;35(4):409–32.

20. Galland BC, Tripp EG, Taylor BJ. The sleep of children with attention deficit hyperactivity disorder on and off methylphenidate: a matched case-control study. J Sleep Res 2010;19(2):366–73.

21. Sonuga-Barke EJ, Coghill D, Wigal T, et al. Adverse reactions to methylphenidate treatment for attention-deficit/hyperactivity disorder: structure and associations with clinical characteristics and symptom control. J Child Adolesc Psychopharmacol 2009;19(6):683–90.

22. Yildiz O, Sismanlar SG, Memik NC, et al. Atomoxetine and methylphenidate treatment in children with ADHD: the efficacy, tolerability and effects on executive functions. Child Psychiatry Hum Dev 2011;42(3):257–69.

23. Schwartz S, Correll CU. Efficacy and safety of atomoxetine in children and adolescents with attention-deficit/hyperactivity disorder: results from a

comprehensive meta-analysis and metaregression. J Am Acad Child Adolesc Psychiatry 2014;53(2):174–87.

24. Fredriksen M, Halmoy A, Faraone SV, et al. Long-term efficacy and safety of treatment with stimulants and atomoxetine in adult ADHD: a review of controlled and naturalistic studies. Eur Neuropsychopharmacol 2013;23(6):508–27.

25. Banaschewski T, Roessner V, Dittmann RW, et al. Non-stimulant medications in the treatment of ADHD. Eur Child Adolesc Psychiatry 2004;13(Suppl 1):I102–16.

26. Leslie LK, Plemmons D, Monn AR, et al. Investigating ADHD treatment trajectories: listening to families' stories about medication use. J Dev Behav Pediatr 2007;28(3):179–88.

27. Turgay A, Goodman DW, Asherson P, et al. Lifespan persistence of ADHD: the life transition model and its application. J Clin Psychiatry 2012;73(2):192–201.

28. Pellow J, Solomon EM, Barnard CN. Complementary and alternative medical therapies for children with attention-deficit/hyperactivity disorder (ADHD). Altern Med Rev 2011;16(4):323–37.

29. Rostain A, Jensen PS, Connor DF, et al. Toward quality care in ADHD: defining the goals of treatment. J Atten Disord 2013. [Epub ahead of print].

30. Steele M, Jensen PS, Quinn DM. Remission versus response as the goal of therapy in ADHD: a new standard for the field? Clin Ther 2006;28(11): 1892–908.

31. Milberger S, Biederman J, Faraone SV, et al. Pregnancy, delivery and infancy complications and attention deficit hyperactivity disorder: issues of gene-environment interaction. Biol Psychiatry 1997;41(1):65–75.

32. Altink ME, Arias-Vasquez A, Franke B, et al. The dopamine receptor D4 7-repeat allele and prenatal smoking in ADHD-affected children and their unaffected siblings: no gene-environment interaction. Journal Child Psychology Psychiatry Allied Disciplines 2008;49(10):1053–60.

33. Buschgens CJ, van Aken MA, Swinkels SH, et al. Differential family and peer environmental factors are related to severity and comorbidity in children with ADHD. J Neural Transm 2008;115(2):177–86.

34. Xue C, Yang Q. The model of traditional Chinese medicine. J Tradit Chin Med 2003;23(4):308–11 [in Chinese].

35. Yan JH. Expert inquiry of TCM preponderant illness and its theoretical origin. Jiangsu J Tradit Chin Med 2001;22(9):1–4 [in Chinese].

36. Cao HX. Strategic consideration and practice of clinical study of TCM preponderant illness. J Tradit Chin Med 2009;50(1):11–2 [in Chinese].

37. National Administration of Traditional Chinese Medicine. Chinese medical diagnosis and treatment project for 105 diseases in 24 majors. Beijing (China): National Administration of Traditional Chinese Medicine; 2012. p. 490–4 [in Chinese].

38. Duan JA, Su SL, Fan XS, et al. Exploration of action patterns and mechanisms of traditional Chinese medicine incompatibility of qi-Qing antagonism and mutual inhibition/restraint based on drug interaction. World Science Technology 2012; 14(3):1547–52 [in Chinese].

39. Li XR, Chen ZJ. Clinical comparative observation on duodongning and Ritalin in treating child hyperkinetic syndrome. Chinese Journal Integrated Traditional Western Medicine 1999;19(7):410–1 [in Chinese].

40. Ding GA, Yu GH, Chen SF. Assessment on effect of treatment for childhood hyperkinetic syndrome by combined therapy of yizhi mixture and Ritalin. Chinese Journal Integrated Traditional Western Medicine 2002;22(4):255–7 [in Chinese].

41. Wang MJ, Wei H, Zhang Y, et al. Clinical observation of Jingling oral liquid combined with methylphenidate in the treatment of ADHD with transient Tic disorder. Chinese Traditional Patent Medicine 2011;33(9):1638–9 [in Chinese].

42. Li JJ, Li ZW, Wang SZ, et al. Ningdong granule: a complementary and alternative therapy in the treatment of attention deficit/hyperactivity disorder. Psychopharmacology 2011;216(4):501–9.

43. Ma RQ. Clinical study of Duodong Ting decoction on the content of serum Pb, Zn, Cu, Mg of children with Attention deficit hyperactivity disorder. Xi'an (China): Shaanxi College of Traditional Chinese Medicine; 2007 [in Chinese].

44. Chen J, Chen YY, Wang XM. Clinical study on treatment of children attention deficit hyperactivity disorder by jiangqian granule. Chinese Journal Integrated Traditional Western Medicine 2002;22(4):258–60 [in Chinese].

45. Zhang L, Lu JF, Chen XR, et al. Clinical observation of Tiaonao Ling in the treatment of children with Attention deficit hyperactivity disorder. Shanghai Journal TCM 2007;41(7):44–5 [in Chinese].

46. Wei XW. Clinical efficacy of Xiaoer Zhili syrup on 60 cases of Attention deficit hyperactivity disorder. Seek Medical Ask Medicine 2011;9(10):173–5 [in Chinese].

47. Li YM. Observation on the curative effect of infantile intelligence syrup for treatment of children with attention deficit hyperactivity disorder. Journal Maternal Child Health Care China 2012;27(28):4481–3 [in Chinese].

48. Chai TQ. Clinical observation of acupuncture in the treatment of 155 cases of attention deficit hyperactivity disorder. J Chin Acupuncture 1999;(1):5–8 [in Chinese].

49. Shi XM. Acupuncture. Beijing (China): Chinese Press of Traditional Chinese Medicine; 2002. p. 154–5 [in Chinese].

50. Wang R, Li PY, Gao Y. Clinical observation of Jingling oral liquid combined with acupuncture in the treatment of ADHD. Chin J Misdiagn 2008;8(36):8880–1 [in Chinese].

51. Wang YL, Shi XP. Observation on the effects of massage on treatment of attention deficit hyperactivity disorder in children. Chinese Journal Tissue Engineering Research 2005;9(4):216–7 [in Chinese].

52. Zhuo Y. Clinical study of tui-na and ear acupoint-sticking in the treatment of ADHD. Jiliin J Tradit Chin Med 2006;26(7):41–2 [in Chinese].

53. Yin F, Wang GY. Yin-yang and deficiency-excess of tai chi chuan and Chinese medicine. Henan J Tradit Chin Med 2004;19(1):20 [in Chinese].

54. Pang J, Yang Y, Tang HL, et al. Chinese medicine regimen methods embodied in Tai Chi chuan. Sichuan J Tradit Chin Med 2007;25(10):46–7 [in Chinese].

55. He YH. Explore of fitness mechanism of tai chi chuan. Journal Sports World 2007;(1):66–7 Academic Edition. [in Chinese].

56. Wen HX. Study of the effect of Taijiquan on children who have a tendency to ADHD. Fuzhou (China): Fujian Normal University; 2009 [in Chinese].

57. Hernandez-Reif M, Field TM, Thimas E. Attention deficit hyperactivity disorder: benefits from tai chi. Journal Bodywork Movement Therapies 2001;5(2):120–3.

58. Ni SM. Diet therapy of traditional Chinese medicine. Beijing (China): Chinese Press of Traditional Chinese Medicine; 2004. p. 217–21 [in Chinese].

59. Boutron I, Guittet L, Estellat C, et al. Reporting methods of blinding in randomized trials assessing nonpharmacological treatments. PLoS Med 2007;4(2):e61.

60. Julliard KN, Citkovitz C, McDaniel D. Towards a model for planning clinical research in Oriental medicine. Explore 2007;3(2):118–28.

61. Liu JP. The composition of evidence body of traditional medicine and recommendations for its evidence grading. Chinese Journal Integrative Medicine 2007;27(12):1061–4.
62. OCEBM Levels of Evidence Working Group. The Oxford 2011 levels of evidence. Oxford (UK): Oxford Centre for Evidence-Based Medicine; 2011.
63. Wang SC, Chen ZG, Xu S, et al. Study on evidence grading system in evidence-based clinical practice guidelines of traditional Chinese medicine. World Science Technology Modernization Traditional Chinese Medicine 2013;15(7):1488–92 [in Chinese].
64. Chinese Medical Association. Prevention and cure guideline for attentional deficit hyperactivity disorder. Beijing (China): Peking University Medical Press; 2007 [in Chinese].
65. Lan Y, Zhang LL, Luo R. Attention deficit hyperactivity disorder in children: comparative efficacy of traditional Chinese medicine and methylphenidate. J Int Med Res 2009;37(3):939–48 [in Chinese].
66. Wong YW, Kim DG, Lee JY. Traditional oriental herbal medicine for children and adolescents with ADHD: a systematic review. Evid Based Complement Alternat Med 2012;2012:520198.
67. Li S, Yu B, Zhou D, et al. Acupuncture for attention deficit hyperactivity disorder (ADHD) in children and adolescents. Cochrane Database Syst Rev 2011;(4):CD007839.
68. May BH, Lu C, Lu Y, et al. Chinese herbs for memory disorders: a review and systematic analysis of classical herbal literature. Journal Acupuncture Meridian Studies 2013;6(1):2–11.
69. Kwon YS, Nabeshima T, Shin EJ, et al. PAP 9704, a Korean herbal medicine attenuates methamphetamine-induced hyperlocomotion via adenosine A2A receptor stimulation in mice. Biol Pharm Bull 2004;27(6):906–9.
70. Chung IW, Moore NA, Oh WK, et al. Behavioural pharmacology of polygalasaponins indicates potential antipsychotic efficacy. Pharmacol Biochem Behav 2002;71(1–2):191–5.
71. Xu W, Towers AD, Li P, et al. Traditional Chinese medicine in cancer care: perspectives and experiences of patients and professionals in China. Eur J Cancer Care 2006;15(4):397–403.
72. Zhu X, Bensoussan A, Zhu L, et al. Primary dysmenorrhoea: a comparative study on Australian and Chinese women. Complement Ther Med 2009;17(3): 155–60.
73. Qu L. Clinical epidemiological study on the type of symptom of Chinese traditional medicine of coronary heart disease of three kinds of race. Changsha (China): Hunan University of TCM; 2011 [in Chinese].
74. Wang XY. Influence of interracial constitution difference to the Chinese medicine formula. Jinagsu J Tradit Chin Med 2009;41(5):12–3 [in Chinese].
75. Wang XY. Influence of interracial constitution difference to the Chinese medicine therapies. J Liaoning Univ TCM 2009;11(1):21–4 [in Chinese].
76. Wang HW. Practical Chinese medicine contraindication. Beijing (China): People's Medical Publishing House; 2009 [in Chinese].
77. Gao XM. Chinese medicine. Beijing (China): Chinese Press of Traditional Chinese Medicine; 2007. p. 30–5.
78. Liu JD. Clinical research on ADHD treatment with Jin's three-needle therapy. Guangzhou (China): Guangzhou University of TCM; 2009 [in Chinese].
79. Dela Pena IC, Young Yoon S, Kim Y, et al. 5,7-Dihydroxy-6-methoxy-4'-phenoxyflavone, a derivative of oroxylin A improves attention-deficit/hyperactivity

disorder (ADHD)-like behaviors in spontaneously hypertensive rats. Eur J Pharmacol 2013;715(1–3):337–44.

80. Yoon SY, Dela Pena I, Kim SM, et al. Oroxylin A improves attention deficit hyperactivity disorder-like behaviors in the spontaneously hypertensive rat and inhibits reuptake of dopamine in vitro. Arch Pharm Res 2013;36(1):134–40.

81. Chen XG, Tian H, Lai DL, et al. Yizhining decoction improves sustained attention deficit and impulsiveness of spontaneous hypertensive rats. Neural Regen Res 2007;2(1):50–3.

82. Lai DL. Clinical and experimental research of Yizhi Ning in the treatment of Attention deficit hyperactivity disorder. Guangzhou (China): Guangzhou University of TCM; 2005 [in Chinese].

83. Zametkin AJ, Rapoport JL. Noradrenergic hypothesis of attention deficit disorder with hyperactivity: a critical review. In: Meltzer HY, editor. Psychopharmacology the Third Generation of Progress. New York: Raven Press; 1987. p. 837–47.

84. Pliszka SR, McCracken JT, Maas JW. Catecholamines in attention-deficit hyperactivity disorder: current perspectives. J Am Acad Child Adolesc Psychiatry 1996;35(3):264–72.

85. Biederman J, Spencer T. Attention-deficit/hyperactivity disorder (ADHD) as a noradrenergic disorder. Biol Psychiatry 1999;46(9):1234–42.

86. Puumala T, Sirvio J. Changes in activities of dopamine and serotonin systems in the frontal cortex underlie poor choice accuracy and impulsivity of rats in an attention task. Neuroscience 1998;83(2):489–99.

87. Swanson JM, Kinsbourne M, Nigg J, et al. Etiologic subtypes of attention-deficit/ hyperactivity disorder: brain imaging, molecular genetic and environmental factors and the dopamine hypothesis. Neuropsychol Rev 2007;17(1):39–59.

88. Han XM, Zhu XK. Clinical study of Anshen Dingzhi Ling in the treatment of 58 children with Attention deficit hyperactivity disorder. J Tradit Chin Med Hebei 2004;26(12):898–9 [in Chinese].

89. Liu CQ, Han XM, Zhu XK, et al. Clinical research of 30 cases of treating ADHD with clearing the heart, calming the liver, reducing phlegm for resuscitation. Journal New Chinese Medicine 2010;42(12):44–6 [in Chinese].

90. Li J. Observation of clinical efficacy of huanglian wendan decoction for ADHD. Journal Guide China Medicine 2010;8(22):240–1 [in Chinese].

91. Kong DR, Huo J, Fu HP, et al. Treatment of sixty cases of attention deficit hyperactivity disorder using Qijudihuang pills. Shandong Chinese Medicine Journal 2007;26(7):445–7 [in Chinese].

92. Qi L. Observation of clinical efficacy of modified Lingjiao Gouteng decoction combined with methylphenidate in the treatment of Attention deficit hyperactivity disorder. Fuzhou (China): Fujian University of TCM.[D]; 2011 [in Chinese].

93. Gao CX. The clinical research about the therapy of attention deficit hyperactivity disorder from heart, liver and kidney. Chengdu (China): Chengdu University of Traditional Chinese Medicine; 2011 [in Chinese].

94. Leng FN, Ling YX, Peng GC, et al. Clinical therapeutics of children with attention deficit hyperactivity Disorder[M]. Beijing (China): People's Military Medical Publisher; 2010 [in Chinese].

95. Han XM. Study of clinical pathway of attention deficit hyperactivity disorder of TCM. Journal Pediatrics TCM 2012;8(5):20–5 [in Chinese].

96. Wang YP, Shi P. Observation of clinical efficacy of Jingling oral liquid in the treatment of ADHD. J Chin Traditional Herbal Drugs 2003;34(2):162–4 [in Chinese].

97. Fan L, Zhang G. Comparison of Chinese medicine and Western medicine in the treatment of the ADHD. Medical Journal Industrial Enterprise 1998;11(3):69 [in Chinese].
98. Zhang JN, Li M, Wang HR, et al. Observation of clinical treatment efficacy of 69 cases of ADHD. Chinese Journal Child Health Care 2004;12(1):22–4 [in Chinese].
99. Yue WZ, Hua N. Clinical observation of treating ADHD with Chinese medicine combined with Western medicine. Chinese Journal Information TCM 2006; 13(3):68–70 [in Chinese].
100. Yue WZ, Xu H. Clinical observation of treating ADHD with Jingling oral liquid combined with Ritalin. J Hubei Traditional Chinese Medicine 2006;28(9):14–5 [in Chinese].
101. Ma R, Li XM, Wei XW, et al. Clinical observation of Yishentianjing method on treating fifty-five children with attention deficit hyperactivity disorder. J Tianjin Univ Trad Chin Med 2007;26(3):122–5 [in Chinese].
102. Mei QX, Wang MJ, Li Y, et al. Clinical analysis of Xiaoer Zhili syrup in the treatment of Attention deficit hyperactivity disorder. Journal Chinese Traditional Patent Medicine 2010;32(7):1272–4 [in Chinese].
103. Zhang LP. Efficacy evaluation of Xiaoer Zhili syrup in the treatment of Attention deficit hyperactivity disorder. Journal Practical Clinical Medicine 2011;12(6): 78–9 [in Chinese].
104. Wang RQ, Zhao XZ, Mou CS, et al. Clinical observation of Xiaoer Zhili syrup in the treatment of Attention deficit hyperactivity disorder. Journal Clinical Rational Drug Use 2011;4(9):64 [in Chinese].
105. China Association of Chinese Medicine. Technical specification of health preservation and prevention of traditional Chinese medicine-massage for children. Beijing (China): Chinese Medicine Press; 2010 [in Chinese].

Nutritional Supplements for the Treatment of ADHD

Michael H. Bloch, MD, MS*, Jilian Mulqueen, BA

KEYWORDS

- Attention-deficit hyperactivity disorder • Omega-3 fatty acids
- Polyunsaturated fatty acids • Zinc • Magnesium • *Gingko biloba*

KEY POINTS

- Polyunsaturated fatty acid supplementation appears to have modest benefit for improving ADHD symptoms.
- Melatonin is effective in improving chronic insomnia in children with ADHD but has little evidence for efficacy in improving core ADHD symptoms.
- Many other supplements are commonly used despite little evidence of efficacy and evidence of possible side-effects.

INTRODUCTION

Attention-deficit/hyperactivity disorder (ADHD) is a common and impairing health condition affecting school-aged children.[1,2] Pharmacotherapies are currently considered the cornerstone of evidence-based treatment for ADHD. More than 70% of children with ADHD respond to psychostimulant medications.[3] Other medications, such as atomoxetine, alpha-2 agonists, bupropion, and tricyclic antidepressants, also have demonstrated efficacy in treating ADHD.[4–6] However, many families elect not to use traditional pharmacotherapies to treat ADHD. This decision is often related to concerns over possible short-term side effects or doubts regarding long-term efficacy or effects on development of these medications.[7–10] Instead, alternative and complementary treatments, such as natural supplements, are often used by families to treat ADHD.[11]

Despite a modest evidence base compared with conventional treatments for ADHD, complementary and alternative treatments are commonly used by children with ADHD. Although few population-based, epidemiologic studies have been performed in the area, current evidence suggests that 12% to 64% of children with ADHD use

Disclosures: The authors have no conflicts of interest to disclose.
Yale Child Study Center, PO BOX 207900, 230 South Frontage Road, New Haven, CT 06520, USA
* Corresponding author.
E-mail address: michael.bloch@yale.edu

Abbreviations	
ADHD	Attention-deficit/hyperactivity disorder
CAP	Child attention problems
EPA	Eicosapentaenoic acid
NHANES	National Health and Nutrition Examination Survey
PUFAs	Polyunsaturated fatty acids

some form of complementary medicine.[12] Examination of adolescent dietary supplement use in the National Health and Nutrition Examination Survey (NHANES), a series of nationally representative surveys of the civilian, noninstitutionalized population in the United States administered by the National Center for Health Statistics, suggested that adolescents with ADHD were roughly 10% more likely to use dietary supplements than adolescents without ADHD.[13]

The goal of this review was to synthesize and evaluate the scientific evidence regarding the potential efficacy and side effects of natural supplements and herbal remedies for ADHD. We additionally will provide clinicians with recommendations regarding their potential use and role in overall ADHD treatment.

METHODS

PubMed and Cochrane Central Register of Controlled Trials was searched on March 24, 2014, using the search strategy "Attention Deficit Disorder with Hyperactivity"[Mesh] AND "Dietary Supplements"[Mesh] OR "Zinc"[Mesh] OR "Magnesium"[Mesh] OR "Iron"[Mesh] OR "Hypericum"[Mesh] OR "Ginkgo biloba"[Mesh] OR "Vitamins"[Mesh]. The search was further limited to clinical trials, reviews, and meta-analyses. Trials were included in this review if they (1) examined treatments for ADHD, and (2) were randomized and (3) placebo-controlled trials. References in reviews and systematic reviews in the area generated by the search strategy were also reviewed for additional eligible trials.[14–24] Trials were additionally required to involve a therapy of interest, which for the sake of this article includes vitamins, minerals, natural supplements, and herbal remedies. Specifically excluded from this review are non–pill-based treatment modalities, such as neurofeedback, behavioral therapies, restriction or food color exclusion diets, and chiropractic interventions.

INTERVENTIONS
Dietary Supplements

Polyunsaturated fatty acids

Polyunsaturated fatty acids (PUFAs) are a well-studied complementary treatment for ADHD. Omega-3 fatty acids cannot be synthesized by humans and are required in our diet. In the Western diet, omega-6 fatty acids or their precursors (eg, linoleic acid) are much more abundant than omega-3 fatty acids or their precursors (eg, alpha-linolenic acid).[25] A high omega-6 to omega-3 ratio can alter cell membrane properties and increase production of inflammatory mediators because arachidonic acid, an omega-6 fatty acid found in cell membranes, is the precursor of inflammatory eicosanoids, such as prostaglandins and thromboxanes.[26] By contrast, omega-3 fatty acids are anti-inflammatory.[26] Therefore, a high dietary omega-6 to omega-3 fatty ratio could promote neuroinflammation. Increased omega-3 fatty acid concentration in the diet also may act by altering central nervous system cell membrane fluidity and phospholipid composition, which may alter the structure and function of the proteins embedded in it.[27] By this mechanism, increased omega-3 fatty acid concentrations in cell membranes have been shown to affect serotonin and dopamine neurotransmission, especially in the frontal cortex and may be of importance in ADHD pathogenesis.[28] Omega-3 fatty acids also may potentially act in reducing oxidative stress, which has been demonstrated to be elevated in ADHD.[29]

An initial meta-analysis involving 10 trials including 699 children with ADHD demonstrated a significant benefit of PUFA supplementation compared with placebo. The benefits of PUFA supplementation were small (compared with the effect sizes observed for conventional pharmacologic treatments for ADHD) but statistically significant.[17] Additionally, meta-regression demonstrated a significant relationship between eicosapentaenoic acid (EPA) dose within supplements and measured efficacy.[17] Two updated systematic reviews using similar methodology have since confirmed the efficacy of PUFA supplementation for ADHD symptoms.[30,31] One of these meta-analyses also confirmed the significant association between EPA dose and measured benefit in the treatment of ADHD.[31]

However, 2 recent systematic reviews have raised questions regarding the benefits of omega-3 supplementation of ADHD.[19,32] The divergent results of these meta-analyses are attributable to methodological differences from the other systematic reviews. A recent Cochrane review in the area failed to demonstrate a significant benefit of omega-3 supplementation on most but not all outcome measures for ADHD.[19] As is traditional for Cochrane reviews, the investigators did not pool results across different study designs (eg, crossover vs parallel-group trials) and this difference in methodology led to comparatively underpowered meta-analyses for many outcomes. Another recent systematic review, by contrast, added additional trials that examined the effects of omega-3 fatty acid supplementation on ADHD symptoms in other clinical populations (eg, children with reading difficulties, developmental coordination disorders, and dyslexia).[32] This meta-analysis found a significant benefit of PUFA supplementation, but also noted evidence of publication bias in the literature that might be inflating effect estimates. Publication bias was detected through asymmetry in the funnel plot. However, the addition of trials involving subjects with primary diagnoses other than ADHD (included only in this meta-analysis) was likely responsible for asymmetry in the funnel plot (as none of the previous ADHD-only meta-analyses detected funnel plot asymmetry). One particular trial examining ADHD symptoms in children with reading disabilities included a larger number of participants (comprised 24% of the total weight of the meta-analysis) and demonstrated a minimal effect of PUFA supplementation in improving ADHD.[33] Inclusion of this large trial is responsible for the funnel plot asymmetry in the meta-analysis. However, it is quite plausible that children with primary reading disabilities would have less benefit from PUFA supplementation in improving ADHD symptoms (because they are secondary to reading difficulties or less severe than in an ADHD clinical population).

Cumulative evidence suggests that there is currently Center for Evidence-Based Medicine (CEBM) level-1 evidence demonstrating the efficacy of omega-3 fatty acids for the treatment of ADHD. Current evidence would recommend supplementation with a dose of 1 to 2 g daily with a substantial content of EPA within the omega-3 formulation. However, evidence supporting supplementation is much less clear when examining ADHD symptoms in children with other primary disorders (such as dyslexia, developmental coordination disorder, and with reading impairments). **Table 1** summarizes the results of randomized, placebo-controlled trials of nutritional supplements in ADHD.

Table 1
Randomized, placebo-controlled trials of natural supplements for ADHD

Author, Year	N	Age Range	Dosing (mg/d)	Duration	Comparison	Result
PUFAs						
Milte,[34] 2012	90	7–12	EPA Enriched: EPA 1109, DHA 108 DHA Enriched: EPA 264, DHA 1032	16 wk	Placebo	EPA = DHA = placebo
Stevens,[35] 2003	50	6–13	EPA 80, DHA 480	16 wk	Placebo	PUFA = placebo
Raz,[36] 2009	63	7–13	LA 960, ALA 120	7 wk	Placebo	EFA = placebo
Sinn,[37] 2007	104	7–12	Fish oil 2400, including EPA 558, DHA	15 wk	Placebo	PUFA > placebo
Voigt,[38] 2001	54	6–12	DHA 345	16 wk	Placebo	DHA = placebo
Richardson,[39] 2005	102	5–12	EPA 558, DHA 174	12 wk	Placebo	PUFA > placebo
Richardson,[40] 2002	41	8–12	EPA 186, DHA 480	12 wk	Placebo	PUFA = placebo (but greater improvement on some ADHD outcomes)
Johnson,[41] 2009	75	8–18	EPA 558, DHA 174	12 wk	Placebo	PUFA = placebo
Belanger,[42] 2009	26	6–11	EPA 500–1000, DHA 200–400 mg	16 wk	Placebo	PUFA = placebo
Gustafsson,[43] 2010	92	7–12	EPA 500, DHA 2.7	15 wk	Placebo	EPA > placebo
Aman,[44] 1987	31	X	Efamol: LA 2160, GLA 270	4 wk	Placebo	EFA = placebo
Manor,[45] 2012	147	6–13	EPA + DHA 120	15 wk	Placebo	PUFA = placebo
Perera,[46] 2012	94	6–12	Omega-3 600, omega-6361 (+MPH)	6 mo	Placebo (+MPH)	PUFA > placebo
Arnold,[47] 1989	18	6–12	Efamol: LA 2160, GLA 270	3 mo	Placebo, D-amphetamine	D-amphetamine > efamol = placebo
Yehuda,[48] 2011	78	9–12	LA 1440; ALA 180	10 wk	Placebo	PUFA > placebo

Zinc						
Zamora et al,[65] 2011	40	7–14	10 (+MPH)	Placebo (+MPH)	6 wk	Zinc = placebo
Arnold et al,[66] 2011	52	6–14	15 or 30	Placebo	8 wk	Zinc = placebo
Bilici et al,[63] 2004	193	6–14	150	Placebo	12 wk	Zinc > placebo
Akhondzadeh et al,[64] 2004	44	5–11	55 (+MPH)	Placebo (+MPH)	6 wk	Zinc > placebo
Iron						
Konofal et al,[58] 2008	23	5–8	80	Placebo	12 wk	Iron > placebo
St. John's Wort: Hypericum perforatum						
Weber,[49] 2008	54	6–17	900	Placebo	8 wk	Hypericum perforatum = placebo
Pycnogenol: Pinus mainus						
Trebatická et al,[78] 2006	61	6–14	1 mg/kg/d	Placebo	4 wk	Pycnogenol > placebo
Tenenbaum et al,[77] 2002	24	24–53	Pycnogenol 1 mg/lb/d	Placebo	3 wk	Pycnogenol = placebo = MPH
Carnitine						
Van Oudheusden & Scholte,[54] 2002	26	6–13	100 mg/kg/d	Placebo	8 wk	L-carnitine = placebo
Abbasi et al,[55] 2011	40	7–13	1000–3000 (+MPH 20–30mg/d)	Placebo (+MPH 20–30 mg/d)	6 wk	ALC = placebo
Arnold et al,[56] 2007	16	5–12	1000–3000	Placebo	16 wk	ALC = placebo
Melatonin						
Van der Heijden et al,[53] 2007	105	6–12	3 or 6	Placebo	4 wk	Improved sleep latency, no effect on ADHD symptoms
Weiss et al,[52] 2006	19	6–14	5	Placebo	10 d	Improved sleep latency, no effect on ADHD symptoms

Abbreviations: ADHD, attention-deficit/hyperactivity disorder; ALA, alpha-linolenic acid; ALC, acetyl-L-carnitine; DHA, docosahexaenoic acid; EPA, eicosapentaenoic acid; GLA, gamma-linolenic acid; LA, linolenic acid; MPH, methylphenidate; PUFA, polyunsaturated fatty acid.

Melatonin

Melatonin is a hormone secreted primarily by the pineal gland in response to variations in the circadian cycle and has been used for the past 2 decades for the treatment of sleep disorders in adults and children. In contrast to most available sleep medications, melatonin has little dependence potential, is not associated with habituation, and typically produces no hangover. Given its reported hypnotic effects, relatively benign side-effect profile, and over-the-counter availability, melatonin has been widely used in the United States.[50] Melatonin has been demonstrated in meta-analysis of randomized placebo-controlled trials to decrease sleep latency, increase total sleep time, and improve sleep quality in both children and adults with primary sleep disorders.[51] Given that sleep problems are common in children with ADHD and are hypothesized to possibly be related to the pathogenesis of the disorder, there remains the possibility that melatonin may help improve both sleep problems and ADHD symptoms in children with both conditions. It has been hypothesized that a subset of children with ADHD experience chronic sleep-onset insomnia that leads to excessive daytime sleepiness associated with disinhibition, hyperarousal, and problems with executive function that mimics ADHD. Two, randomized placebo-controlled trials of melatonin have been conducted in children with ADHD and sleep problems. An initial crossover study in 27 stimulant-treated children with ADHD and sleep-onset insomnia demonstrated a significant benefit of melatonin in improving sleep outcomes (decreased sleep onset latency) but not ADHD symptoms.[52] The second trial that examined the efficacy of melatonin in reducing sleep problems in 105 children with ADHD and chronic sleep onset insomnia demonstrated a significant benefit of melatonin on primary sleep measures (decreased time to sleep onset and increased total sleep time) but demonstrated no effect on ADHD symptoms.[53] Taken together, these trials and meta-analyses suggest that melatonin has CEBM level-1 evidence for reducing sleep-onset latency in children with chronic sleep-onset insomnia (regardless of a comorbid diagnosis of ADHD) but there is no evidence to suggest melatonin improves ADHD symptoms. Melatonin should be prescribed in a single, nighttime dose of 3 to 6 mg (depending on child's weight) approximately 30 minutes before bedtime.

Carnitine

Carnitine is a small molecule necessary for energy production, specifically involved in oxidation and transport of fatty acids. An initial randomized, double-blind, placebo-controlled crossover trial of L-carnitine in 24 children with ADHD failed to demonstrate a significant difference compared with placebo.[54] Similarly, 2 other randomized, placebo-controlled trials of acetyl-L-carnitine in children with ADHD also have failed to demonstrate any evidence of efficacy in treating children with ADHD.[55,56] Based on currently available trial data in children with ADHD, there is no evidence to suggest carnitine is a more effective treatment for ADHD than placebo.

Minerals

Iron

Iron is a cofactor for tyrosine hydroxylase, the rate-limiting enzyme of monoamine synthesis and thus is critical for dopamine and norepinephrine production. In a recent meta-analysis of case control studies, patients with ADHD have been demonstrated to have lower serum ferritin levels compared with healthy controls.[57] A small, pilot, randomized, placebo-controlled trial in 23 children with ADHD and abnormally low serum ferritin levels demonstrated a significant improvement in ADHD symptoms in children randomized to ferrous sulfate (80 mg/d) compared with placebo.[58] Further trials are needed to establish whether iron supplementation has any clinical utility beyond patients with ADHD with evidence of iron deficiency.

Zinc

Zinc is a cofactor for enzymes that are important for cell membrane stabilization, and in the metabolism of neurotransmitters, melatonin, and prostaglandins. Zinc has indirect effects on dopamine metabolism and antioxidant functions.[15] Chinese children with zinc deficiency have demonstrated impaired neuropsychological function and growth that improved with zinc repletion.[59] Symptoms of zinc deficiency can include inattention, jitters, and delayed cognitive development, which mimic the symptoms of ADHD. Zinc intake is primarily from the diet and its main sources include red meat, poultry, beans, fortified breakfast cereals, and dairy products. Zinc deficiencies can be due to insufficient dietary intake or malabsorption (diarrhea, lack of intestinal absorption, liver or kidney disease, sickle-cell anemia, or other chronic disease). Zinc deficiency is fairly common in some areas of the developing world but is uncommon in the United States. Case-control trials in several areas of the world (Israel, Turkey, and Poland) have demonstrated lower zinc levels in children diagnosed with ADHD compared with healthy controls.[60–62] These results have not been replicated in samples in the United States, although overall meta-analysis suggests a significant association between low zinc levels and a diagnosis of ADHD.[15,16,57]

Randomized, placebo-controlled trials of zinc supplementation either as an adjunct to psychostimulant treatment or as monotherapy have provided conflicting evidence of efficacy. These discrepant results are likely related to differences in underlying study quality and prevalence of zinc deficiency in the study populations.[15] A completer's analysis of 193 (of 400 randomized) Turkish children with ADHD demonstrated a significant benefit of 150 mg zinc sulfate per day compared with placebo after 12 weeks of treatment.[63] However, these positive results need to be treated with an abundance of caution given the high-drop rate and the non–intention-to-treat analysis. A small, randomized, placebo-controlled trial of zinc sulfate 55 mg per day demonstrated that zinc augmentation of methylphenidate (1 mg/d) was more effective than placebo augmentation in 44 Iranian children with ADHD after 6 weeks.[64] A more recent randomized, placebo-controlled trial examined the addition of zinc sulfate 10 mg per day (compared with placebo) as an adjunct to methylphenidate (0.3 mg/kg/d) in 40 Chilean children with ADHD.[65] This trial demonstrated no significant differences between zinc supplementation and placebo on attentional measures but did demonstrate a trend toward greater improvement with zinc supplementation on Connor's attentional measures that did not reach statistical significance. Zinc plasma levels were normal in the sample at baseline and decreased throughout the trial in both the placebo and zinc supplementation groups. A randomized, placebo-controlled trial examining the efficacy of zinc glycinate (15–30 mg/d) monotherapy over 8 weeks in 52 American children with ADHD[66] failed to demonstrate any benefit of zinc supplementation over the 8 weeks of treatment on any ADHD rating scales. Additionally, measures of zinc were not appreciably affected by supplementation. However, when children were given D-amphetamine over the next 5 weeks of the trial, lower doses of D-amphetamine (37% reduction compared to placebo) were needed to achieve the same clinical effects in the zinc supplementation group.

Taken together, these data suggest zinc supplementation may be a reasonable treatment option in areas where zinc deficiencies are common, and in patients with demonstrated (or at high risk) for zinc deficiency. However, evidence is insufficient to recommend zinc supplementation in American children where zinc deficiencies are rare and trial results have been negative. Also, the dosing and form of zinc supplementation has varied widely between trials, so an optimal dosing strategy is not apparent.

Magnesium

No randomized, placebo-controlled trials have demonstrated the efficacy of magnesium supplementation compared with placebo. Currently there exists only CEBM level-4 evidence based on controlled cohort studies suggesting magnesium supplementation may be beneficial in treating ADHD. Furthermore, there is significant evidence that at high doses (>10 mg/kg/d) magnesium can be toxic, so magnesium supplementation if used should be given only at moderate doses (<200 mg/d).[16] The side effects of magnesium supplementation at appropriate doses can include nausea, diarrhea, and cramps. Magnesium overdoses are potentially fatal. A recent systematic review in this area expands on the evidence regarding magnesium supplementation more in depth.[14]

The rationale for use of magnesium supplementation comes from a few case-control trials that have demonstrated reduced serum levels of magnesium in patients with ADHD compared with healthy controls.[67–69] The association between lower magnesium levels and ADHD has not been consistently found and overall meta-analysis of case-control studies does not suggest an association with ADHD.[57,70,71] Magnesium is a cofactor for many enzymes and has been demonstrated to interact with many monoamine receptors relevant in ADHD pathophysiology (serotonin 5-HT1A, 5-HT2A, and 5-HT2C), noradrenergic (alpha1 and alpha 2) and dopamine (D1 and D2) receptors in mouse models.[72] A single, double-blind placebo-controlled trial demonstrated that psychostimulants increased serum magnesium levels in ADHD after 3 weeks of treatment.[73] Multiple, uncontrolled trials have demonstrated a reduction in magnesium levels in children with ADHD compared with controls and that the deficiency in magnesium and ADHD symptoms improved after a few months of magnesium supplementation (typically 6 mg/kg/d of Mg along with 0.6 mg/kg/d of vitamin B6). However, randomized, blinded trials in the area are lacking.

Herbal Supplements

Gingko biloba

Gingko biloba is a natural supplement proposed to promote brain blood flow and inhibit platelet activation.[16] G biloba has been touted as a treatment for dementia and memory impairment, although systematic reviews assessing the efficacy of G biloba for improving cognitive function have not been supportive of these claims.[74] A single, 6-week, randomized, methylphenidate-controlled trial in children with ADHD demonstrated the superiority of methylphenidate to G biloba in terms of improving ADHD symptoms.[75] Although significantly worse than methylphenidate, the improvement over time with G biloba was nontrivial (pre-post effect size = 0.5). Thus, although it is clear that G biloba is less effective than conventional pharmacologic treatment for ADHD, it remains unanswered whether G biloba has any benefit compared with placebo. Increased bleeding risk with G biloba treatment makes its current use for ADHD unadvised.[16]

St John's Wort: Hypericum perforatum

St John's Wort is a natural supplement that has been demonstrated to inhibit reuptake of serotonin, norepinephrine, and dopamine.[76] The potential mechanism of action of St John's Wort is similar to 2 commonly used ADHD medications: atomoxetine (a norepinephrine reuptake inhibitor) and bupropion (a norepinephrine and dopamine reuptake inhibitor).[76] A well-designed, randomized, placebo-controlled trial of 54 children with ADHD failed to demonstrate a significant benefit or a trend toward benefit in children taking St John's Wort compared with placebo over 8 weeks of treatment.[24] Therefore, despite a plausible biological rationale for efficacy of

St John's Wort for ADHD, current evidence suggests that St John's Wort is no better than placebo. St John's Wort further has significant interactions with medications (SSRIs, tricyclic antidepressants, MAOIs, etc) commonly prescribed for ADHD, depression and anxiety that has caused serotonin syndrome in rare cases. Additionally, sun sensitivity is a known side effect of St John's Wort.

Pycnogenol: Pinus mainus

Pycnogenol is a standardized extract from the bark of the French maritime pine. The potential mechanism of action of Pycnogenol is unclear but case reports and case series have suggested that its use is associated with improvements in ADHD symptoms as a monotherapy or as an adjunct to psychostimulant medications. An initial, randomized, placebo-controlled and methylphenidate- controlled crossover trial of Pycnogenol failed to demonstrate a significant benefit of Pycnogenol compared with placebo. The results of this trial were more consistent with a failed trial rather than convincing evidence of inefficacy given that (1) the trial also failed to demonstrate a benefit of methylphenidate and (2) the trial demonstrated a medium, albeit nonsignificant, benefit of Pycnogenol in improving inattention symptoms of ADHD.[77] A subsequent, 4-week randomized, placebo-controlled trial of 61 children with ADHD randomized to either Pycnogenol (1 mg/kg/d) or placebo in a 2.5:1.0 ratio demonstrated a significant benefit of Pycnogenol in improving ADHD symptoms on Child Attention Problems (CAP) teacher rating scale.[78] Pycnogenol did not significantly reduce ADHD symptoms according to Connor's Parent and Teacher Ratings but by and large the trends for improvement were in the same direction as the CAP. Lower catecholamines also were demonstrated in the urine of the patients prescribed Pycnogenol in the trial, suggesting that Pycnogenol may act by affecting catecholamine formation or metabolism. Further research is needed to definitively evaluate the safety and efficacy of this compound before use in patients with ADHD could be recommended.

SUMMARY

Table 2 provides an appraisal of available evidence and recommendations regarding use for supplements contained in this review. Two dietary supplements, omega-3 fatty acids in treating ADHD symptoms and melatonin in treating sleep-onset insomnia in children with ADHD (but not primary ADHD symptoms), have strong supportive evidence of efficacy. However, many other dietary and herbal supplements have widespread use in the United States for ADHD despite minimal evidence of efficacy. Some herbal remedies, such as *G biloba* and St John's Wort, are fairly frequently used to treat ADHD despite nonexistent to negative evidence of efficacy and clear evidence for possible side effects. Given the widespread use of many dietary supplements by families of children with ADHD (and possible interactions with many traditional medications), it remains imperative that clinicians inquire about their use with families and coordinate pharmacologic management of ADHD with them. Polyunsaturated fatty acids, especially omega-3 fatty acids, have fairly convincing evidence of efficacy in treating ADHD across a sizable number of randomized, controlled trials. That being said, the efficacy of omega-3 fatty acids for ADHD appears well below the treatment gains achieved from traditional medications for ADHD, such as psychostimulant medications. The use of omega-3 fatty acids in the treatment of ADHD should generally be reserved for mild cases of ADHD and as an adjunctive treatment in more severe ADHD cases. Melatonin appears to be an excellent option to treat sleep problems in ADHD (stimulant-induced or not) if behavioral treatments have been unsuccessful and reducing or adjusting psychostimulant medication use is not feasible.

Table 2
Current evidence supporting use of natural supplements in attention-deficit/hyperactivity disorder (ADHD)

Treatment	Dosing Recommendations	Duration	Comment
Level 1 evidence for efficacy (based on systematic review of randomized controlled trials)			
Omega-3 fatty acids	1–2 g/d (>400 mg eicosapentaenoic acid)	12–16 wk	Smaller treatment benefits compared with psychostimulants.
Level 2 evidence for efficacy (based on multiple randomized controlled trials)			
Melatonin (for sleep)	3–6 mg (30 min before bed)	As needed	Effective in reducing sleep-onset latency. No evidence of benefit in ADHD.
Level 3 evidence for efficacy (based on nonrandomized studies or single randomized controlled trial prone to possible bias)			
Zinc	30–150 mg/d	8–12 wk	Limited evidence in US and Western European populations. Some evidence of efficacy in areas with prevalent zinc deficiency.
Iron	10 mg/d (prevent deficiency) – 80 mg/d (repletion)	12 wk	Indicated for patients with ADHD with evidence of iron deficiency.
Pycnogenol	1 mg/kg/d	12 wk	Small, positive, placebo-controlled randomized controlled trial. Unclear biological mechanism of action.
Ningdong	5 mg/kg/d	8 wk	Small, underpowered trial without statistical separation from MPH. No placebo-controlled trials.
Level 4 evidence for efficacy (case series and mechanism-based reasoning)			
Magnesium	100–350 mg/d	12 wk	Toxic in high doses.
Best available evidence suggests ineffective with potential adverse effects			
St. John's Wort: Hypericum perforatum			
G biloba			
Carnitine			

Abbreviation: MPH, methylphenidate.

FUTURE DIRECTIONS

Rigorous, randomized, placebo-controlled clinical trials examining the efficacy of dietary supplements in the treatment of ADHD are needed. Many of these supplements are commonly used by families despite a lack of convincing evidence of efficacy. The dearth of quality clinical trials in this area highlights an area of need for future federally and foundation-funded research.

ACKNOWLEDGMENTS

M.H. Bloch gratefully acknowledges support from the National Institute of Mental Health K23MH091240, support of the Trichotillomania Learning Center, the Yale Child Study Center Research Training Program T32MH01826830, the National Institutes of Health 1K23MH091240, the AACAP/Eli Lilly Junior Investigator Award, NARSAD, and UL1 RR024139 from the National Center for Research Resources, a component of the National Institutes of Health, and NIH Roadmap for Medical Research. Connecticut also provided resource support via the Abraham Ribicoff Research Facilities at the Connecticut Mental Health Center.

REFERENCES

1. Clinical practice guideline: diagnosis and evaluation of the child with attention-deficit/hyperactivity disorder. American Academy of Pediatrics. Pediatrics 2000; 105(5):1158–70.
2. Goldman LS, Genel M, Bezman RJ, et al. Diagnosis and treatment of attention-deficit/hyperactivity disorder in children and adolescents. Council on Scientific Affairs, American Medical Association. JAMA 1998;279(14):1100–7.
3. Spencer T, Biederman J, Wilens T, et al. Pharmacotherapy of attention-deficit hyperactivity disorder across the life cycle. J Am Acad Child Adolesc Psychiatry 1996;35(4):409–32.
4. Schachter HM, Pham B, King J, et al. How efficacious and safe is short-acting methylphenidate for the treatment of attention-deficit disorder in children and adolescents? A meta-analysis. CMAJ 2001;165(11):1475–88.
5. Connor DF, Fletcher KE, Swanson JM. A meta-analysis of clonidine for symptoms of attention-deficit hyperactivity disorder. J Am Acad Child Adolesc Psychiatry 1999;38(12):1551–9.
6. Cheng JY, Chen RY, Ko JS, et al. Efficacy and safety of atomoxetine for attention-deficit/hyperactivity disorder in children and adolescents—meta-analysis and meta-regression analysis. Psychopharmacology (Berl) 2007;194(2): 197–209.
7. Coyle JT. Psychotropic drug use in very young children. JAMA 2000;283(8): 1059–60.
8. Dunnick JK, Hailey JR. Experimental studies on the long-term effects of methylphenidate hydrochloride. Toxicology 1995;103(2):77–84.
9. Klein RG, Landa B, Mattes JA, et al. Methylphenidate and growth in hyperactive children. A controlled withdrawal study. Arch Gen Psychiatry 1988;45(12): 1127–30.
10. Nasrallah HA, Loney J, Olson SC, et al. Cortical atrophy in young adults with a history of hyperactivity in childhood. Psychiatry Res 1986;17(3):241–6.
11. Chan E, Gardiner P, Kemper KJ. At least its natural: herbs and dietary supplements in ADHD. Contemp Pediatr 2000;17:116–30.

12. Chan E, Rappaport LA, Kemper KJ. Complementary and alternative therapies in childhood attention and hyperactivity problems. J Dev Behav Pediatr 2003; 24(1):4–8.
13. Gardiner P, Buettner C, Davis RB, et al. Factors and common conditions associated with adolescent dietary supplement use: an analysis of the National Health and Nutrition Examination Survey (NHANES). BMC Complement Altern Med 2008;8:9.
14. Ghanizadeh A. A systematic review of magnesium therapy for treating attention deficit hyperactivity disorder. Arch Iran Med 2013;16(7):412–7.
15. Arnold LE, DiSilvestro RA. Zinc in attention-deficit/hyperactivity disorder. J Child Adolesc Psychopharmacol 2005;15(4):619–27.
16. Arnold LE, Hurt E, Lofthouse N. Attention-deficit/hyperactivity disorder: dietary and nutritional treatments. Child Adolesc Psychiatr Clin N Am 2013;22(3): 381–402, v.
17. Bloch MH, Qawasmi A. Omega-3 fatty acid supplementation for the treatment of children with attention-deficit/hyperactivity disorder symptomatology: systematic review and meta-analysis. J Am Acad Child Adolesc Psychiatry 2011; 50(10):991–1000.
18. Ghanizadeh A, Berk M. Zinc for treating of children and adolescents with attention-deficit hyperactivity disorder: a systematic review of randomized controlled clinical trials. Eur J Clin Nutr 2013;67(1):122–4.
19. Gillies D, Sinn J, Lad SS, et al. Polyunsaturated fatty acids (PUFA) for attention deficit hyperactivity disorder (ADHD) in children and adolescents. Cochrane Database Syst Rev 2012;(7):CD007986.
20. Hurt EA, Arnold LE, Lofthouse N. Dietary and nutritional treatments for attention-deficit/hyperactivity disorder: current research support and recommendations for practitioners. Curr Psychiatry Rep 2011;13(5):323–32.
21. Rucklidge JJ, Johnstone J, Kaplan BJ. Nutrient supplementation approaches in the treatment of ADHD. Expert Rev Neurother 2009;9(4):461–76.
22. Sarris J, Kean J, Schweitzer I, et al. Complementary medicines (herbal and nutritional products) in the treatment of attention deficit hyperactivity disorder (ADHD): a systematic review of the evidence. Complement Ther Med 2011; 19(4):216–27.
23. Skokauskas N, McNicholas F, Masaud T, et al. Complementary medicine for children and young people who have attention deficit hyperactivity disorder. Curr Opin Psychiatry 2011;24(4):291–300.
24. Weber W, Newmark S. Complementary and alternative medical therapies for attention-deficit/hyperactivity disorder and autism. Pediatr Clin North Am 2007;54(6):983–1006, xii.
25. Simopoulos AP. Omega-3 fatty acids in health and disease and in growth and development. Am J Clin Nutr 1991;54(3):438–63.
26. Simopoulos AP. Omega-3 fatty acids in inflammation and autoimmune diseases. J Am Coll Nutr 2002;21(6):495–505.
27. Freeman MP, Rapaport MH. Omega-3 fatty acids and depression: from cellular mechanisms to clinical care. J Clin Psychiatry 2011;72(2):258–9.
28. Chalon S. Omega-3 fatty acids and monoamine neurotransmission. Prostaglandins Leukot Essent Fatty Acids 2006;75(4–5):259–69.
29. Joseph N, Zhang-James Y, Perl A, et al. Oxidative stress and ADHD: a meta-analysis. J Atten Disord 2013. [Epub ahead of print].
30. Sonuga-Barke EJ, Brandeis D, Cortese S, et al. Nonpharmacological interventions for ADHD: systematic review and meta-analyses of randomized controlled

trials of dietary and psychological treatments. Am J Psychiatry 2013;170(3): 275–89.

31. Hawkey E, Nigg JT. Omega-3 fatty acids and ADHD: blood level analysis and meta-analytic extension of supplementation trials. Clin Psychol Rev, in press.

32. Puri BK, Martins JG. Which polyunsaturated fatty acids are active in children with attention-deficit hyperactivity disorder receiving PUFA supplementation? A fatty acid validated meta-regression analysis of randomized controlled trials. Prostaglandins Leukot Essent Fatty Acids 2014;90(5):179–89.

33. Richardson AJ, Burton JR, Sewell RP, et al. Docosahexaenoic acid for reading, cognition and behavior in children aged 7–9 years: a randomized, controlled trial (the DOLAB Study). PLoS One 2012;7(9):e43909.

34. Milte CM, Parletta N, Buckley JD, et al. Eicosapentaenoic and docosahexaenoic acids, cognition, and behavior in children with attention-deficit/hyperactivity disorder: a randomized controlled trial. Nutrition 2012;28(6):670–7.

35. Stevens L, Zhang W, Peck L, et al. EFA supplementation in children with inattention, hyperactivity, and other disruptive behaviors. Lipids 2003;38:1007–21.

36. Raz R, Carasso RL, Yehuda S. The influence of short-chain essential fatty acids on children with attention-deficit/hyperactivity disorder: a double-blind placebo-controlled study. J Child Adolesc Psychopharmacol 2009;19:167–77.

37. Sinn N, Bryan J. Effect of supplementation with polyunsaturated fatty acids and micronutrients on learning and behavior problems associated with child ADHD. J Dev Behav Pediatr 2007;28:82–91.

38. Voigt RG, Llorente AM, Jensen CL, et al. A randomized, double-blind, placebo-controlled trial of docosahexaenoic acid supplementation in children with attention-deficit/hyperactivity disorder. J Pediatr 2001;139:189–96.

39. Richardson AJ, Montgomery P. The Oxford-Durham study: a randomized, controlled trial of dietary supplementation with fatty acids in children with developmental coordination disorder. Pediatrics 2005;115:1360–6.

40. Richardson AJ, Puri BK. A randomized double-blind, placebo-controlled study of the effects of supplementation with highly unsaturated fatty acids on ADHD-related symptoms in children with specific learning difficulties. Prog Neuropsychopharmacol Biol Psychiatry 2002;26:233–9.

41. Johnson M, Ostlund S, Fransson G, et al. Omega-3/omega-6 fatty acids for attention deficit hyperactivity disorder: a randomized placebo-controlled trial in children and adolescents. J Atten Disord 2009;12:394–401.

42. Belanger SA, Vanasse M, Spahis S, et al. Omega-3 fatty acid treatment of children with attention-deficit hyperactivity disorder: a randomized, double-blind, placebo-controlled study. Paediatr Child Health 2009;14:89–98.

43. Gustafsson PA, Birberg-Thornberg U, Duchen K, et al. EPA supplementation improves teacher-rated behaviour and oppositional symptoms in children with ADHD. Acta Paediatr 2010;99:1540–9.

44. Aman MG, Mitchell EA, Turbott SH. The effects of essential fatty acid supplementation by Efamol in hyperactive children. J Abnorm Child Psychol 1987;15:75–90.

45. Manor I, Magen A, Keidar D, et al. The effect of phosphatidylserine containing Omega3 fatty-acids on attention-deficit hyperactivity disorder symptoms in children: a double-blind placebo-controlled trial, followed by an open-label extension. Eur Psychiatry 2012;27(5):335–42.

46. Perera H, Jeewandara KC, Seneviratne S, et al. Combined omega3 and omega6 supplementation in children with attention-deficit hyperactivity disorder (ADHD) refractory to methylphenidate treatment: a double-blind, placebo-controlled study. J Child Neurol 2012;27(6):747–53.

47. Arnold LE, Kleykamp D, Votolato NA, et al. Gamma-linolenic acid for attention-deficit hyperactivity disorder: placebo-controlled comparison to D-amphetamine. Biol Psychiatry 1989;25:222–8.

48. Yehuda S, Rabinovitz-Shenkar S, Carasso RL. Effects of essential fatty acids in iron deficient and sleep-disturbed attention deficit hyperactivity disorder (ADHD) children. Eur J Clin Nutr 2011;65(10):1167–9.

49. Weber W, Vander Stoep A, McCarty RL, et al. Hypericum perforatum (St John's wort) for attention-deficit/hyperactivity disorder in children and adolescents: a randomized controlled trial. JAMA 2008;299(22):2633–41.

50. Bliwise DL, Ansari FP. Insomnia associated with valerian and melatonin usage in the 2002 National Health Interview Survey. Sleep 2007;30(7):881–4.

51. Ferracioli-Oda E, Qawasmi A, Bloch MH. Meta-analysis: melatonin for the treatment of primary sleep disorders. PLoS One 2013;8(5):e63773.

52. Weiss MD, Wasdell MB, Bomben MM, et al. Sleep hygiene and melatonin treatment for children and adolescents with ADHD and initial insomnia. J Am Acad Child Adolesc Psychiatry 2006;45(5):512–9.

53. Van der Heijden KB, Smits MG, Van Someren EJ, et al. Effect of melatonin on sleep, behavior, and cognition in ADHD and chronic sleep-onset insomnia. J Am Acad Child Adolesc Psychiatry 2007;46(2):233–41.

54. Van Oudheusden LJ, Scholte HR. Efficacy of carnitine in the treatment of children with attention-deficit hyperactivity disorder. Prostaglandins Leukot Essent Fatty Acids 2002;67(1):33–8.

55. Abbasi SH, Heidari S, Mohammadi MR, et al. Acetyl-L-carnitine as an adjunctive therapy in the treatment of attention-deficit/hyperactivity disorder in children and adolescents: a placebo-controlled trial. Child Psychiatry Hum Dev 2011;42(3): 367–75.

56. Arnold LE, Amato A, Bozzolo H, et al. Acetyl-L-carnitine (ALC) in attention-deficit/hyperactivity disorder: a multi-site, placebo-controlled pilot trial. J Child Adolesc Psychopharmacol 2007;17(6):791–802.

57. Scassellati C, Bonvicini C, Faraone SV, et al. Biomarkers and attention-deficit/hyperactivity disorder: a systematic review and meta-analyses. J Am Acad Child Adolesc Psychiatry 2012;51(10):1003–19.e20.

58. Konofal E, Lecendreux M, Deron J, et al. Effects of iron supplementation on attention deficit hyperactivity disorder in children. Pediatr Neurol 2008;38(1): 20–6.

59. Sandstead HH, Penland JG, Alcock NW, et al. Effects of repletion with zinc and other micronutrients on neuropsychologic performance and growth of Chinese children. Am J Clin Nutr 1998;68(Suppl 2):470S–5S.

60. Toren P, Eldar S, Sela BA, et al. Zinc deficiency in attention-deficit hyperactivity disorder. Biol Psychiatry 1996;40(12):1308–10.

61. Kozielec T, Kaszczyk-Kaczmarek K, Kotkowiak L, et al. The level of calcium, magnesium, zinc and copper in blood serum in children and young people between 5 and 18 years of age. Przegl Lek 1994;51(9):401–5 [in Polish].

62. Bekaroglu M, Aslan Y, Gedik Y, et al. Relationships between serum free fatty acids and zinc, and attention deficit hyperactivity disorder: a research note. J Child Psychol Psychiatry 1996;37(2):225–7.

63. Bilici M, Yildirim F, Kandil S, et al. Double-blind, placebo-controlled study of zinc sulfate in the treatment of attention deficit hyperactivity disorder. Prog Neuropsychopharmacol Biol Psychiatry 2004;28(1):181–90.

64. Akhondzadeh S, Mohammadi MR, Khademi M. Zinc sulfate as an adjunct to methylphenidate for the treatment of attention deficit hyperactivity disorder in

children: a double blind and randomized trial [ISRCTN64132371]. BMC Psychiatry 2004;4:9.

65. Zamora J, Velasquez A, Troncoso L, et al. Zinc in the therapy of the attention-deficit/hyperactivity disorder in children. A preliminary randomized controlled trial. Arch Latinoam Nutr 2011;61(3):242–6 [in Spanish].

66. Arnold LE, Disilvestro RA, Bozzolo D, et al. Zinc for attention-deficit/hyperactivity disorder: placebo-controlled double-blind pilot trial alone and combined with amphetamine. J Child Adolesc Psychopharmacol 2011;21(1):1–19.

67. Mahmoud MM, El-Mazary AA, Maher RM, et al. Zinc, ferritin, magnesium and copper in a group of Egyptian children with attention deficit hyperactivity disorder. Ital J Pediatr 2011;37:60.

68. Archana E, Pai P, Prabhu BK, et al. Altered biochemical parameters in saliva of pediatric attention deficit hyperactivity disorder. Neurochem Res 2012;37(2): 330–4.

69. Nogovitsina OR, Levitina EV. Neurological aspect of clinical symptoms, pathophysiology and correction in attention deficit hyperactivity disorder. Zh Nevrol Psikhiatr Im S S Korsakova 2006;106(2):17–20 [in Russian].

70. Irmisch G, Thome J, Reis O, et al. Modified magnesium and lipoproteins in children with attention deficit hyperactivity disorder (ADHD). World J Biol Psychiatry 2011;12(Suppl 1):63–5.

71. Antalis CJ, Stevens LJ, Campbell M, et al. Omega-3 fatty acid status in attention-deficit/hyperactivity disorder. Prostaglandins Leukot Essent Fatty Acids 2006;75(4–5):299–308.

72. Cardoso CC, Lobato KR, Binfare RW, et al. Evidence for the involvement of the monoaminergic system in the antidepressant-like effect of magnesium. Prog Neuropsychopharmacol Biol Psychiatry 2009;33(2):235–42.

73. Schmidt ME, Kruesi MJ, Elia J, et al. Effect of dextroamphetamine and methylphenidate on calcium and magnesium concentration in hyperactive boys. Psychiatry Res 1994;54(2):199–210.

74. Canter PH, Ernst E. Ginkgo biloba is not a smart drug: an updated systematic review of randomised clinical trials testing the nootropic effects of G. biloba extracts in healthy people. Hum Psychopharmacol 2007;22(5):265–78.

75. Salehi B, Imani R, Mohammadi MR, et al. Ginkgo biloba for attention-deficit/hyperactivity disorder in children and adolescents: a double blind, randomized controlled trial. Prog Neuropsychopharmacol Biol Psychiatry 2010;34(1):76–80.

76. Muller WE, Rolli M, Schafer C, et al. Effects of hypericum extract (LI 160) in biochemical models of antidepressant activity. Pharmacopsychiatry 1997; 30(Suppl 2):102–7.

77. Tenenbaum S, Paull JC, Sparrow EP, et al. An experimental comparison of Pycnogenol and methylphenidate in adults with attention-deficit/hyperactivity disorder (ADHD). J Atten Disord 2002;6(2):49–60.

78. Trebatická J, Kopasova S, Hradecna Z, et al. Treatment of ADHD with French maritime pine bark extract, Pycnogenol. Eur Child Adolesc Psychiatry 2006; 15(6):329–35.

Healthy Body, Healthy Mind?
The Effectiveness of Physical Activity to Treat ADHD in Children

Jeffrey M. Halperin, PhD[a],*, Olga G. Berwid, PhD[b],
Sarah O'Neill, PhD[c]

KEYWORDS

- Physical activity • Exercise • Attention-deficit/hyperactivity disorder • ADHD
- Children • Intervention • Treatment • Evidence-based

KEY POINTS

- Structured physical activity has the potential to be an effective treatment of ADHD in children.
- Incontrovertible data from animal studies indicate that exercise enhances brain development and behavioral functioning.
- Studies suggest that, acutely, physical activity may lead to gains in neuropsychological functioning, including processing speed and some executive functions.
- After long-term (ie, ≥5 weeks) moderate–vigorous exercise interventions, research suggests that children's ADHD-related behaviors may be less severe and improvements in performance on measures of neuropsychological function may be observed.
- Physical activity may offer benefits over and above psychostimulant use.
- The current literature is predominated with small, unblinded pilot studies. The field needs methodologically robust, blinded, randomized controlled trials to determine the efficacy of physical activity as a treatment of children's ADHD.

This work was supported by grant #'s R01 MH68286 and R33MH085898 from the National Institute of Mental Health to J.M. Halperin. The content is solely the responsibility of the authors and does not necessarily represent the official view of the National Institute of Mental Health.
Disclosure Statement: The authors report no conflicts of interest.
[a] Psychology Department, Queens College, The City University of New York (CUNY), 65-30 Kissena Boulevard, Flushing, NY 11367, USA; [b] York College, The City University of New York (CUNY), 94-20 Guy R. Brewer Boulevard, Jamaica, NY 11451, USA; [c] Psychology Department, The City College, The City University of New York (CUNY), 160 Convent Avenue, New York, NY 10031, USA
* Corresponding author.
E-mail address: Jeffrey.halperin@qc.cuny.edu

Abbreviations	
ADHD	Attention-deficit/hyperactivity disorder
ASER	Acoustic startle eyeblink response
ASQ	Conners Abbreviated Symptom Questionnaire
BDNF	Brain-derived neurotrophic factor
BMI	Body mass index
Bpm	Beats per minute
CBCL	Child Behavior Checklist
CPT-II	Conners Continuous Performance Test, Second Edition
DA	Dopamine
HR	Heart rate
HRmax	Maximum heart rate
LD	Learning disorder
MPH	Methylphenidate
MVPA	Moderate–vigorous physical activity
RCT	Randomized controlled trial
RPE	Ratings of perceived exertion
SSRS	Social Skills Rating System
Vo_2	Oxygen consumption per unit time
Vo_{2max}	Maximum oxygen consumption
WCST	Wisconsin Card Sorting Test
WISC-R	Wechsler Intelligence Scale for Children-Revised
YSR	Youth Self Report

INTRODUCTION/BACKGROUND

Target of Treatment

Emerging research suggests considerable potential for enhanced physical activity, in particular regular moderately intensive aerobic exercise, to be beneficial to the core inattentive and hyperactive/impulsive symptoms of ADHD, an array of neuropsychological deficits associated with the disorder, and perhaps academic difficulties. In addition, improved physical health and fitness that results from such exercise programs may increase status with peers and, in turn, improve peer relations.

Need for Treatment

At present, there are 2 well-established evidence-based treatment strategies for childhood ADHD: medication and behavior modification. As such, one may ask, why is anything else needed? Current evidence-based interventions, however, although providing symptomatic relief to many patients, have several significant limitations, making them far from a panacea.

Recent estimates from the Centers for Disease Control and Prevention indicate that as many as 6.1% (3.5 million) of American youth between the ages of 4 and 17 years are being treated with medication for ADHD.[1] This reflects both the high prevalence of ADHD in the population and that, relative to other interventions, medication, in particular psychostimulants, are generally safe and provide the greatest symptomatic relief.[2,3] Yet, treatment with medication has several well-known limitations, including that some children do not respond or experience side effects precluding their use; many parents and children are not comfortable with medication as an ongoing intervention for children; a substantial portion of individuals have only a partial response to treatment, leaving them still highly symptomatic; and despite that ADHD is considered a chronic disorder, a majority of individuals prescribed medication stop taking it within the first year,[4,5] and once medication is terminated, symptoms typically return the next day. In addition, despite its efficacy for treating inattention, impulsiveness, and overactivity, medication is less effective for treating associated features, such as poor social skills[6] and executive function deficits.[7]

Most psychosocial treatments of ADHD train parents and/or teachers to use an array of contingency management techniques to help manage the behavioral difficulties of their children and/or students. Data suggest that psychosocial interventions are not as effective as medication for reducing core ADHD symptoms,[2,8] yet they seem effective for improving associated impairments, such as oppositional behavior and defiance.[8] Psychosocial treatments are difficult to use, however, and are often expensive. Furthermore, beneficial effects tend not to generalize beyond the setting in which the intervention is used. Finally, like medication, once the active phase of the intervention ends, benefits rapidly subside and there seems little or no long-term benefit to children with ADHD.[9]

Thus, current interventions provide short-term benefits to children with ADHD, but as soon as treatment ends, symptoms and associated impairments rapidly return. It could be argued that patients should continue taking medication throughout development and into early adulthood or as long as they remain symptomatic. This might work, but unfortunately, few patients, for a variety of reasons, remain on medication for more than a year.[4,5] Because few, if any, medical or psychosocial treatments are maintained over extended periods of time for this chronic disorder, alternative approaches are warranted. The authors propose the implementation of lifestyle changes in the form of physical exercise that is incorporated into daily routines early in life. This may not yield the dramatic acute symptom relief characteristic of medication, but it has the potential for flattening the adverse trajectory of the disorder and improving long-term outcomes.[10]

PHYSICAL ACTIVITY AS AN INTERVENTION FOR ADHD
Theoretic Overview

Data paint a picture of ADHD as an etiologically heterogeneous neurodevelopmental disorder that varies with regard to behavioral phenotypes as well as underlying genetic and neural substrates. Children with ADHD present with an array of executive[11] and nonexecutive[12] neurocognitive deficits with differing patterns of weaknesses across children.[13–15] Consistent with neurocognitive data, structural neuroimaging data indicate that youth with ADHD have smaller overall brain size[16] and delays in cortical development that are most prominent in prefrontal regions but present throughout the cerebral cortex.[17,18] Similarly, functional neuroimaging data suggest that in many respects, children with ADHD have neural responses to stimuli that are similar to younger typically developing children.[19] Thus, considerable data indicate that as a group, children with ADHD have delayed or diminished brain development compared with their typically developing peers and that neural and neurocognitive deficits are pervasive and not limited to a single brain region or neurocognitive domain. Furthermore, emerging data suggest that clinical improvement over development may be associated with neurocognitive improvements[20,21] as well as normalization in cortical development[22,23] and enhanced thalamocortical functional connectivity[24] relative to those with persisting ADHD symptoms. Although these longitudinal data are correlational in nature and causal inferences must be made with caution, they suggest a direct link between brain development and symptom remission across the lifespan.[25,26] As such, it has been suggested that environmental influences that enhance brain development could have long-term beneficial effects on ADHD outcomes.[10,27]

The notion that environmental factors influence brain development is not new. In the 1940s, Hebb[28] demonstrated that synapses were strengthened by repeated use, and in the 1960s Rosenzweig and Bennett[29,30] showed that environmental manipulations affect brain weight, cortical thickness, the structure of dendrites, and cognitive functioning. Hubel and Weisel's[31] Nobel prize winning work demonstrated that environmental influences alter neurodevelopment in the visual system, and through a series of studies in the 1970s, Greenough and colleagues[32–34] demonstrated the impact of environmental enhancements on a range of neural processes, including dendritic branching, spine density, synaptogenesis, angiogenesis, and gliogenesis. More recent research in nonhuman species has consistently shown that environmental enrichment promotes brain growth (for review, see Halperin and Healey[27]).

Physical exercise is one environmental factor that influences the trajectory of neural development. Two hundred years ago, Spurzheim (1815, as cited by Rosenzweig[29[p321]]) proposed that it was likely that "the organs [of the brain] increase by exercise." Compelling evidence from nonhuman animal research and emerging human literature suggest that Spurzheim was accurate. Physical exercise is defined as an increase in energy expenditure resulting from musculoskeletal movement for the purposes of increasing physical fitness. Physical exercise can be categorized into 2 types: anaerobic and aerobic, which are differentiated by the energy transfer systems that fuel them. Anaerobic exercise is typically characterized as brief (60–180 seconds), high-intensity exertion. When immediate energy stores in muscle become depleted, the continuation of physical exertion requires more sustained energy in the form of aerobic metabolism, which is mediated through increased oxygen consumption via increased overall blood flow (ie, cardiac output) and respiration. With repeated aerobic training, the efficiency of aerobic metabolic functions to fulfill energy needs is facilitated, resulting in the quicker onset of the aerobic kinetic response, a greater capacity for oxygen consumption, and smaller demands on the anaerobic system.[35]

Other physical adaptations occur with repeated aerobic training that have positive impacts physical health, including the reduction of body mass and body fat, a more favorable body fat distribution, stronger skeleton and musculature, enhanced physical functioning (eg, greater endurance), and reductions in risk for a variety of health problems, including cardiovascular disease, type 2 diabetes and metabolic syndrome, and some cancers.[36] In light of these health implications, the US Department of Health and Human Services[37] has published age-based guidelines outlining the minimum amount and intensity of physical activity in which individuals should engage. Children and adolescents are recommended to get at least 60 minutes of exercise per day, most of which should be at moderate–vigorous intensity.

Evidence for the potential utility of exercise in the treatment of ADHD is derived from several disparate lines of research: (1) experimental evidence, primarily in animals, demonstrating the impact of exercise on neural functioning and development; (2) experimental data indicating that exercise has positive effects on cognitive/executive control both in adults and typically developing children; and (3) preliminary evidence that exercise improves behavior and cognitive functioning in children with ADHD.

Animal studies

A substantial body of research conducted primarily in rodents provides strong evidence that physical exercise promotes up-regulation of neurotrophic factors that regulate neural development, including the survival, growth, and differentiation of neurons[38,39]; synaptogenesis and myelination[40]; neurogenesis[41,42] and angiogenesis[43,44] (for review see[45–47]). In rats, physical exercise results in increased levels of synaptic proteins,[48–50] glutamate receptors,[51] brain-derived neurotrophic factor (BDNF[52]), and insulin-like growth factor-1.[53] Acute physical exercise also promotes monoamine neurotransmission, by increasing levels of serotonin,[54,55] DA,[56,57] and norepineph-rine.[54,55] The effects of exercise on brain structure and function seem more pro-nounced in younger animals as the capacity for exercise-induced neuroplasticity decreases with age.[58,59]

In concert with these biological changes, physical exercise has been shown to result in improvements in spatial learning,[42,60–63] passive avoidance memory,[64] and motor velocity and balance[56] in normoactive rat species. In addition, several studies provide evidence that exercise may remediate neurocognitive deficits in the spontaneously hy-pertensive rat (SHR), a commonly used animal model of ADHD.[65] After exercise, reduc-tions in locomotion,[63,66] improved spatial learning,[63] reduced responsiveness (ie, orienting) to behaviorally irrelevant stimuli,[66–68] and improvements in social behavior[66–68] have been reported. These effects in rodents were more pronounced in adolescence than in young adulthood[66] and were approximately equivalent in magni-tude to those shown for animals administered MPH and atomoxetine.[67] Finally, consis-tent with literature regarding the suspected mechanisms by which exercise exerts its impact on neurocognition, Kim[63] showed that although tyrosine hydroxylase, the rate-limiting enzyme in the synthesis of DA, and BDNF expression in the substantia nigra and hippocampus were significantly decreased in nonexercising SHRs, they were both increased in exercising SHR rats after 20 days of daily exercise on a treadmill.

Studies in healthy humans

Consistent with findings in animals, physical exercise has been shown to have both direct and indirect effects in humans on neural systems believed to play a role in neu-rocognitive functioning and the pathophysiology of ADHD.[69–71] Physical exercise has been reported to enhance catecholaminergic neurotransmission, which was related to changes in executive performance immediately after exercise.[72] It also produces in-creases in blood flow to the brain[73] and increases in BDNF,[74,75] which plays a role in the differentiation and survival of DA neurons.[76,77]

Accumulating data suggest that exercise exerts a beneficial impact on a variety of cognitive functions in humans across development, including, notably, speed of responding, executive functions, and memory and learning. It seems, however, that the exercise-cognition relationship is complicated by a multitude of moderating fac-tors, including (1) whether outcomes are measured acutely versus after a more extended intervention, consisting of regular repeated bouts of exercise aimed at improving overall fitness over the course of weeks or months; (2) the intensity of the exercise; (3) age; (4) the specific cognitive functions measured; and individual differ-ences in both (5) baseline cognitive functioning and (6) aerobic fitness.[78,79]

Recent meta-analyses have determined that, acutely, exercise confers benefits to overall cognitive functioning across all developmental levels.[78–80] Studies in young adults predominate the literature, and although several studies and reviews have concluded that exercise has an acutely beneficial impact in children, particularly in ex-ecutive functioning,[81–86] some suggest that exercise may be more beneficial to young adults.[79] In young adults, exercise results in faster response times[87,88] and improved performance on objective measures of inhibitory control and working memory.[79,80] A more recent meta-analysis,[80] which focused exclusively on executive function out-comes, indicated that at least in the domain of inhibition/interference control, moderate-intensity exercise is acutely beneficial to preadolescent children, adoles-cents, and young adults, with effect sizes in the moderate range and no differences among the age groups.

Experimentally controlled chronic exercise interventions in typically developing humans have been conducted less frequently. Chronic exercise improves attention, processing speed, working memory and other executive functions, and memory in older adults.[89] Findings from this age group are of limited relevance to ADHD, however, given the early onset of ADHD and evidence that functional impairment declines with age. In younger populations, there are preliminary data suggesting that chronic exercise is beneficial to cognition. Correlational studies indicate that in children, physical fitness, ostensibly a result of long-term exercise, is positively associated with performance on cognitive tasks as well as neurophysiological indices of neurocognitive functioning.[86,90] Causal inferences from correlational studies cannot, however, be made.

Only a few experimental studies examining the impact of chronic exercise interventions on neurocognitive functioning have been conducted in typically developing children.[91–97] These studies provide preliminary evidence that prolonged periods of repeated physical activity may improve some measures of executive functioning, notably spatial span and working memory, in addition to changes in neurophysiologic measures of cortical functioning in areas of the brain underlying cognitive control. One review[98] concluded that chronic exercise improves dual task coordination and shifting; whether it benefits performance on complex tasks that tax multiple higher-order cognitive functions is less clear.

Two recent meta-analyses examined the impact of exercise on academic achievement.[99,100] Consistent with the conclusions of prior systematic reviews,[84,101] both concluded that increases in physical activity resulted in small, but significant improvements in children's academic performance. One large-scale study showed that this benefit was present even when time was reassigned from academic instruction.[102]

Finally, several studies have provided evidence that exercise enhances attention, concentration, and social functioning in the classroom, with greater effects in children exhibiting disruptive behaviors (for review, see Trudeau and Shephard[101]). In-class physical activity and frequent recess breaks in school have been found to increase children's time on task right after completing these physical activities.[103–105] Longer-term sustained effects of the interventions on behavior, however, were not examined. One meta-analysis[106] concluded that exercise reduces disruptive behavior and aggression in typically developing children and adults. This is notable in light of the high comorbidity between ADHD and disruptive behaviors.[107]

In sum, compelling evidence indicates that physical exercise facilitates brain development in animals and, in geriatric populations, regular physical exercise delays age-related and pathologic declines in neural integrity and cognitive functioning. Furthermore, preliminary evidence indicates that physical exercise may improve cognitive functioning in healthy children and young adults. Because exercise seems to enhance brain development and function across a wide array of domains, and ADHD is associated with delayed brain development[17,18] and immature brain function,[19] it is possible that exercise has the potential to promote recovery in children with ADHD.[27,81] Given the heterogeneity of ADHD, however, it is possible that exercise may work for some individuals and not for others and/or that different individuals may respond differently to various exercise types and intensities.

EMPIRICAL SUPPORT FOR THE USE OF EXERCISE IN CHILDREN WITH ADHD

Several preliminary studies have been published throughout the past decade examining both the acute and chronic effects of exercise on children with ADHD (**Table 1**). Studies examining acute effects have typically had participants walk or run on a treadmill or pedal on a cycle ergometer, so that exercise intensity could be well controlled. Studies examining chronic exercise interventions have varied widely

Table 1
Studies examining the impact of exercise on children with ADHD

Study	Participants (N [Boys])	Study Design	Exercise and Control Groups	Measures	Outcome
Ahmed & Mohamed,[119] 2011	84 (50) With ADHD (investigators report children randomly assigned to 3 equal groups) 11–16 y Meds use not reported (discussion alludes to medication treatment).	Between-subjects (exercise vs control); repeated measures pre–post exercise (each group analyzed separately, rather than in a single mixed ANOVA)	Exercise: mod aerobic— (intensity reported by investigators; not measured). 3×/wk for 10 wk; week 1–4: 40 min week 5–10: 50 min + 30-min walk in weekend from week 6 Control: activities of control group not reported	Based on teacher report the interviewer completed the behavior rating scale: attention, motor skills, task orientation, emotional and oppositional behavior, academic and classroom behavior	Exercise group: sig improvement in attention, motor skills, and academic and classroom behavior Control group: no significant changes from pre–post intervention
Bernard-Brak et al,[123] 2011	17,565 (~50%) from community-based sample K–1st grade Meds use not reported	Longitudinal	Exercise: physical education classes within curriculum; intensity not reported Control: N/A	Derived from parent and teacher ratings: physical activity composite and ADHD severity	Sig negative relation between physical activity in K and ADHD severity in 1st grade

(continued on next page)

Table 1
(continued)

Study	Participants (N [Boys])	Study Design	Exercise and Control Groups	Measures	Outcome
Chang et al,[110] 2012	40 (37) All with ADHD 8–13 y 10 Children in exercise gp and 10 children in control gp taking medicine	2 (Group: exercise, control) × 2 (time: pre-, postexercise) with repeated measures over time	Exercise: single bout of 30-min treadmill running; mod intensity (50%–70% HR reserve; RPE 12–15) Control: watched an exercise-related video for 30 min	Stroop test: color, word, color-word (time to complete, seconds) WCST: total correct, perseverative responses, perseverative errors, nonperseverative errors, conceptual level response, categories completed	Stroop Color–Word: sig group × time interaction—both groups faster at post-test, but exercise group faster than controls WCST non-perseverative errors and categories completed: group × time interaction—time effect for exercise group not seen in controls, pretest group differences not observed post-test. WCST total correct, perseverative responses, perseverative errors and conceptual level responses: ME time (improvement post-test) but no ME group and no group × time interaction.

Study	Sample	Design	Intervention	Measures	Results
Craft,[108] 1983	31 (31) Hyperactive 31 (31) Controls 7–10 y Medication naive	Within-subjects—order of cycling sessions randomized	Exercise: cycle ergometer; physical work capacity HR = 170 bpm; 3 × single sessions lasting for 1, 5, and 10 min. Control: no active control condition—1-, 5-, and 10-min cycling compared with rest	WISC-R Digit Span, WISC-R Coding B, Illinois Test of Psycholinguistic Abilities—Visual Sequential Memory	Digit Span, Coding, and Visual Sequential Memory: group ME (non-hyperactive boys performed better than hyperactive boys). No session ME. No group × session interactions
Gapin & Etnier,[126] 2010	18 (18) ADHD 8–12 y 18 Taking MPH or amph 2 Melatonin; 3 omega-3 All taking medication as prescribed during testing	Correlational	Exercise: not manipulated—"naturally occurring" MVPA recorded over a 7-d period (eg, swimming, skateboarding, biking) Control: N/A	Time in MVPA (from accelerometer and self-reported daily physical activity logs) Children's Color Trails Tests 1 and 2—time to completion Digit Span—total scaled score Tower of London—total move score Total correct score Total execution time	Greater time spent in MVPA predictor of lower TOL total move score and faster total execution time (both indicative of better performance)

(continued on next page)

Table 1
(continued)

Study	Participants (N [Boys])	Study Design	Exercise and Control Groups	Measures	Outcome
Kang et al,[125] 2011	32 (32) ADHD Randomly assigned to medicine + sports therapy, medicine + education intervention (M [SD] age = 8.4 ± 0.9 y) or medicine + education intervention (M [SD] age = 8.6 ± 1.2 y) 32 ppts started at 10 mg MPH; titrated to 20–40 mg first week. Dose maintained for intervention	2 (Intervention: medicine + sports therapy, medicine + education) × 2 (time: pre, post) with repeated measures over time	Exercise: moderate aerobic (eg, shuttle runs) and goal-directed exercise (eg, throwing tennis ball at a target) and jump rope 2 × 90-min sessions per week for 6 wk Control: medicine + education sessions about behavioral control (12 sessions over 6 wk)	Parent ratings on Korean version of DuPaul's ADHD rating scale: inattention; hyperactivity/ impulsivity; total score Teacher ratings on SSRS: self-control; cooperativeness; verbal assertion Digit Symbol test of the KEDI-WISC Trail Making Test B	Parent-rated inattention and total scores: group × time interaction—sport group showed greater improvement pre–post treatment than education group. Parent-rated hyperactivity: no sig differences in change in score between groups Teacher-rated cooperativeness: greater increase in scores from pre–post intervention for sports group than for education group Teacher-rated self-control and verbal assertiveness: no sig differences in change in score between groups Digit symbol test: sig improvement from pre–post treatment of sport group; no change for education group Trail making test B: greater reduction in time to complete task from pre–post treatment of sport group than education group

| Katz et al,[127] 2010 | 1214 (593) from community-based sample 2nd–4th grade Schools randomly assigned to physical activity (PA) intervention group or control group PA group: n = 655 (326 boys); 21% taking medicine for ADHD Controls: n = 559 (267 boys); 14% taking medicine for ADHD | 2 (Group: PA group, controls) × 2 (time: pre, post) with repeated measures over time | Exercise: activity bursts, comprising warm-up (stretch, light aerobic exercise), core strength, or aerobic activities (eg, squats), and cool down (stretch, low-intensity exercise). Intensity not measured. Aim was for at least 30 min cumulative total time per day spent in activity bursts. Duration of intervention = 6 mo Control: normal curricular activities | Anthropometric and physical fitness: weight; BMI; endurance; strength; flexibility; Vo_{2max} Medication use: asthma and ADHD Classroom behavior: work and social skills on the independence school district (ISD) progress report card Student attitudes toward physical activity: school physical activity and nutrition questionnaire Academic performance: classroom grades (communication arts and math components of the ISD progress report card); last quarter grades; Missouri Academic Performance (MAP) scores | Anthropometric and physical fitness: sig decline in weight and BMI for controls but not PA ppts; greater gains in right side flexibility for controls than PA group; greater gains in abdominal and upper body strength, and trunk extensor Medication use: sig decrease asthma meds and trend for decrease in ADHD meds by PA group Classroom behavior and student attitudes toward physical activity: no sig group differences in change in ISD work and social skills or attitudes to physical activity Academic performance: no sig group differences in change in MAP reading or math achievement; greater ppn controls improved math and reading (using ISD progress report) than in PA group |

(continued on next page)

Table 1
(continued)

Study	Participants (N [Boys])	Study Design	Exercise and Control Groups	Measures	Outcome
Kiluk et al,[122] 2009	65 (40) ADHD 32 (16) LD 6–14 y Medication status not reported	Retrospective, cross-sectional design	Exercise: number of sports and time spent playing sports as reported by parents on the CBCL (children classified as having played 0–2 sports or 3+ sports) Intensity not measured Control: N/A	CBCL: anxious/depressed subscale	4 Separate analyses: ADHD boys and girls; LD boys and girls, controlling for CBCL social and school scores For both boys and girls with ADHD, lower anxious/depressed scores in children whose parents reported them playing 3+ sports compared with children playing 0–2 sports For boys or girls with an LD, no diff in anxious/depressed scores as a function of number sports
Lufi & Parish-Plass,[117] 2011	15 (15) ADHD 17 (17) Other behavioral problems 8–13.5 y Medication naive	2 (Group: ADHD, other behavioral problems) × 3 (time: pre-exercise, post-exercise, 1-y follow-up), with repeated measures over time	Exercise: individual PA (eg, relay races); group-based PA (eg, soccer, basketball) Intensity not measured; 20 90-min sessions comprising individual (20–30 min) and group-based (30–40 min) PA and 25–40 min discussion	Parents-rated ASQ-P and CBCL Child-rated YSR CBCL and YSR scales: withdrawn, aggression, anxiety, attention, delinquency, social, somatic, thoughts, internalizing,	ASQ-P: ME time—scores decreased over time (no posthocs performed); ME group not reported; no group × time interaction CBCL: ME time for aggression, anxiety, attention, social, externalizing, and

Study	Sample	Design	Intervention	Measures	Results
			Control: no active control—post-exercise and 1-y follow-up compared with pre-exercise	externalizing, and total	total—scores decreased over time (no posthocs performed); ME group not reported; no group × time interaction YSR: ME time for anxiety, somatic, internalizing, and total scales—scores decreased over time (posthocs not performed); ME group not reported; no group × time interaction
McKune et al,[124] 2003	19 (13) ADHD all taking MPH Ppts assigned (but not randomly) to exercise (n = 13; 10 boys; M ± SD age = 10.8 ± 1.9 y) or Control (n = 6; 3 boys M ± SD age = 11.2 ± 1.5 y)	2 (Group: exercise, control) × 3 (time: pre, during, after intervention) with repeated measures over time	Exercise: 15-min warm-up, 30-min aerobic activity (eg, skipping), 10-min cool-down 50%–75% HRmax—aim to be exercising at target HR at least 20 min; 5×/wk for 5 wk Control: no active control, during and post-ex vs pre-ex	Modified Conners Parent Rating Scale: total behavior, attention, emotional, motor skills, task orientation, oppositional behavior	No significant findings emerged when data analyzed as a function of group and time Data collapsed across group and investigated using repeated measures across time Significant improvements seen in total behavior, attention, emotional and motor skills but not task orientation or oppositional behavior, from pre-intervention to post-intervention

(continued on next page)

Table 1
(continued)

Study	Participants (N [Boys])	Study Design	Exercise and Control Groups	Measures	Outcome
Medina et al,[113] 2010	25 (25) ADHD 7–15 y 16 Boys taking MPH (withheld 48 h prior to testing)	Between-subjects (non-user vs MPH) Within-subjects (treadmill vs stretching)—order of conditions not stated	Exercise: high-intensity treadmill; single 30-min session of 10 × 2-min intervals, with 1-min rest between each interval Control: 1-min of stretching (quadriceps and triceps bilaterally each for 15 s)	CPT-II: omissions, commissions, Hit RT, Hit SE, variability of SE, d', Response Style (B), Perseveration, Hit RT Block Change, Hit SE Block Change Hit RT Interstimulus (ISI) Change, Hit SE ISI change, confidence index (CI)	No difference on any of the 13 CPT-II measures post-ex as a function of medication status. Data collapsed across medication status and within-subjects comparison of CPT-II performance after ex compared with stretching. Compared with stretching, after ex sig improvement in Hit RT, Hit SE, Hit RT ISI change, perseveration, and CI
Pontifex et al,[109] 2013	20 (14) ADHD 20 (14) Controls 8–10 y No medication for at least 1 mo prior to study	2 (Group: ADHD, controls) × 2 (session: treadmill, reading), with repeated measures over session Order of treadmill and reading sessions counterbalanced	Exercise: single 20-min session on treadmill at 65%–75% HRmax Control: reading	Flanker task: accuracy, median RT, post-error median RT P3 amplitude, latency ERN WRAT3 Reading Comprehension, Arithmetic, and Spelling	Flanker: accuracy—improved after exercise for both ADHD and controls relative to reading; median RT—no sig ME or interactions; post-error median RT—group × session interaction with greater post-error slowing after exercise relative to reading for ADHD group

					P3: amplitude—larger for both groups after ex relative to reading; latency—shorter after ex for both groups relative to reading ERN—smaller in ADHD after reading; no between-group differences after ex WRAT3 reading comp, arithmetic—both ADHD and controls improved after exercise relative to reading; spelling—no sig ME or interactions.
Reza & Hamid,[118] 2011	20 ADHD (gender breakdown not reported) 7-11 y Investigators state, "subjects … underwent to drug treatment"—no other details.	Within-subjects; repeated measures over time (pre-exercise, post-exercise, and 2-wk follow-up).	Exercise: 10-min warm-up; 15 min with ball; 5-min cool-down 30-min cycle. Intensity not reported. 2 × 60-min sessions per week for 16 wk Control: no active control Post-ex and 2-wk FU vs pre-ex	Parent- and teacher-rated Child Symptom Inventory (CSI-4)—attention and hyperactivity/impulsivity severity	CSI-4 attention and hyp/imp severity—ME time. For both parent and teacher, sig decrease from pre-exercise to post-exercise, maintained at 2-wk follow-up (post-exercise and follow-up not sig different)

(continued on next page)

Table 1
(continued)

Study	Participants (N [Boys])	Study Design	Exercise and Control Groups	Measures	Outcome
Smith et al,[120] 2013	14 (6) At risk for ADHD (had 4+ hyp/imp *DSM-IV* symptoms using parent and teacher reports on the Disruptive Behavior Disorders rating scale) 5.2–8.7 y Medication naïve	Within-subjects; repeated measures over time (pre-, post-intervention). For weekly and daily measures, first half of the program compared with second half of the program.	Exercise: MVPA aerobic activity (eg, skipping, crab walking) 30-min sessions (of which at least 26 min spent in MVPA) every school day for 8 wk Control: no active control condition. Post-exercise compared with pre-exercise	Pre-post: Bruininks-Oseretsky Test of Motor Proficiency-2 (BOT-2); Motor Timing; Shape School A–D; WPPSI-R/WISC-III Mazes; WRAML2 Finger Windows and Sentence Memory WJ III Cog Numbers Reversed Weekly: Simon says and red light/green light—ppn inhibition failures; Pittsburgh Modified Conners Teacher Rating Scale: Abbreviated Conners, Iowa inattention/overactivity, Iowa oppositional/defiant, peer interactions scale Daily: observations of neg. behaviors: not speaking nicely, interrupting, intentional aggression, unintentional aggression, not following adult directions Post-program: ratings of perceived improvement by parent, teacher, staff	Significant improvement pre–post intervention seen on BOT-2, Shape School Condition B (response inhibition), red light/green light proportion of inhibition failures, abbreviated Conners score, Iowa inattention/overactivity score, Iowa oppositional/defiant score, and behavioral observations of interrupting Global ratings of overall improvement—% of children rated as improved by • Parent = 69% • Teacher = 64% • Staff = 71%

Study	Sample	Method	Measures	Results
Tantillo et al,[115] 2002	18 (10) ADHD 25 (11) Controls 8–12 y All children with ADHD taking MPH—stopped 24 h before testing	2 (Group: ADHD, controls) × 2 (gender: male, female) × Condition (VO_2 peak, 65%–75% VO_2 peak, quiet rest) × 2 (time: pre-, post-condition), repeated measures over condition and time High-intensity ex always first; submax exercise and quiet rest counterbalanced	Exercise: treadmill Two exercise sessions: 1. VO_2 peak exercise test (duration 5–25 min to reach max) 2. 65%–75% VO_2 peak (duration matched to individual's maximal test) Control: quiet rest	STAIC—state anxiety Rate of spontaneous eyeblinks ASER: amplitude and latency Motor Impersistence Battery (MIB)	State anxiety: no effects observed Spontaneous eyeblink: ADHD boys faster blink rate after max exercise, no change after quiet rest or submax ex. ADHD girls and controls—little change in spontaneous eyeblinks across time ASER amplitude: increase in ASER in ADHD girls after submax ex. After quiet rest, increase in ASER for control boys but decrease for control girls ASER latency: ADHD boys—decrease in latency after max ex, little change after submax ex and quiet rest; ADHD girls—decrease in latency after submax ex, little change after max ex and quiet rest; controls—no change over time or conditions MIB: ADHD boys—better scores after max ex, no diff after submax ex or rest; controls—no effects

(continued on next page)

Table 1
(continued)

Study	Participants (N [Boys])	Study Design	Exercise and Control Groups	Measures	Outcome
Verret et al,[121] 2012	21 (19) ADHD participants assigned (but not randomly) to PA program (n = 10; 9 boys) or control group (n = 11; 10 boys) 7–12 y 11 Controls and 3 children in the PA program taking stimulant meds. Asked not to take medicine the day before testing.	2 (Group: PA, controls) × 2 (time: pre, post) with repeated measures over time	Exercise: aerobic, muscular and motor skills exercises MVPA (average HR measured during PA program = 154 bpm, 77% HRmax) 45-min sessions 3×/wk for 10 wk Control: no exercise	Anthropometric and fitness measures: weight, BMI, percentile BMI, push-ups (max #), sit-ups (#/60 s), flexibility, resting HR, Bruce running time, Bruce percentile Test of gross motor development 2: locomotor; object control; total motor control Test of everyday attention (Tea-Ch): sky search (visual search), score (auditory sustained attent.), sky search DT (divided attent), walk don't walk (response inh) CBCL—parent, teacher: anx-dep, withdrawn-depression, somatic, social probs, thought probs, attent probs, rule breaking; aggressive; internalized probs, externalized probs, total probs	ANCOVA used to compare between PA and control groups on post-test scores, adjusted for differences in pre-test scores. Anthropometric and fitness: PA group carried out more push-ups than the control group; no other differences. Motor skills: PA group higher locomotor and total motor scores than controls Tea-Ch: only sig difference was on score pondered; PA group demonstrated better auditory sustained attention than controls. CBCL—parent: PA group sig lower than controls on social, thought, attention, and total probs CBCL—teacher: no sig diff between groups post-intervention

| Wigal et al,[116] 2003 | 10 (10) ADHD-Combined; (8) controls 7–12 y Medication naive | 2 (Group: ADHD vs controls) × 4 (time: pre-exercise; peak exercise; 30-min post-exercise; 60-min post-exercise), with repeated measures over time | Exercise: cycle ergometry Intensity = 50% of the difference between anaerobic or lactate threshold and peak V_{O_2}; single 30-min session comprising 10 × 2-min intervals, with 1-min rest between each interval Control: no active control. Peak and post-exercise vs pre-exercise | Blood samples taken pre-exercise, during last 2 min of exercise, and 30 min and 60 min after exercise to yield radioactive metabolites DA, NE, EP, and plasma lactate | DA: sig increase for controls but not ADHD children during exercise NE: ADHD children lower than controls pre-ex. In response to ex, NE increased for both groups, but greater increase in controls than ADHD children Plasma lactate, EP: group × time interaction—plasma lactate and EP increased for both groups during exercise; greater increase in controls compared with ADHD at peak exercise |

Abbreviations: ADHD, attention-deficit/hyperactivity disorder; amph, amphetamine; ANCOVA, analysis of covariance; ANOVA, analysis of variance; anx-dep, anxious-depressed; ASER, acoustic startle eyeblink response; ASQ-P, Conners Abbreviated Symptom Questionnaire-Parent; attent, attention; B, response style; BMI, body mass index; BOT-2, Bruininks-Oseretsky Test of Motor Proficiency-2; bpm, beats per minute; CBCL, Child Behavior Checklist; CI, confidence index; CPT-II, Conners Continuous Performance Test, Second Edition; CSI-4, Child Symptom Inventory, Fourth Edition; d, day; d′, detectability; DA, dopamine; DSM-IV, Diagnostic and Statistical Manual of Mental Disorders, 4th Edition; EP, epinephrine; ERN, error-related negativity; ex, exercise; FU, follow-up; gp, group; h, hour; HR, heart rate; HRmax, maximum heart rate; hyp/imp, hyperactive/impulsive; inh, inhibition; ISD, interstimulus interval; ISI, interstimulus interval; KEDI-WISC, Korean Educational Development Institute–Wechsler Intelligence Scale for Children; LD, learning disorder; M, mean; MAP, Missouri Academic Performance; max, maximal; ME, main effect; meds, medication; mg, milligram; MIB, Motor Impersistence Battery; min, minutes; mo, months; mod, moderate; MPH, methylphenidate; MVPA, moderate–vigorous physical activity; N/A, not applicable; NE, norepinephrine; neg, negative; PA, physical activity; ppn, proportion; ppts, participants; probs, problems; RPE, ratings of perceived exertion; RT, reaction time; s, second; SD, standard deviation; SE, standard error; sig, significant; SSRS, Social Skills Rating System; STAIC, State-Trait Anxiety Inventory for Children; submax, submaximal; Tea-Ch, Test of Everyday Attention; TOL, Tower of London; V_{O_2}, oxygen consumption per unit time; $V_{O_{2max}}$, maximum oxygen consumption; WCST, Wisconsin Card Sorting Test; WISC-III, Wechsler Intelligence Scale for Children, Third Edition; WISC-R, Wechsler Intelligence Scale for Children-Revised; WJ III Cog, Woodcock-Johnson III Tests of Cognitive Abilities; wk, week; WPPSI-R, Wechsler Preschool and Primary Scale of Intelligence, Revised; WRAML2, Wide Range Assessment of Memory and Learning, Second Edition; WRAT3, Wide Range Achievement Test, 3rd edition; y, year; YSR, Youth Self Report; #, number.

in the types of exercise, the frequency and duration of exercise sessions, and program duration. For the most part, chronic interventions have taken place in schools. Games and rewarding incentives have been used to engage and motivate children. Furthermore, many studies have used interventions in a social context in which groups of children exercise together, guided by instructors on site, to keep children motivated and to encourage compliance with exercise intervention programs.

Acute Exercise Interventions in Children with ADHD

Studies are reviewed that examined acute effects of exercise in children with ADHD on measures of cognitive functioning, academic performance, and catecholaminergic response. These studies are generally nonrandomized cohort studies, case-control studies, or studies that used a within-subjects design without an adequate control group; none was an RCT.

Cognitive and academic functioning

Craft[108] conducted one of the earliest studies to examine the impact of acute exercise in children with ADHD. They investigated the effect of exercise on cognitive performance in 7- to 10-year-old hyperactive (n = 31) and nonhyperactive boys (n = 31) as identified by a school psychologist. Boys pedaled a cycle ergometer at an individually tailored level of resistance to sustain HR at approximately 170 bpm (vigorous intensity) for 0, 1, 5, or 10 minutes in random order on 4 different days. Each day, children completed the WISC-R Digit Span subtest, the WISC-R Coding B subtest, and the Illinois Test of Psycholinguistic Abilities—Visual Sequential Memory immediately after cycling. Hyperactive boys performed more poorly on all tests than nonhyperactive boys, but no effect of exercise duration and no hyperactivity × exercise duration interaction was observed. The duration of exercise in this early study was much shorter than that used in more recent studies; longer periods of exercise may be required for cognitive benefits to be observed.

Approximately, 30 years later, Pontifex and colleagues[109] compared the impact of 20 minutes of moderate-intensity physical activity (ie, treadmill walking at 65%–75% of HRmax) in 20 8- to 10-year-old unmedicated children with ADHD to that of a group of well-matched typically developing controls. Using a repeated-measures design, they compared exercise to a control condition (ie, reading), counterbalancing order of conditions. Both groups experienced benefits in reading comprehension and arithmetic performance after exercise compared with the control condition, but no differential benefit was seen in children with ADHD. Improvement in accuracy during a flanker task as well as P3 amplitude, and latency was observed for all children after exercise. Children with ADHD experienced differential benefits to post-error slowing (a self-regulatory response) after treadmill walking relative to reading, which was not observed in the typically developing children. Findings suggest that a short, single session of moderate-intensity aerobic exercise may confer benefits to academic performance and cognitive processing in all children and differential self-regulatory benefits in children with ADHD.

Treadmill walking was also used by Chang and colleagues[110] in their examination of moderate-intensity exercise and children's neuropsychological functioning. Forty children with ADHD, aged 8 to 13 years, were randomly assigned to exercise or control groups. Children in the exercise group completed 30 minutes of treadmill running at 50% to 70 % of HR reserve[111] and children's Borg RPE ranging from 12 to 15 (ie, somewhat hard). The control group watched a running/exercise-related video. Children were administered the Stroop task and a computerized version of the WCST[112] at the beginning and end of each session. Acute exercise improved performance in the Stroop Color–Word condition, and reduced non-perseverative errors and increased categories completed on the WCST; no changes were noted in the control group.

Beneficial effects of exercise on cognition were also observed by Medina and colleagues,[113] who examined whether physical activity differentially had an impact on physiologic and cognitive measures in 7- to 15-year-old boys with ADHD who did (n = 16) and did not (n = 9) take MPH. The boys were administered the CPT-II[114] on 3 occasions: at diagnosis, after a 30-min high intensity aerobic tread-mill session, and after a 1-min stretching control session. For boys taking MPH, medication was withheld for 48 hours prior to each testing session. No significant differences in cognitive performance were seen between the treated and untreated groups. Collapsing across treatment groups, treadmill, but not stretching, resulted in significantly faster response speed, lower response speed variability, improvements in vigilance and impulsivity, and marginal ($P = .08$) improvements in stimulus discriminability. The investigators concluded that physical activity may improve children's cognitive functioning irrespective of psychostimulant use. This conclusion must be tempered because medication was withheld for 48 hours prior to testing, but this question is important and warrants further investigation (discussed later).

Catecholaminergic function
That exercise increases DA concentration, thus potentially redressing the purported DA deficiency in children with ADHD, is one hypothesized mechanism by which exercise may exert beneficial effects. Therefore, investigators have sought to examine catecholaminergic response to exercise in children with ADHD.

Tantillo and colleagues[115] examined the impact of both moderate (ie, approximately 65%–75% peak V_{O_2}) and vigorous (ie, graded maximal exercise to determine peak V_{O_2}) intensity aerobic exercise in 8- to 12-year-old children with (n = 18; 10 boys) and without (n = 25; 11 boys) ADHD. The investigators matched the durations of a submaximal and a rest condition with the duration of each child's maximal exercise test. Pre–post changes in state anxiety and several behaviors conceptualized as DA probes (ie, rate of spontaneous eyeblinks; ASER amplitude and latency; and motor impersistence) were examined each session. Control children did not show change on any of the parameters, but boys with ADHD showed increased spontaneous eye-blink rate, decreased ASER latency, and improved motor impersistence after maximal intensity exercise. Girls with ADHD, however, showed decreased ASER latency and increased ASER amplitude after submaximal exercise and no changes in motor imper-sistence. In addition, control girls decreased, but control boys increased ASER ampli-tude after quiet rest. Although the sample size was small, and findings differed for boys and girls depending on exercise intensity, findings suggest that exercise may enhance DA response.

In contrast, Wigal and colleagues[116] observed a blunted DA response to exercise in children with ADHD relative to controls. They compared the catecholaminergic response to moderate-intensity exercise during ten 2-minute intervals, each separated by 1 minute, in 10 treatment-naïve 7- to 12-year-old boys with ADHD to 8 age- and gender-matched controls. Blood samples were taken pre-exercise, during the last 2 minutes of exercise (peak exercise), 30 minutes after exercise, and 60 mi-nutes after exercise to yield radiolabeled metabolites of epinephrine, norepinephrine, and DA as well as plasma lactate. At baseline, only norepinephrine was significantly lower in the ADHD group. Although exercise resulted in increases in all metabolites in controls, they found no increase in DA in children with ADHD. The investigators concluded that it was not clear whether lack of DA response in the periphery in ADHD is related to a systemic DA deficit or, alternatively, simply to less stimulation of the adrenals in response to exercise.

Summary of acute effects of exercise

These few data suggest that exercise of at least moderate intensity and sufficient duration (≥20 minutes) may acutely exert positive impact on a range of cognitive functions. Improvements have been seen in measures of interference control, post-error slowing, set shifting, consistency in response speed, vigilance, and impulse control. Together, findings suggest greater top-down control over behavior after a single session of exercise. Although some findings[116] suggest that the mechanism by which these improvements occur is not likely a result of increases in the release of catecholaminergic neurotransmitters, at least as measured in the periphery, others[115] suggest that increased DA innervation may partially account for the findings, although these latter findings are complicated by different responses for boys and girls.

Chronic Exercise Interventions in Children with ADHD

Several studies have examined the impact of regular aerobic exercise in children with ADHD across multiple domains of functioning, including the core symptoms of ADHD as well as associated behavioral and emotional difficulties, neuropsychological functioning, and academic achievement.

Lufi and Parish-Plass[117] investigated the effect of group-based physical activity in 8 to 13.5-year-old medication-naïve boys with ADHD (n = 15) or other behavioral or social problems (n = 17). Children received 20 90-min weekly group therapy sessions, of which 50 minutes were spent in individual sporting activity (eg, running or obstacle courses) and team sports. Behavioral strategies, such as prompting and token economies, were used throughout the sessions. No untreated comparison group was included. Behavioral functioning was assessed at pretreatment, post-treatment, and 1-year follow-up using the Youth Self Report (YSR) and parent-completed CBCL and the ASQ. Scores declined from pretreatment in both groups on YSR anxiety and somatic scales and for the ASQ parent-rated ADHD symptoms and CBCL aggression, anxiety, delinquency, social, externalizing, and total scores. Sports therapy in conjunction with behavioral management techniques may be useful for several emotional and behavioral difficulties, including ADHD.

Similarly, Reza and Hamid[118] conducted an open clinical study to examine the effects of cycling on inattention and hyperactivity in 7- to 11-year-old children with ADHD. Children completed two 1-hour exercise sessions per week for 16 weeks. Sessions comprised a warm-up, 30 minutes of cycling, and a warm-down. Preintervention, postintervention, and 2-week follow-up evaluations were completed using parent and teacher ratings. Compared with preintervention scores, significant declines in parent and teacher-rated inattention and hyperactivity were observed postintervention that were maintained at 2-week follow-up. Thus, cycling may help reduce ADHD symptoms, but again, a more rigorous study design is necessary to have greater confidence in findings.

Ahmed and Mohamed[119] investigated the effect of an aerobic exercise intervention, delivered in school, not only on children's behavior and emotional functioning but also on cognition, motor skills, and academics. Children (N = 84; 11–16 years) were assigned to either an exercise group or a nonexercising control group. Exercise sessions took place 3 times per week for 10 weeks, with session duration increasing from 40 minutes in weeks 1 to 4 to 50 minutes for weeks 5 to 10. From weeks 6 through 10, parents were encouraged to take a 30-minute walk with their children during the weekend. Pre to post changes on a teacher-completed behavior rating scale were assessed. Children who completed the exercise program were reported to show significantly improved attention, motor skills, academic performance, and classroom behavior. Task orientation and emotional and oppositional behavior were not significantly altered. No significant differences in pre to post outcomes were seen in the control group. Findings suggest that aerobic exercise over a 10-week period may be associated with positive change across many domains of adaptive behavior. Teachers were not blind to children's exercise status, however, which may have influenced findings.

A more comprehensive assessment of the effect of physical activity on neuropsychological function was carried out by Smith and colleagues.[120] They conducted an open trial in 17 children, ages 5 through 8, who exhibited at least 4 parent and/or teacher-endorsed symptoms of hyperactivity/impulsivity on a behavioral rating scale. Thirty-minute exercise sessions were held each morning before school started during which children spent at least 26 minutes engaging in MVPA. Children completed their exercises in groups of approximately 5. Eight sessions were completed over a 9-week period. Compliance was good (12/14 children met or exceeded 75% attendance rate). Pre- and post-intervention assessments were completed, using several objective and informant-reported measures of behavior, cognition, social functioning, and motor skills. Significant improvement in motor proficiency (Cohen d = 0.96), as measured by the Bruininks-Osteretsky Test of Motor Proficiency, was observed. Furthermore, response inhibition improved (Cohen d = 0.96), as measured by Shape School Condition B and during weekly games of red light/green light. No gains were observed on other domains of cognitive and motor functioning. Children's ADHD behavior also improved, as measured using Conners rating scales and behavioral observations of interrupting behavior. Results suggest that long-term treatment comprising physical activity in a social context may be helpful for young children with ADHD, particularly in the realm of response inhibition. Again, this was an open trial and teachers were not blind to treatment.

Verret and colleagues[121] tested the hypothesis that a moderate-to-high intensity exercise intervention would improve cognition, fitness, and behavior of 7- to 12-year-old children with ADHD (n = 21). Ten children were assigned to an exercise group (3 of whom were taking MPH) and the remaining 11 children were assigned to the control group (all were taking MPH). Sessions comprising warm up, aerobic, muscular, and motor skills exercises, and a cool down were held for 45 minutes over lunch, 3 times per week for 10 weeks. Parent and teacher ratings of behavior, measures of children's fitness and motor skills, and attention and executive functioning were collected pre- and post-intervention. Compared with children in the control group, those completing the exercise program showed greater improvement in motor skills despite modest fitness gains. Parents reported that children who completed the exercise program had lower total problems score, as well as attention, social, and thought problems scores than control children on the CBCL. Teachers noted significant decline in anxiety/depression and nonsignificant trends in the direction of improvement for all other teacher scales for children in the exercise group only. Finally, compared with controls, children who exercised showed better-sustained auditory attention and a trend for faster visual search. This exploratory study suggests that long-term exercise intervention may be beneficial for children with ADHD. An RCT is necessary, however, to overcome limitations, including nonrandom assignment to group, differential medication treatment across groups, and unblind parent and teacher reports.

Shedding some light on the relation between exercise and symptom severity in children with ADHD, Kiluk and colleagues[122] examined anxious/depressed scores on parent-rated CBCL as a function of the number of sports parents reported that their children played (0–2 or 3+). Participants were 6- to 14-year-old clinically referred children with ADHD (n = 65) and a comparison group of children diagnosed with a LD (n = 32). For children with ADHD, anxious/depressed T scores were significantly negatively correlated with number of sports played; no relations were seen for children with LD. It was concluded that physical activity may improve psychological functioning in children with ADHD. The retrospective/cross-sectional design (ie, anxious/depressed children might play fewer sports), however, and use of convenience measures are significant limitations.

A correlational study by Bernard-Brak and colleagues[123] used structural equation modeling to predict parent- and teacher-rated ADHD severity in first grade from the amount of time spent in physical education in kindergarten in a sample of 17,565 children. A significant negative relation between physical activity during kindergarten and ADHD 1 year later was found while controlling for the relation between physical activity from time 1 to time 2, and the relation between ADHD from time 1 to time 2. Results suggest that structured physical activity embedded in the school curriculum may be associated with lower levels of ADHD symptom expression. This study is correlational, however, and included only 2 time points.

At present the first-line treatment of ADHD in school-aged children is medication. Thus, a critical question is whether exercise confers additional benefits to children over and above the effects of medication. At present, 4 studies provide data that shed some light on this question. McKune and colleagues[124] investigated the effectiveness of a 5-week moderate-intensity exercise program on ADHD behavior in 19 children (5–13 years) who were taking MPH. Participants were from a special education school and assigned (not randomly) to an exercise group and a nonexercise control group. Children in the exercise group participated in 60-minute sessions, comprising a 15-minute warm-up, a 30-minute exercise phase (running, plyometrics, and obstacle courses), and a 10-minute cool-down. Exercise sessions were completed each day after school. Parents completed the Conners Parent Rating Scale 1 week prior to the program start, midway through the program, and after the program had been completed. No significant between-group differences were found. These findings question the usefulness of exercise as an intervention for ADHD over and above the use of medication.

In contrast, Kang and colleagues[125] reported benefits of sports therapy over and above those provided by medication in a sample of Korean children with ADHD. Children were randomly assigned to a medication plus sports therapy treatment group (n = 16; mean [SD] age = 8.4 [0.9] years) or a medication plus education control group (n = 16; mean [SD] age = 8.6 [1.2] years). All children were titrated to 20 to 40 mg MPH during week 1 of the intervention and the therapeutic dose was maintained over the 6-week study. Children in the sports therapy group took part in 90-minutes of sports twice per week; these sessions included rope jumping, aerobic exercise, and goal-directed exercise (throwing tennis balls and magnetic darts at a target); children in the education control group received information about behavioral control. Parents completed the Korean version of an ADHD rating scale. Children completed the Digit Symbol test from the Korean WISC and the Trail Making Test Part B. Finally, teachers completed the SSRS. Parent-rated total and inattention, but not hyperactivity/impulsivity, scores, showed greater improvement for children in the sports therapy group compared with the education group. Furthermore, children in the sports therapy group, but not the education group, showed significant improvement on Digit Symbol test, and the sports therapy group showed greater reduction in time to complete the Trail Making Test than the education group. Teacher-rated SSRS cooperativeness scores improved for children in the sports therapy group but not for children in the education group. No change in teacher-rated verbal assertion or self-control was seen for either group. Thus, in contrast to the findings of McKune and colleagues,[124] these findings suggest that exercise may augment the benefits of medication, leading to a reduction in symptom severity, improvements in social functioning, and gains in processing speed and cognitive flexibility.

A correlational study in 8- to 12-year-old boys diagnosed with ADHD by Gapin and Etnier[126] may also shed some light on the impact of physical activity on cognitive functioning in medicated children with ADHD. Eighteen stimulant-treated boys completed 4 neuropsychological tasks designed to measure working memory (WISC-IV Digit Span), planning (Tower of London-2), inhibition (CPT-II), and processing speed (Children's Color Trails Test). Over the following 7 days, children wore an accelerometer and completed a daily physical activity log. Data from both measures were integrated to calculate average minutes per day spent in MVPA. More time spent in MVPA was significantly associated with fewer and faster moves on the Tower of London. Although not significant, associations between greater time spent in MVPA and better executive function test performance were observed for 5 of the remaining 6 measures. The small sample size likely limited ability to see significant relations among variables of interest, and the severity of children's ADHD was not assessed, so it is unclear if this affected outcomes. Furthermore, the correlational design prohibits causal interpretations. In spite of these limitations, the findings are consistent with the notion that exercise may confer benefits on neuropsychological functioning in children with ADHD over and above medication treatment.

One final piece of information related to the impact of exercise on children treated with medication for ADHD can potentially be gleaned from a study by Katz and colleagues,[127] who investigated the effect of a classroom-based physical activity program on physical fitness, academic performance, classroom behavior, and health outcomes of elementary school students. This 6 month–long program had teachers make use of down time in the class to implement an activity burst, comprised of a warm-up, physical activity (eg, jumping jacks or a strength activity, such as lunges), and a warm-down. The aim was that over the course of a day, the activity bursts would add up to at least 30 minutes. Children in grades 2 to 4 (N = 1214) recruited from 5 schools were randomly assigned to receive either the intervention or a control condition consisting of regular academic activities. No differences in classroom behavior or academic performance were observed as a function of treatment condition. Children who received the intervention, however, showed significant improvement in physical fitness and decreased use of asthma medication as well as a nonsignificant trend ($P = .07$) for a decrease in the use of ADHD medications compared with the children attending the control schools. These data, from a sample not recruited to test explicit questions about the effect of exercise on children with ADHD, suggest that exercise may be associated with a reduction in medication usage.

Summary of chronic exercise effects

In general, studies investigating longer-term interventions show that physical activity is associated with a reduction in the severity of ADHD behaviors, although whether ADHD behaviors were normalized is unclear. Anxiety and low mood, commonly associated with ADHD, also seem to lessen after long-term exercise interventions. Neuropsychological changes pre- to post-treatment were evaluated across several different domains. Despite the variability in outcome measures, a pattern emerged suggesting that chronic exercise may be particularly beneficial to children's motor skills and response inhibition, although improvement was also seen in processing speed, set shifting, and auditory attention. Findings are mixed, making it less clear whether the beneficial effects of physical activity are seen over and above those derived from stimulant medication.

Most of the children in the studies described previously were between the ages of 7 and 13 years. No study has investigated the utility of physical exercise for preschoolers with ADHD. It may be that using exercise interventions earlier in the lifespan will yield even greater improvements in children's outcomes than if these same interventions were implemented in later childhood. Such intervention aimed at preschoolers with ADHD may set the stage for changes in lifestyle that promote brain growth and development and subsequently bring benefits to children's physical health, behavior, and neuropsychological functioning. Furthermore, additive effects of earlier positive change on longer-term outcomes are possible. That is, the younger children are when these interventions are started, the greater the cumulative effect of benefits over time.[10] Of course, this is speculation; these are empirical questions that await further study.

Although the findings in this area are encouraging, the current literature is marred by severe methodological weaknesses. In a 2012 review of the literature on the efficacy of physical activity as a treatment of ADHD, Berwid and Halperin[81] stated:

Taken together, these…pilot studies—although each limited by small sample size, unblind status of the researchers and raters of behavior, and/or either lack of or poorly designed control conditions—provide preliminary evidence of the potential for exercise interventions to improve both the behavioral symptoms and neuropsychological functioning of school-aged children with ADHD.

Two years later, the state of the literature is largely the same. Although several additional studies have been published, similar limitations in methodology are observed. Structured physical activity seems to have potential as a treatment of ADHD, either on its own or in conjunction with medication. The field needs double-blind RCTs to overcome the weaknesses identified in the literature.

CLINICAL DECISION MAKING
Who Is Most Likely to Respond?

Research into the efficacy of aerobic exercise as an intervention for ADHD is in its infancy. As such, determinations, such as "who is most likely to respond," are little more than speculations. Because it is likely that a program of exercise is most beneficial if it becomes part of a lifestyle change, family involvement and certain family characteristics might be important. Studies in childhood obesity, which might be informative, point to the effectiveness of family-based interventions. Involving parents in interventions is associated with greater benefits than child-only interventions[128] and control treatments[129–131] that persist 5 and 10 years later.[130] With family-based interventions, change in parent BMI predicts change in child BMI, both during treatment and 2 years later.[132] It has been suggested that parents are the mediators of change for their children's eating, activity level, and caloric intake.[129,133] If such findings generalize to children with ADHD, the extent to which a parent or the entire family is willing to actively engage in active exercise together not only mutually reinforces such behaviors[134] but also has the potential to reduce tension within the family unit. Conversely, more hostile, critical, and less engaged parents, as well as those with lower parenting efficacy or more negative attributions about children's behavior, may sabotage such efforts.[135,136] Consistent with this, parents' support for children's physical activity, principally through encouragement and involvement, is positively related to typically developing children's physical activity levels (for review, see Gustafson and Rhodes[137]). To the extent that it is important for exercise to become a family activity, adjunctive parent management training might be an important component for some families.[138,139]

What Outcomes Are Most Likely to Be Affected by Treatment?

Although promising evidence exists, it is too soon to determine whether engagement in ongoing aerobic exercise will have a lasting impact on the core inattentive and hyperactive/impulsive symptoms of ADHD. Nevertheless, initial findings suggest that underlying cognitive mechanisms believed to contribute to both the core symptoms and associated impairments of ADHD do benefit from such routines. The most compelling evidence exists for improved processing speed,[113,125] motor proficiency/skills,[119,120] and inhibitory control,[109,110,113,120] suggesting that benefits span both executive and nonexecutive neurocognitive domains. If, as posited by Barkley,[140] inhibitory control is the core deficit that leads to ADHD, this should in turn have substantial positive benefits on symptom severity. From another perspective, recent diffusion modeling data derived from reaction time paradigms suggest that nonexecutive processing speed deficits, as measured by drift rate, are central to the pathophysiology of ADHD[141–143] and may mediate relations between ADHD and inhibitory control and working memory deficits.[142] If exercise has an impact on processing speed, it could substantially improve functioning in children with ADHD. Because most data indicate that ADHD is highly heterogeneous with regard to core neurocognitive weaknesses (see Nigg and colleagues[13] and Sonuga-Barke[14]), an intervention that has broad and diverse effects on brain development and neurocognitive impairments might be particularly appealing.

Beyond the potential effects of exercise on neurocognitive functioning, it is likely that as children exercise, not only will their physical health improve but also their self-confidence, self-esteem, and peer relationships.[144,145] Children with greater athletic abilities tend to be held in higher esteem by their peers, a relation observed among typically developing children[146] and children with ADHD.[147] For example, among 6- to 12-year-old children with ADHD who completed a summer treatment program, athletic performance was positively associated with being liked and negatively related to being rejected by peers. As children get older, engagement in positive aerobic activities (eg, running, biking, and swimming) with peers is likely to foster healthy lifestyles that are counter to substance use, truancy, and other adverse outcomes. Engagement in such positive activities is also likely to reduce parental stress. Thus, even if core symptoms of ADHD are reduced only minimally, lifestyle changes that incorporate regular physical exercise is likely to yield a wide array of benefits to children and their families.

Contraindications

In general, aerobic exercise is good for just about everyone, not only children with ADHD. As such, there are few contraindications. Accommodations and adaptations need to be made for children with physical disabilities where deficits in muscular strength, balance, and motor coordination are common.[148] With appropriate modifications, however, most children with physical disabilities should be able to engage in some form of aerobic exercise.

Medical clearance should not be necessary for most children prior to the institution of an exercise routine. For those with known medical conditions that could be adversely affected by rigorous exercise, however, collaboration with a specialist prior to initiating the program, along with periodic monitoring, is advised. For example, caution is necessary when using a regimen of physical exercise in children with known cardiovascular and/or respiratory disease.[148] Furthermore, children with diabetes may need to be cautioned to snack prior to exercise and to check blood sugar levels prior to, during, and after exercise. Finally, children with ADHD are highly accident prone. As such, particularly for younger children, adult supervision is likely necessary as is careful monitoring to ensure that appropriate safety gear (eg, bicycle helmets) and safe practices are followed.

Potential Adverse Effects of Physical Activity

A well-designed program of aerobic exercise is unlikely to have serious adverse effects. Potential adverse effects fall into 3 categories: physical, emotional, and use of time. Like any exercise, particularly when first initiated, muscle soreness is possible and perhaps likely. Potential soreness can typically be averted or reduced through the gradual implementation of the program. Over time, intensity and duration can be gradually increased.

Although physical exercise and improved cardiovascular function and physical health are likely to benefit overall emotional adjustment in most children, negative emotional effects are possible in children who are overweight, clumsy, or awkward or who have comorbid developmental coordination disorder. Such children may get frustrated or feel stigmatized as they see themselves struggling with exercise routines and lower performance levels relative to peers and other family members or if they are teased or bullied by peers while carrying out physical activity. Teasing or bullying may lead to children avoiding physical activity.[149,150]

Finally, a strong routine of aerobic exercise takes time that could potentially be used for other beneficial activities (eg, studying and socializing). Research with typically developing student populations suggests that regular physical education classes, as part of a school's curriculum, is not deleterious to children's academic performance[151]; whether this is the case for children with ADHD is not known. With respect to social functioning, Kang and colleagues[125] observed improvements in children's social competence when physical exercise was carried out in a social context. Thus, participating in team-based sports or class-based physical education may lead to improved peer relationships. These are questions for future research.

Integrating Physical Activity with Other Treatments

It is too early to know how exercise should be sequenced or integrated with other treatments of ADHD. Limited data[121,125] suggest that exercise yields additional benefits in children concurrently treated with stimulant medication. It is not known whether the implementation of exercise could allow for discontinuation of medication or reduction in dose.

It is also unknown whether parent management training or other types of family-based intervention might work well with an exercise routine in children with ADHD. Data derived from diet and exercise programs with obese children suggest that parental knowledge of contingency management techniques can be helpful.[138,139] Particularly in young children, parents need the requisite skills to get their children engaged in such activities, and as such, some form of psychosocial intervention might be helpful.

FUTURE DIRECTIONS

Collectively, the findings from extant studies are promising, but methodologically robust RCTs that more rigorously assess the utility of exercise as a treatment of children with ADHD are needed. Key unanswered questions remain around the intensity and duration of exercise required to yield clinical benefits, the magnitude and persistence of improvements to core ADHD symptoms, and whether improvements span behavioral, emotional, social, cognitive, and academic function. Furthermore, it is unknown whether exercise confers benefits over and above medication and/or behavioral treatments, and whether concurrent use of one or both of these treatment modalities would moderate the effectiveness of an exercise intervention.

SUMMARY

Data from animal studies provide convincing evidence that physical exercise enhances brain development and neurobehavioral functioning in areas believed to be impaired in children with ADHD, and studies in patients with dementia demonstrate clear evidence of exercise-related benefits in neurocognitive functioning. To a lesser but still compelling extent, results from studies in typically developing children and adults indicate beneficial effects of exercise on neurocognitive functions that are impaired in children with ADHD. These data provide a clear rationale for why a program of physical exercise may serve as an effective intervention for children with ADHD. Research into the efficacy and effectiveness of exercise as a treatment of ADHD is in its infancy, however, and despite encouraging findings from several preliminary studies, no RCTs have been conducted. As such, exercise as an intervention for ADHD remains at best a level 3 intervention as defined by the Oxford Centre for Evidence-Based Medicine 2011 Levels of Evidence. Specifically, that indicates that nonrandomized controlled cohort studies support the efficacy of the intervention, but no RCTs have been conducted. If, over time, more rigorous trials provide support for exercise as an evidence-based intervention for ADHD, the challenge will become to develop strategies to increase the likelihood that engagement in these activities will not be limited to brief periods (eg, weeks to months) during which children are engaged in an active treatment program. Rather, the goal will be to inject regular physical exercise into a child's routines and lifestyle, starting from a young age. Research suggests that physical activity levels decline across development,[152,153] but one of the most consistent predictors of continued engagement in physical activity is past engagement in physical activity.[154–156] Thus, the authors propose that if initiated early and with enthusiasm, such activities might get incorporated into a child's life as an important frequent activity and this will increase the likelihood that the child will continue engaging in exercise throughout development and into adulthood. As such, even if exercise only has acute benefits similar to other interventions, persistence over time has the potential to yield long-term gains. Yet, it is also possible that many of the beneficial effects of exercise on brain development may persist even if the activity is eventually discontinued.

Recommendations for Clinicians

- Emerging evidence suggests a positive relation between acute (single session ≥20 min duration) and chronic interventions (≥5 wk) of MVPA and improvements in ADHD children's behavior and/or neuropsychological functioning.
- At present, the strength of evidence supporting these relations is not high. The conclusions are largely based on small, unblinded pilot studies, many of which lack a suitable control group.
- Given the lack of RCTs using blind assessments, clinicians should continue to adhere to current best-practice guidelines for the treatment of ADHD
- Clinicians may, however, choose to recommend regular sessions of at least 30 minutes of MVPA as an adjunct to interventions already in place. Even if benefits are not seen on children's ADHD behaviors per se or ADHD's associated

difficulties, regular exercise confers significant benefits on children's physical health. There is no evidence to suggest such a practice would be harmful to a child with ADHD.

- For children with ADHD who have cardiovascular and/or respiratory conditions or who experience motor difficulties, adaptations to the exercise program may need to be made.
- Physical activity interventions may be more likely to be complied with if parents are involved in their implementation

REFERENCES

1. Visser SN, Blumberg SJ, Danielson ML, et al. State-based and demographic variation in parent-reported medication rates for attention-deficit/hyperactivity disorder, 2007-2008. Prev Chronic Dis 2013;10:E09.
2. MTA Cooperative Group. A 14-month randomized clinical trial of treatment strategies for attention-deficit/hyperactivity disorder. Multimodal Treatment Study of Children with ADHD. Arch Gen Psychiatry 1999;56:1073–86.
3. Pliszka S. Practice parameter for the assessment and treatment of children and adolescents with attention-deficit/hyperactivity disorder. J Am Acad Child Adolesc Psychiatry 2007;46:894–921.
4. Perwien A, Hall J, Swensen A, et al. Stimulant treatment patterns and compliance in children and adults with newly treated attention-deficit/hyperactivity disorder. J Manag Care Pharm 2004;10:122–9.
5. Sanchez RJ, Crismon ML, Barner JC, et al. Assessment of adherence measures with different stimulants among children and adolescents. Pharmacotherapy 2005;25:909–17.
6. Hoza B, Gerdes AC, Mrug S, et al. Peer-assessed outcomes in the multimodal treatment study of children with attention deficit hyperactivity disorder. J Clin Child Adolesc Psychol 2005;34:74–86.
7. Biederman J, Seidman LJ, Petty CR, et al. Effects of stimulant medication on neuropsychological functioning in young adults with attention-deficit/hyperactivity disorder. J Clin Psychiatry 2008;69:1150–6.
8. Van der Oord S, Prins PJ, Oosterlaan J, et al. Efficacy of methylphenidate, psychosocial treatments and their combination in school-aged children with ADHD: a meta-analysis. Clin Psychol Rev 2008;28:783–800.
9. Chronis AM, Fabiano GA, Gnagy EM, et al. An evaluation of the summer treatment program for children with Attention-Deficit/Hyperactivity Disorder using a treatment withdrawal design. Behav Ther 2004;35:561–85.
10. Halperin JM, Bedard AC, Curchack-Lichtin JT. Preventive interventions for ADHD: a neurodevelopmental perspective. Neurotherapeutics 2012;9:531–41.
11. Willcutt EG, Doyle AE, Nigg JT, et al. Validity of the executive function theory of attention-deficit/hyperactivity disorder: a meta-analytic review. Biol Psychiatry 2005;57:1336–46.
12. Frazier TW, Demaree HA, Youngstrom EA. Meta-analysis of intellectual and neuropsychological test performance in attention-deficit/hyperactivity disorder. Neuropsychology 2004;18:543–55.
13. Nigg JT, Willcutt EG, Doyle AE, et al. Causal heterogeneity in attention-deficit/hyperactivity disorder: do we need neuropsychologically impaired subtypes? Biol Psychiatry 2005;57:1224–30.
14. Sonuga-Barke EJ. The dual pathway model of AD/HD: an elaboration of neurodevelopmental characteristics. Neurosci Biobehav Rev 2003;27:593–604.

15. Sonuga-Barke EJ, Halperin JM. Developmental phenotypes and causal pathways in attention deficit/hyperactivity disorder: potential targets for early intervention? J Child Psychol Psychiatry 2010;51:368–89.

16. Castellanos FX, Lee PP, Sharp W, et al. Developmental trajectories of brain volume abnormalities in children and adolescents with attention-deficit/hyperactivity disorder. JAMA 2002;288:1740–8.

17. Shaw P, Eckstrand K, Sharp W, et al. Attention-deficit/hyperactivity disorder is characterized by a delay in cortical maturation. Proc Natl Acad Sci U S A 2007;104:19649–54.

18. Shaw P, Malek M, Watson B, et al. Development of cortical surface area and gyrification in attention-deficit/hyperactivity disorder. Biol Psychiatry 2012;72:191–7.

19. Casey BJ, Castellanos FX, Giedd JN, et al. Implication of right frontostriatal circuitry in response inhibition and attention-deficit/hyperactivity disorder. J Am Acad Child Adolesc Psychiatry 1997;36:374–83.

20. Rajendran K, Rindskopf D, O'Neill S, et al. Neuropsychological functioning and severity of ADHD in early childhood: a four-year cross-lagged study. J Abnorm Psychol 2013;122:1179–88.

21. Rajendran K, Trampush JW, Rindskopf D, et al. Association between variation in neuropsychological development and trajectory of ADHD severity in early childhood. Am J Psychiatry 2013;170:1205–11.

22. Shaw P, Lerch J, Greenstein D, et al. Longitudinal mapping of cortical thickness and clinical outcome in children and adolescents with attention-deficit/hyperactivity disorder. Arch Gen Psychiatry 2006;63:540–9.

23. Shaw P, Malek M, Watson B, et al. Trajectories of cerebral cortical development in childhood and adolescence and adult attention-deficit/hyperactivity disorder. Biol Psychiatry 2013;74:599–606.

24. Clerkin SM, Schulz KP, Berwid OG, et al. Thalamo-cortical activation and connectivity during response preparation in adults with persistent and remitted ADHD. Am J Psychiatry 2013;170:1011–9.

25. Giedd JN, Rapoport JL. Structural MRI of pediatric brain development: what have we learned and where are we going? Neuron 2010;67:728–34.

26. Halperin JM, Schulz KP. Revisiting the role of the prefrontal cortex in the pathophysiology of attention-deficit/hyperactivity disorder. Psychol Bull 2006;132:560–81.

27. Halperin JM, Healey DM. The influences of environmental enrichment, cognitive enhancement, and physical exercise on brain development: can we alter the developmental trajectory of ADHD? Neurosci Biobehav Rev 2011;35:621–34.

28. Hebb DO. The organization of behavior: a neuropsychological theory. New York: John Wiley & Sons; 1949.

29. Rosenzweig MR. Environmental complexity, cerebral change, and behavior. Am Psychol 1966;21:321–32.

30. Rosenzweig MR, Bennett EL. Effects of differential environments on brain weights and enzyme activities in gerbils, rats, and mice. Dev Psychobiol 1969;2:87–95.

31. Hubel DH, Wiesel TN. The period of susceptibility to the physiological effects of unilateral eye closure in kittens. J Physiol 1970;206:419–36.

32. Greenough WT, Volkmar FR, Juraska JM. Effects of rearing complexity on dendritic branching in frontolateral and temporal cortex of the rat. Exp Neurol 1973;41:371–8.

33. Greenough WT, Volkmar FR. Pattern of dendritic branching in occipital cortex of rats reared in complex environments. Exp Neurol 1973;40:491–504.

34. Greenough WT, West RW, DeVoogd TJ. Subsynaptic plate perforations: changes with age and experience in the rat. Science 1978;202:1096–8.

35. McArdle WD, Katch FI, Katch VL, editors. Exercise physiology: nutrition, energy, and human performance. Baltimore (MD): Lippincott Williams & Wilkins; 2010.
36. Centers for Disease Control and Prevention. Physical activity and health. 2011. Available at: http://www.cdc.gov/physicalactivity/everyone/health. Accessed June 23, 2014.
37. U.S.Department of Health and Human Services. 2008 Physical Activity Guidelines for Americans. 2014. Available at: http://www.health.gov/paguidelines/guidelines/. Accessed June 23, 2014.
38. Vaynman S, Gomez-Pinilla F. Revenge of the "sit": how lifestyle impacts neuronal and cognitive health through molecular systems that interface energy metabolism with neuronal plasticity. J Neurosci Res 2006;84:699–715.
39. van Praag H, Kempermann G, Gage FH. Running increases cell proliferation and neurogenesis in the adult mouse dentate gyrus. Nat Neurosci 1999;2:266–70.
40. Bobinski F, Martins DF, Bratti T, et al. Neuroprotective and neuroregenerative effects of low-intensity aerobic exercise on sciatic nerve crush injury in mice. Neuroscience 2011;194:337–48.
41. Gregoire CA, Bonenfant D, Le NA, et al. Untangling the influences of voluntary running, environmental complexity, social housing and stress on adult hippocampal neurogenesis. PLoS One 2014;9:e86237.
42. Li H, Liang A, Guan F, et al. Regular treadmill running improves spatial learning and memory performance in young mice through increased hippocampal neurogenesis and decreased stress. Brain Res 2013;1531:1–8.
43. Ding YH, Li J, Zhou Y, et al. Cerebral angiogenesis and expression of angiogenic factors in aging rats after exercise. Curr Neurovasc Res 2006; 3:15–23.
44. Swain RA, Harris AB, Wiener EC, et al. Prolonged exercise induces angiogenesis and increases cerebral blood volume in primary motor cortex of the rat. Neuroscience 2003;117:1037–46.
45. Cotman CW, Berchtold NC, Christie LA. Exercise builds brain health: key roles of growth factor cascades and inflammation. Trends Neurosci 2007;30:464–72.
46. Dishman RK, Berthoud HR, Booth FW, et al. Neurobiology of exercise. Obesity (Silver Spring) 2006;14:345–56.
47. van Praag H. Exercise and the brain: something to chew on. Trends Neurosci 2009;32:283–90.
48. Ding Q, Vaynman S, Akhavan M, et al. Insulin-like growth factor I interfaces with brain-derived neurotrophic factor-mediated synaptic plasticity to modulate aspects of exercise-induced cognitive function. Neuroscience 2006;140: 823–33.
49. Tong L, Shen H, Perreau VM, et al. Effects of exercise on gene-expression profile in the rat hippocampus. Neurobiol Dis 2001;8:1046–56.
50. Vaynman SS, Ying Z, Yin D, et al. Exercise differentially regulates synaptic proteins associated to the function of BDNF. Brain Res 2006;1070:124–30.
51. Farmer J, Zhao X, van PH, et al. Effects of voluntary exercise on synaptic plasticity and gene expression in the dentate gyrus of adult male Sprague-Dawley rats in vivo. Neuroscience 2004;124:71–9.
52. Berchtold NC, Chinn G, Chou M, et al. Exercise primes a molecular memory for brain-derived neurotrophic factor protein induction in the rat hippocampus. Neuroscience 2005;133:853–61.
53. Trejo JL, Carro E, Torres-Aleman I. Circulating insulin-like growth factor I mediates exercise-induced increases in the number of new neurons in the adult hippocampus. J Neurosci 2001;21:1628–34.

54. Bailey SP, Davis JM, Ahlborn EN. Neuroendocrine and substrate responses to altered brain 5-HT activity during prolonged exercise to fatigue. J Appl Physiol (1985) 1993;74:3006–12.

55. Elam M, Svensson TH, Thoren P. Brain monoamine metabolism is altered in rats following spontaneous, long-distance running. Acta Physiol Scand 1987;130: 313–6.

56. Petzinger GM, Walsh JP, Akopian G, et al. Effects of treadmill exercise on dopaminergic transmission in the 1-methyl-4-phenyl-1,2,3,6-tetrahydropyridine-lesioned mouse model of basal ganglia injury. J Neurosci 2007;27:5291–300.

57. Foley TE, Fleshner M. Neuroplasticity of dopamine circuits after exercise: implications for central fatigue. Neuromolecular Med 2008;10:67–80.

58. Adlard PA, Perreau VM, Cotman CW. The exercise-induced expression of BDNF within the hippocampus varies across life-span. Neurobiol Aging 2005;26:511–20.

59. Kim YP, Kim H, Shin MS, et al. Age-dependence of the effect of treadmill exercise on cell proliferation in the dentate gyrus of rats. Neurosci Lett 2004;355:152–4.

60. Fordyce DE, Farrar RP. Physical activity effects on hippocampal and parietal cortical cholinergic function and spatial learning in F344 rats. Behav Brain Res 1991;43:115–23.

61. Fordyce DE, Wehner JM. Effects of aging on spatial learning and hippocampal protein kinase C in mice. Neurobiol Aging 1993;14:309–17.

62. Grace L, Hescham S, Kellaway LA, et al. Effect of exercise on learning and memory in a rat model of developmental stress. Metab Brain Dis 2009;24:643–57.

63. Kim H, Heo HI, Kim DH, et al. Treadmill exercise and methylphenidate ameliorate symptoms of attention deficit/hyperactivity disorder through enhancing dopamine synthesis and brain-derived neurotrophic factor expression in spontaneous hypertensive rats. Neurosci Lett 2011;504:35–9.

64. Samorajski T, Delaney C, Durham L, et al. Effect of exercise on longevity, body weight, locomotor performance, and passive-avoidance memory of C57BL/6J mice. Neurobiol Aging 1985;6:17–24.

65. Sagvolden T, Russell VA, Aase H, et al. Rodent models of attention-deficit/hyperactivity disorder. Biol Psychiatry 2005;57:1239–47.

66. Robinson AM, Hopkins ME, Bucci DJ. Effects of physical exercise on ADHD-like behavior in male and female adolescent spontaneously hypertensive rats. Dev Psychobiol 2011;53:383–90.

67. Robinson AM, Eggleston RL, Bucci DJ. Physical exercise and catecholamine reuptake inhibitors affect orienting behavior and social interaction in a rat model of attention-deficit/hyperactivity disorder. Behav Neurosci 2012;126:762–71.

68. Hopkins ME, Sharma M, Evans GC, et al. Voluntary physical exercise alters attentional orienting and social behavior in a rat model of attention-deficit/hyperactivity disorder. Behav Neurosci 2009;123:599–606.

69. del Campo N, Chamberlain SR, Sahakian BJ, et al. The roles of dopamine and noradrenaline in the pathophysiology and treatment of attention-deficit/hyperactivity disorder. Biol Psychiatry 2011;69:e145–57.

70. Volkow ND, Wang GJ, Newcorn JH, et al. Motivation deficit in ADHD is associated with dysfunction of the dopamine reward pathway. Mol Psychiatry 2011;16: 1147–54.

71. Arnsten AF. Fundamentals of attention-deficit/hyperactivity disorder: circuits and pathways. J Clin Psychiatry 2006;67(Suppl 8):7–12.

72. McMorris T, Collard K, Corbett J, et al. A test of the catecholamines hypothesis for an acute exercise-cognition interaction. Pharmacol Biochem Behav 2008;89: 106–15.

73. Querido JS, Sheel AW. Regulation of cerebral blood flow during exercise. Sports Med 2007;37:765–82.
74. Ferris LT, Williams JS, Shen CL. The effect of acute exercise on serum brain-derived neurotrophic factor levels and cognitive function. Med Sci Sports Exerc 2007;39:728–34.
75. Rasmussen P, Brassard P, Adser H, et al. Evidence for a release of brain-derived neurotrophic factor from the brain during exercise. Exp Physiol 2009; 94:1062–9.
76. Hyman C, Hofer M, Barde YA, et al. BDNF is a neurotrophic factor for dopaminergic neurons of the substantia nigra. Nature 1991;350:230–2.
77. Knusel B, Winslow JW, Rosenthal A, et al. Promotion of central cholinergic and dopaminergic neuron differentiation by brain-derived neurotrophic factor but not neurotrophin 3. Proc Natl Acad Sci U S A 1991;88:961–5.
78. Lambourne K, Tomporowski P. The effect of exercise-induced arousal on cognitive task performance: a meta-regression analysis. Brain Res 2010;1341:12–24.
79. Chang YK, Labban JD, Gapin JI, et al. The effects of acute exercise on cognitive performance: a meta-analysis. Brain Res 2012;1453:87–101.
80. Verburgh L, Konigs M, Scherder EJ, et al. Physical exercise and executive functions in preadolescent children, adolescents and young adults: a meta-analysis. Br J Sports Med 2014;48(12):973–9.
81. Berwid OG, Halperin JM. Emerging support for a role of exercise in attention-deficit/hyperactivity disorder intervention planning. Curr Psychiatry Rep 2012; 14:543–51.
82. Tomporowski PD, Davis CL, Miller PH, et al. Exercise and children's intelligence, cognition, and academic achievement. Educ Psychol Rev 2008;20:111–31.
83. Tomporowski PD, Lambourne K, Okumura MS. Physical activity interventions and children's mental function: an introduction and overview. Prev Med 2011; 52(Suppl 1):S3–9.
84. Sibley BA, Etnier JL. The relationship between physical activity and cognition in children. Pediatr Exerc Sci 2003;15:243–56.
85. Best JR. Effects of physical activity on children's executive function: contributions of experimental research on aerobic exercise. Dev Rev 2010;30:331–551.
86. Hillman CH, Kamijo K, Scudder M. A review of chronic and acute physical activity participation on neuroelectric measures of brain health and cognition during childhood. Prev Med 2011;52(Suppl 1):S21–8.
87. McMorris T, Sproule J, Turner A, et al. Acute, intermediate intensity exercise, and speed and accuracy in working memory tasks: a meta-analytical comparison of effects. Physiol Behav 2011;102:421–8.
88. McMorris T, Hale BJ. Differential effects of differing intensities of acute exercise on speed and accuracy of cognition: a meta-analytical investigation. Brain Cogn 2012;80:338–51.
89. Smith PJ, Blumenthal JA, Hoffman BM, et al. Aerobic exercise and neurocognitive performance: a meta-analytic review of randomized controlled trials. Psychosom Med 2010;72:239–52.
90. Centers for Disease Control and Prevention. The association between school-based physical activity, including physical education, and academic performance. 2010. Available at: http://www.cdc.gov/healthyyouth/health_and_academics/pdf/pa-pe_paper.pdf. Accessed June 23, 2014.
91. Fisher A, Boyle JM, Paton JY, et al. Effects of a physical education intervention on cognitive function in young children: randomized controlled pilot study. BMC Pediatr 2011;11:97.

92. Kamijo K, Pontifex MB, O'Leary KC, et al. The effects of an afterschool physical activity program on working memory in preadolescent children. Dev Sci 2011; 14:1046–58.
93. Davis CL, Tomporowski PD, McDowell JE, et al. Exercise improves executive function and achievement and alters brain activation in overweight children: a randomized, controlled trial. Health Psychol 2011;30:91–8.
94. Davis CL, Tomporowski PD, Boyle CA, et al. Effects of aerobic exercise on overweight children's cognitive functioning: a randomized controlled trial. Res Q Exerc Sport 2007;78:510–9.
95. Chaddock-Heyman L, Erickson KI, Voss MW, et al. The effects of physical activity on functional MRI activation associated with cognitive control in children: a randomized controlled intervention. Front Hum Neurosci 2013;7:72.
96. Monti JM, Hillman CH, Cohen NJ. Aerobic fitness enhances relational memory in preadolescent children: the FITKids randomized control trial. Hippocampus 2012;22:1876–82.
97. Castelli DM, Hillman CH, Hirsch J, et al. FIT kids: time in target heart zone and cognitive performance. Prev Med 2011;52(Suppl 1):S55–9.
98. Barenberg J, Berse T, Dutke S. Executive functions in learning processes: do they benefit from physical activity? Educ Res Rev 2011;6:208–22.
99. Lees C, Hopkins J. Effect of aerobic exercise on cognition, academic achievement, and psychosocial function in children: a systematic review of randomized control trials. Prev Chronic Dis 2013;10:E174.
100. Fedewa AL, Ahn S. The effects of physical activity and physical fitness on children's achievement and cognitive outcomes: a meta-analysis. Res Q Exerc Sport 2011;82:521–35.
101. Trudeau F, Shephard RJ. Relationships of physical activity to brain health and the academic performance of schoolchildren. Am J Lifestyle Med 2010;4:138–50.
102. Shephard RJ. Habitual physical activity and academic performance. Nutr Rev 1996;54:S32–6.
103. Kibbe DL, Hackett J, Hurley M, et al. Ten Years of TAKE 10! (R): integrating physical activity with academic concepts in elementary school classrooms. Prev Med 2011;52(Suppl 1):S43–50.
104. Mahar MT, Murphy SK, Rowe DA, et al. Effects of a classroom-based program on physical activity and on-task behavior. Med Sci Sports Exerc 2006;38: 2086–94.
105. Mahar MT. Impact of short bouts of physical activity on attention-to-task in elementary school children. Prev Med 2011;52(Suppl 1):S60–4.
106. Allison DB, Faith MS, Franklin RD. Antecedent exercise in the treatment of disruptive behavior: a meta-analytic review. Clin Psychol 1995;2:279–304.
107. Wilens TE, Biederman J, Spencer TJ. Attention deficit/hyperactivity disorder across the lifespan. Annu Rev Med 2002;53:113–31.
108. Craft DH. Effect of prior exercise on cognitive performance tasks by hyperactive and normal young boys. Percept Mot Skills 1983;56:979–82.
109. Pontifex MB, Saliba BJ, Raine LB, et al. Exercise improves behavioral, neurocognitive, and scholastic performance in children with attention-deficit/hyperactivity disorder. J Pediatr 2013;162(3):543–51.
110. Chang YK, Liu S, Yu HH, et al. Effect of acute exercise on executive function in children with attention deficit hyperactivity disorder. Arch Clin Neuropsychol 2012;27:225–37.
111. American College of Sports Medicine. ASCM's guidelines for exercise testing and prescription. New York: Lippincott, Williams & Wilkins; 2010.

112. Heaton RK. WCST: computer version 4-research edition. Lutz (FL): Psychological Assessment Resources; 2008.
113. Medina JA, Netto TL, Muszkat M, et al. Exercise impact on sustained attention of ADHD children, methylphenidate effects. Atten Defic Hyperact Disord 2010;2: 49–58.
114. Conners CK, Staff MH. Continuous performance test II (CPTII) computer programs for Windows technical guide. North Tonawada (NY): Multi-Health Systems; 2000.
115. Tantillo M, Kesick CM, Hynd GW, et al. The effects of exercise on children with attention-deficit hyperactivity disorder. Med Sci Sports Exerc 2002;34: 203–12.
116. Wigal SB, Nemet D, Swanson JM, et al. Catecholamine response to exercise in children with attention deficit hyperactivity disorder. Pediatr Res 2003;53: 756–61.
117. Lufi D, Parish-Plass J. Sport-based group therapy program for boys with ADHD or with other behavioral disorders. Child Fam Behav Ther 2011;33:217–30.
118. Reza AB, Hamid F. Biological effects of cycling exercise on reducing symptoms of children's attention deficit hyperactivity disorder. Ann Biol Res 2011;2:617–23.
119. Ahmed GM, Mohamed S. Effect of regular aerobic exercises on behavioral, cognitive and psychological response in patients with attention deficit-hyperactivity disorder. Life Science Journal 2011;8:366–71.
120. Smith AL, Hoza B, Linnea K, et al. Pilot physical activity intervention reduces severity of ADHD symptoms in young children. J Atten Disord 2013;17:70–82.
121. Verret C, Guay MC, Berthiaume C, et al. A physical activity program improves behavior and cognitive functions in children with ADHD: an exploratory study. J Atten Disord 2012;16:71–80.
122. Kiluk BD, Weden S, Culotta VP. Sport participation and anxiety in children with ADHD. J Atten Disord 2009;12:499–506.
123. Bernard-Brak L, Davis T, Sulak T, et al. The association between physical education and symptoms of attention deficit hyperactivity disorder. J Phys Act Health 2011;8:964–70.
124. McKune AJ, Pautz J, Lombard J. Behavioural response to exercise in children with attention-deficit/hyperactivity disorder. South African Journal of Sports Medicine 2003;15:17–21.
125. Kang KD, Choi JW, Kang SG, et al. Sports therapy for attention, cognitions and sociality. Int J Sports Med 2011;32:953–9.
126. Gapin J, Etnier JL. The relationship between physical activity and executive function performance in children with attention-deficit hyperactivity disorder. J Sport Exerc Psychol 2010;32:753–63.
127. Katz DL, Cushman D, Reynolds J, et al. Putting physical activity where it fits in the school day: preliminary results of the ABC (Activity Bursts in the Classroom) for fitness program. Prev Chronic Dis 2010;7:A82.
128. Golan M, Weizman A, Apter A, et al. Parents as the exclusive agents of change in the treatment of childhood obesity. Am J Clin Nutr 1998;67:1130–5.
129. Beech BM, Klesges RC, Kumanyika SK, et al. Child- and parent-targeted interventions: the Memphis GEMS pilot study. Ethn Dis 2003;13:S40–53.
130. Epstein LH, Valoski A, Wing RR, et al. Ten-year follow-up of behavioral, family-based treatment for obese children. JAMA 1990;264:2519–23.
131. Janicke DM, Sallinen BJ, Perri MG, et al. Comparison of parent-only vs family-based interventions for overweight children in underserved rural settings: outcomes from project STORY. Arch Pediatr Adolesc Med 2008;162:1119–25.

132. Wrotniak BH, Epstein LH, Paluch RA, et al. Parent weight change as a predictor of child weight change in family-based behavioral obesity treatment. Arch Pediatr Adolesc Med 2004;158:342–7.
133. Garn SM, Clark DC. Trends in fatness and the origins of obesity Ad Hoc Committee to Review the Ten-State Nutrition Survey. Pediatrics 1976;57: 443–56.
134. Bandura A. Social learning theory of aggression. J Commun 1978;28:12–29.
135. Pelham WE, Gnagy EM, Greiner AR, et al. Behavioral versus behavioral and pharmacological treatment in ADHD children attending a summer treatment program. J Abnorm Child Psychol 2000;28:507–25.
136. Hoza B, Owens JS, Pelham WE, et al. Parent cognitions as predictors of child treatment response in attention-deficit/hyperactivity disorder. J Abnorm Child Psychol 2000;28:569–83.
137. Gustafson SL, Rhodes RE. Parental correlates of physical activity in children and early adolescents. Sports Med 2006;36:79–97.
138. Epstein LH, Paluch RA, Gordy CC, et al. Decreasing sedentary behaviors in treating pediatric obesity. Arch Pediatr Adolesc Med 2000;154:220–6.
139. Hills AP, Parker AW. Obesity management via diet and exercise intervention. Child Care Health Dev 1988;14:409–16.
140. Barkley RA. Behavioral inhibition, sustained attention, and executive functions: constructing a unifying theory of ADHD. Psychol Bull 1997;121:65–94.
141. Huang-Pollock CL, Karalunas SL, Tam H, et al. Evaluating vigilance deficits in ADHD: a meta-analysis of CPT performance. J Abnorm Psychol 2012;121:360–71.
142. Karalunas SL, Huang-Pollock CL, Nigg JT. Is reaction time variability in ADHD mainly at low frequencies? J Child Psychol Psychiatry 2013;54:536–44.
143. Metin B, Roeyers H, Wiersema JR, et al. ADHD performance reflects inefficient but not impulsive information processing: a diffusion model analysis. Neuropsychology 2013;27:193–200.
144. Slutzky CB, Simpkins SD. The link between children's sport participation and self-esteem: exploring the mediating role of sport self-concept. Psychol Sport Exerc 2009;10:381–9.
145. Tremblay MS, Inman JW, Willms D. The relationship between physical activity, self-esteem, and academic achievement in 12-year-old children. Pediatr Exerc Sci 2000;12:312–23.
146. Weiss MR, Duncan SC. The relationship between physical competence and peer acceptance in the context of children's sports participation. J Sport Exerc Psychol 1992;14:177–91.
147. Lopez-Williams A, Chacko A, Wymbs BT, et al. Athletic performance and social behavior as predictors of peer acceptance in children diagnosed with Attention-Deficit/Hyperactivity Disorder. J Emot Behav Disord 2005;13:173–80.
148. Riner WF, Sellhorst SH. Physical activity and exercise in children with chronic health conditions. J Sport Health Sci 2013;2:12–20.
149. Jensen CD, Cushing CC, Elledge AR. Associations between teasing, quality of life, and physical activity among preadolescent children. J Pediatr Psychol 2014;39:65–73.
150. Verschuren O, Wiart L, Hermans D, et al. Identification of facilitators and barriers to physical activity in children and adolescents with cerebral palsy. J Pediatr 2012;161:488–94.
151. Sallis JF, McKenzie TL, Kolody B, et al. Effects of health-related physical education on academic achievement: project SPARK. Res Q Exerc Sport 1999; 70:127–34.

152. Dumith SC, Gigante DP, Domingues MR, et al. Physical activity change during adolescence: a systematic review and a pooled analysis. Int J Epidemiol 2011; 40:685–98.

153. Kimm SY, Glynn NW, Kriska AM, et al. Decline in physical activity in black girls and white girls during adolescence. N Engl J Med 2002;347:709–15.

154. Janz KF, Dawson JD, Mahoney LT. Tracking physical fitness and physical activity from childhood to adolescence: the muscatine study. Med Sci Sports Exerc 2000;32:1250–7.

155. Sallis JF, Prochaska JJ, Taylor WC. A review of correlates of physical activity of children and adolescents. Med Sci Sports Exerc 2000;32:963–75.

156. Telama R, Yang X, Viikari J, et al. Physical activity from childhood to adulthood: a 21-year tracking study. Am J Prev Med 2005;28:267–73.

Restriction and Elimination Diets in ADHD Treatment

Joel T. Nigg, PhD[a],*, Kathleen Holton, PhD, MPH[b]

KEYWORDS

- ADHD • Food elimination diet • Alternative treatment • Few foods diet

KEY POINTS

- Food elimination diets come in different forms; the most restrictive or "few foods" diet eliminates a wide range of foods for a temporary period, adding foods back in one by one in an attempt to identify symptomatic triggers.
- Use of elimination diets to treat attention deficit and hyperactivity disorder (ADHD) has been proposed and studied for nearly 40 years and frequently reviewed and discussed.
- A consensus has emerged among most reviewers that an elimination diet produces a small aggregate effect but may have greater benefit among some children.
- Very few studies enable proper evaluation of the likelihood of response in children with ADHD who are not already preselected based on prior diet response. This critical question should be the focus of future studies.
- Future studies should be accompanied by examination of moderators of response (which children respond) and mediators (mechanisms, particularly physiologic mechanisms).

The numerous "alternative" or "nonmedical" treatments that have been proposed for attention deficit and hyperactivity disorder (ADHD) over the years include several kinds of dietary interventions, including single nutrient supplements,[1] multinutrient supplements,[2,3] supplementation with omega-3 fatty acids,[4–7] and others. Among the most enduring ideas has been the use of a food restriction or food elimination diet, hereafter referred to simply as an elimination diet.

ELIMINATION DIETS AND HEALTH

The concept of an elimination diet to improve health was first proposed by Albert Rowe[8] in 1926 in regards to food allergies and spelled out in his subsequent book. The concept of "Allergy of the Nervous System" dates back to 1934, when Lapage[9] mentions the use of Rowe's elimination diet. Subsequently, hundreds of papers

[a] Department of Psychiatry, Oregon Health & Science University, 3181 SW Sam Jackson Park Road, Portland, OR 97239, USA; [b] School of Education, Teaching and Health, Center for Behavioral Neuroscience American University, 4400 Massachusetts Avenue, NW, Washington, DC 20016, USA
* Corresponding author.
E-mail address: niggj@ohsu.edu

Child Adolesc Psychiatric Clin N Am 23 (2014) 937–953
http://dx.doi.org/10.1016/j.chc.2014.05.010
1056-4993/14/$ – see front matter © 2014 Elsevier Inc. All rights reserved.

childpsych.theclinics.com

have been written on the general topic area of allergy, food, and the nervous system. In 1976, Hall[10] referenced the use of an elimination diet for the treatment of "behavioral disturbances including headaches, convulsions, learning disabilities, schizophrenia, and depression" related to allergy of the nervous system. It was around this same time that the Feingold diet was introduced as treatment of hyperkinetic syndrome, as detailed herein. Therefore, the idea of an elimination diet to help child or adult mood, attention, or behavior is not new, but has regained renewed interest in recent years.

The focus of elimination diets is to remove specific foods from the diet in an effort to eliminate potential allergens that occur naturally in food (eg, eggs, wheat, dairy, soy) or artificial ingredients that may have allergenic or even toxicant effects (eg, synthetic food additives: artificial colors, flavors, sweeteners, as well as flavor enhancers [like monosodium glutamate (MSG)] and preservatives). These diets are used to attempt to diagnose and treat food allergies and intolerances.

Food elimination diets vary in their specific content, but take 3 main forms. A single food exclusion diet excludes one suspected food, such as eggs. A multifood exclusion diet, such as the 6-food elimination diet, eliminates the most common food allergens: cow-milk protein, soy, wheat, eggs, peanuts, and seafood. A "few foods diet" (also called an oligoantigenic diet) restricts a person's diet to only a few less commonly consumed foods (eg, lamb/venison, quinoa/rice, pear, and others with low allergenic potential). The "few foods diet" must be overseen by a properly qualified professional (eg, dietitian) to avoid nutritional deficiency, but is effective at identifying multiple food allergies in an individual.[11] Much of the use of these diets in the medical literature is targeted at single specific food allergies (eg, cow's milk[12] or physical symptoms thought to potentially be related to food allergies, such as esophagitis).[13,14]

Other specific elimination diets exist, such as a gluten-free diet and the Kaiser Permanente (or Feingold) diet. The gluten-free diet is currently the only successful treatment for patients with celiac disease[15] and is also being used to treat nonceliac gluten sensitivity.[16] Gluten is the protein found in wheat, rye, and barley, and thus, any item in the diet containing these grains (including some food additives) must be removed. A gluten and casein-free diet is also being tested in autism.[17] The Feingold diet eliminates food colorings and sometimes certain preservatives and foods with naturally occurring salicylates.[18] The Feingold diet was later adapted to only exclude artificial colorings and preservatives, which Feingold came to think were the pertinent factors in ADHD.

All elimination diets use the same 2-step process, wherein the diet is followed for a period of time; then, if symptoms remit, foods (or food additives) are reintroduced one at a time to test for a return of symptoms. When using the "few foods diet," this process is lengthy, because many foods must be tested until enough foods have been identified to reinstate a healthy balanced diet without allergens. When food allergy is suspected, skin prick allergy testing can accompany dietary treatment. More commonly, the dietary intervention is purely "empirical" in that foods are eliminated and reintroduced while symptoms are monitored.

Allergists define *food allergy* as an immunologic response in the body after exposure to a food item. Common manifestations of food allergy include skin responses (uticaria), sensitivity/swelling in the mouth, rhinitis, breathing difficulties, and gastrointestinal issues ranging from vomiting to diarrhea; less well-known neurologic symptoms, like headache, anxiety, confusion, nervousness, and lethargy, have also been reported.[19]

On the other hand, *food intolerance* is defined by allergists as a nonimmunological (ie, nonallergic) response to a food item, which may be due to enzyme deficiency (eg, lactose intolerance) or another nonimmunological hypersensitivity reaction such as to food additives.[20] Food intolerances can also cause gastrointestinal difficulties, but often also result in other symptoms, which can range from headache and blurred vision to mood changes, fatigue, and pain. Pelsser and colleagues[21] hypothesized that ADHD involves food hypersensitivity (intolerance). This type of food intolerance is often considered to be a toxicologic or pharmacologic response to chemicals found in food. However, intolerance is difficult to verify because the idea of intolerance proposes that reaction may occur after a substantial time period; furthermore, the mechanisms of such intolerance are not necessarily demonstrated for most additives.

However, some examples have been compelling. A well-known example is tetrodotoxin, which is a neurotoxin found in Fugu fish commonly consumed in Japan.[22] Another is the common food additive, MSG, which may have excitotoxic effects in the nervous system.[23]

To illustrate the latter effect, an excitotoxin elimination diet was tested in a group of fibromyalgia patients who also suffered from irritable bowel syndrome. Fibromyalgia is characterized by a constellation of neurologic symptoms including widespread muscle pain, cognitive dysfunction, headache, paresthesias, difficulty sleeping, balance issues, and fatigue. Those who improved on the diet (defined as >30% of their symptoms remitting) were challenged with MSG in a crossover placebo-controlled double-blind manner. A significant return of symptoms was seen with MSG as compared with placebo.[24] It is important to note that fibromyalgia patients tend to suffer from cognitive difficulties, including problems with attention.[25] This toxicologic response to MSG therefore may be of importance in ADHD, because, similar to fibromyalgia, disordered glutamatergic neurotransmission has also been implicated in ADHD.[26–28] At least one study has examined the effects of MSG in children with ADHD, although in combination with removal of other additives.[29] Furthermore, other research has demonstrated that artificial food colors may act synergistically with MSG,[30] a possibility yet to be examined in relation to ADHD.

ADHD APPLICATIONS

As mentioned earlier, the specific hypothesis that synthetic food colorings influence ADHD (at that time, hyperkinetic reaction), via either allergenic or pharmacologic mechanisms, was introduced in the 1970s by Feingold.[31–33] Feingold was an allergist, so his predisposition was to evaluate for potential allergens in patients. He suggested initially that children who are allergic to aspirin (which contains salicylates) may be reactive to synthetic food colors as well as naturally occurring salicylates, although he later focused in particular on food color additives. He proposed a diet free of foods with a natural salicylate radical and all synthetic colors and flavors to treat hyperactivity. This diet is also referred to as the Kaiser Permanente diet. This approach is still promoted today by the organization he founded (https://www.feingold.org/). A narrower approach simply restricts synthetic food colors, although these are sometimes also restricted as part of more general diets.

In the 1970s and 1980s, various versions of the Feingold diet were heavily studied in the United States, but more recently this type of diet has been investigated primarily in Europe. In 1982, the National Institutes of Health convened a consensus development conference on defined diets and childhood hyperactivity, which recommended further study.[34] In the subsequent 30 years, several major reviews have been attempted, albeit on a persistently weak literature. Those reviews are summarized in **Table 1**. Herein, their insights and a few others are briefly highlighted.

An initial meta-analysis in 1983[35] included 23 studies of varying quality regarding the efficacy of the Feingold diet; the authors concluded that the composite effect

Authors, Year	Focus	Method	Conclusion
Kavale & Forness,[35] 1983	Feingold diet	Meta-analysis	ES = 0.11 (ns)
Breakey,[59] 1997	Diet generally	Qualitative	Some children
Schab & Trinh,[36] 2004	Food colors	Meta-analysis	ES = 0.21* (parent)
Stevens et al,[41] 2011	Diet generally	Qualitative	Some promise
Pelsser et al,[39] 2011	Restriction	Meta-analysis	ES = 1.2*
Nigg et al,[42] 2012	Restriction	Meta-analysis	ES = 0.30*
Nigg et al,[42] 2012	Food colors	Meta-analysis	ES = 0.22*
Sonuga-Barke et al,[6] 2013	Restriction	Meta-analysis	ES = 0.51 (ns)
Sonuga-Barke et al,[6] 2013	Food colors	Meta-analysis	ES = 0.42*
Arnold et al,[60] 2013	Diet generally	Qualitative	Some promise
Stevenson et al,[46] 2014	Diet generally	Qualitative	Some promise

Table 1
Major reviews of ADHD and restriction/elimination diets

Abbreviation: ES, effect size.
  * p<.05

size ($d = 0.11$) was too small to be important, setting the tone for 2 decades of professional skepticism as to the value of elimination diets. More recently, however, in 2004, Schab and Trinh[36] reviewed 15 higher quality studies, which were all double-blind, placebo-controlled studies focused on food color elimination or challenge, plus 6 others for a supplemental analysis. They concluded that there was a reliable effect ($d = 0.28$) linking synthetic colors to ADHD symptoms in parent ratings, but not in teacher or observer ratings. The effects seemed to be similar whether or not children were initially selected to be hyperactive. Although the results were equivocal (failure to see a reliable effect in teacher or observer ratings, least prone to hidden failure of study blinding), they spurred new interest.

About that same time, a widely publicized population-based study conducted in England[37] concluded that food additives contribute to hyperactivity, prompting the European Union Parliament recently to require warning labels on foods containing 6 colors (not all of which are approved for use in the United States by the US Food and Drug Administration, FDA[38]). The FDA has approved 9 synthetic colors for use in food subject to batch certification: FD&C Blue number 1 (brilliant blue), FD&C Blue number 2 (Indigotine), FD&C Green number 3 (Green S; fast green), Orange B, Citrus Red number 2 (Amaranth), FD&C Red number 3 (Erythrosine), FD&C Red number 40 (Allura Red), FD&C Yellow number 5 (Tartrazine), and FD&C Yellow number 6 (Sunset Yellow). All but Orange B are also approved for use in Europe, but in Europe, warning labels are now required on FD&C Red number 40 (Allura Red AC), FD&C Yellow number 5 (Tartrazine), FD&C Yellow number 6 (Sunset Yellow), and 3 colors used in Europe but not the United States: Quinoline Yellow, Carmoisine, and Ponceau. That study did not examine a restriction/elimination diet, however. Rather, they challenged typically developing children selected from the community with a drink containing a measured dose of food colors and a sodium benzoate preservative. The children were a cohort of 3 year olds (n = 153) and a cohort of 8 year olds (n = 144). The results were complicated by the use of 2 different formulations of active drink plus placebo, and the finding that in the 2 age groups different formulations influenced ADHD symptoms. Nonetheless, given the absence of nutritional benefit of the food additives and a precautionary stance, European regulators took action. This study seemed to support, indirectly, that an elimination diet therefore might help children with ADHD.

Another large European study, conducted in the Netherlands, also attracted considerable attention and some controversy. Pelsser and colleagues[39] conducted a double-blind crossover study of an elimination diet. They randomized 50 children with ADHD to an individually designed few foods diet and 50 to healthy diet counseling. Responders to the elimination diet were then given a challenge using high-inflammatory or low-inflammatory foods on the basis of each child's individual IgG blood test result. Thirty children (60%) had a positive response to the restriction/elimination diet, but only 19 of 30 had symptom relapse on the challenge foods. The authors concluded that their restriction/elimination diet was effective for ADHD but that the use of IgG blood test to determine who should be treated was not useful. Although findings appeared to be impressive, a critical flaw in the design was that the authors relied on clinician ratings for the primary findings, and clinicians in turn relied on parent reports—but parents were, of course, not blind to the interventions. Those same authors reported a brief review of prior trials of restriction diets in ADHD and identified a large effect of d = 1.2. However, that effect relied on including nonblind, open-label trials.

Controversy continued in North America. In 2008, the Center for Science in the Public Interest, a consumer advocacy organization, petitioned the FDA to regulate food color additives. They provided an unpublished literature review arguing that colorings contributed to behavior problems and contended there was little justification for incurring any health risks, because food colors provide no health benefits.[40] The FDA subsequently commissioned its own unpublished, qualitative review, which concluded in 2011 that the evidence fell short of a causal association for food colors that are approved in the United States. However, that same year a major published qualitative review by Stevens and colleagues[41] (see **Table 1**) concluded that a subgroup of children with ADHD is sensitive to synthetic color additives, flavors, or salicylates and could benefit from a restriction/elimination diet. Thus, they highlighted not only the issue of differential response across different children but also the idea that restriction/elimination diets have value, and food coloring per se may not be the main culprit.

To further investigate all this quantitatively, Nigg and colleagues[42] conducted a meta-analysis of both restriction/elimination diet effects and food coloring effects on ADHD. They identified 6 restriction diet studies that used either a placebo-controlled diet challenge or a crossover design,[29,39,43–45] which in aggregate examined 195 children for improvement in hyperactive symptoms. However, one study[39] had questionable blinding of participants and was also a statistical outlier that fully accounted for heterogeneity of effects. Effects therefore were interpreted with the remaining 5 studies. These studies yielded a summed response rate (response being defined variously across studies) of greater than 35% (95% confidence interval [CI], 19%–52%; n = 164). Because of the variable definition of responder across studies, the aggregate effect size on symptom change was examined. Pooling across all informants (parents, teachers, observers), the 5-study effect was g = 0.29 (Standard error = 0.12 [95% CI, 0.16–0.52]; P = .014) with almost no variation across studies.

Sonuga-Barke and colleagues[6] identified a somewhat larger effect size in their meta-analysis by restricting studies to children who had a clear diagnosis of ADHD, as noted in **Table 1**. Stevenson and colleagues[46] distinguished between restriction elimination diet generally and elimination of food coloring. They concluded that both interventions might work, but that well-conducted large trials were lacking (foreshadowing the present authors' own conclusion to an extent).

When putting together both studies of restriction/elimination diets generally and studies of food color elimination specifically, effects sizes across the best studies therefore appear to range from d = 0.2 to d = 0.4 depending on study selection, with the possibility that effects are somewhat larger in children with ADHD. However, the finding of larger mean symptom changes in children with ADHD is difficult to interpret, because those children by definition have more extreme symptom scores and therefore less restriction of range in their scores in response to intervention. In addition, if food colors are not the main culprit in dietary effects, then challenge studies of food colors will underestimate the effects of an elimination diet. Carter and colleagues[47] challenged children who had responded to an elimination diet with foods to identify what caused their symptoms to worsen. During these challenges, a wide range of foods provoked reactions, including typical allergenic foods (wheat, eggs, milk, cheese), chocolate, and additive-containing foods. Only a small minority of children seemed to react primarily to artificial colorings.

Furthermore, and crucially, the mean symptom change is of little interest when it comes to clinical decision-making: more important is likelihood of positive response. What percentage of children might respond? If responses are heterogeneous, then the mean symptom change may obscure a strong response in some children and no response in the others. This topic is discussed again below.

Thus, as should be apparent, a key challenge in evaluating this literature is that different reviewers do not agree on what the relevant set of studies is for a given question, simply because variation in study methodology is so vast. Evaluating response to diet is also complicated by a wide range of study designs and questions asked. The studies in the literature have asked the following questions and arrived at the following answers.

First, many studies simply asked, when an open-label few foods diet is given with no attempt to blind raters to the diet, what percentage of parents or other observers think their child has improved after a few weeks? Nigg and colleagues[42] pooled studies on this question and answered, "49%" as shown in modified form in **Table 2**. However,

Table 2
Open-label, non-blind trials of restriction/elimination diet of any type (colors only, few foods, other) on variously defined symptom response rate of children with ADHD

Study Name, Year	N	Rate (%)	LL (%)	UL (%)	P Value
Cook & Woodhill,[61] 1976	10/15	67	41	85	.206
Rapp,[62] 1978	12/23	52	32	71	.835
Conners (Ch 3),[63] 1980	27/63	43	31	55	.258
Conners et al (Ch 4),[70] 1980	14/37	38	24	54	.143
Conners et al (Ch 5),[71] 1980	38/54	70	57	81	.004
Holborow et al,[64] 1981	29/344	8	6	12	.000
Egger et al,[43] 1985	62/76	82	71	89	.000
Loblay,[65] 1985	6/14	43	21	68	.594
Rowe,[66] 1988	14/55	25	16	39	.001
Sarantinos et al,[67] 1990	9/13	69	41	88	.177
Breakey et al,[68] 1991	281/516	54	50	59	.043
Carter et al,[47] 1993	50/130	38	31	47	.009
Boris & Mandel,[69] 1994	19/26	73	53	87	.024
Rowe & Rowe,[48] 1994	150/800	19	16	22	.000
Pelsser et al,[21] 2009	11/15	73	47	90	.083
Pelsser et al,[39] 2011	32/50	64	50	76	.051
Total	764/2231	49	36	63	.924

this number is not the number of randomly selected children with ADHD who will respond to diet—many of these studies drew children from specialty clinics for parents of children who either were interested in dietary intervention or already had suspected dietary problems. Others examined normal, nonhyperactive youth.

Two of these studies are considered in detail for the purpose of illustration. Rowe and Rowe[48] had 800 children referred for problems with hyperactivity. Of these 800, they selected 200 whose parents suspected that problems were related to diet (it was not clear if more than 200 parents suspected this, so a conservative estimate is that at least 25% of the parents thought diet might be affecting their child's symptoms). These 200 then underwent an open-label, nonblind trial of a diet free of food colorings; fully 75% (150) of them saw improvement. Of these, 54 agreed to a double-blind, placebo-controlled trial in which 24 of 54 seemed to respond. From this study, it seems clear that some children respond to dietary intervention, but the prior probability of response for a given child with ADHD is very difficult to gauge. It is not 24 of 54, because many nonresponders were already screened out. An alternative inference might be that 150 of 800 were responders by parent report on open label, and that half of these were "genuine," leading to an estimated true dietary response rate in the total ADHD population of 75 of 800 or about 9% to 10%, rather than the 49% in **Table 2**.

Carter and colleagues[47] provide another example. They selected 130 children referred to a specialty clinic for diet and hyperactivity (many already on special diets to address their ADHD). Each child was then placed on an individualized, open-label, nonblinded few foods diet for 2 to 3 weeks, with dietary adjustments made to maximize chances of improvement. Only 78 (60%) were able to tolerate the 2- to 3-week few foods trial and continued. For 59 of them, parents thought there was meaningful improvement, suggesting an open-label response rate of 45% (59/130), but 9 of these were unable to continue the diet after the trial, leading to an open-label success rate of 38% even in children for whom parents suspected a dietary problem ahead of time. Foods were then reintroduced in an effort to identify offending substances or foods, again in a nonblind, open-trial fashion. Finally, 19 children who had been responders were given a double-blind, placebo-controlled trial with and without offending foods. This trial was done by disguising offending foods or food colors into the food. For 14 of 19 (73%) children, behavior was "better" on placebo, although size of the effect required to identify a change was unclear. From this study, it would be inferred that perhaps 28% (38% × 73%) of children whose parents suspect a dietary influence will have a true positive response to diet in regards to a reduction in ADHD symptoms, again less than the 49% implied in **Table 2**.

Second, then, is the question of a true double-blind trial to look at response rate. Because most studies have been preoccupied with mean symptom change, only a few studies meet the criteria of using an elimination diet, maintaining at least a single-blind (observers or raters are not aware of the diet) or a double-blind (parents, children, and observers are unaware of the diet), and also enable a count of percentage of responders by some definition. Nevertheless, these are the most informative if heterogeneity of response is assumed.

As noted earlier, Nigg and colleagues[42] concluded that the handful of available studies in this vein suggested a response rate that could be 25% to 30%. A conservative set of such studies is summarized in **Table 3**. (**Table 3** excludes some studies that purported to be double-blind but which were judged not to be double-blind.) **Table 3** suggests a response rate of about 26% of ADHD children to various forms of restriction diet. The authors considered these studies a bit more closely to scrutinize

Table 3
Summary of 5 double-blind randomized trials of elimination or challenge diet in children with ADHD not preselected to be diet responsive

Authors, Year	Δ Criterion (%)	N	Rate (%)	LL (%)	UL (%)
Conners et al,[72] 1978	25	15	26.7	10.4	53.3
Harley et al,[44] 1978	10	23	22.8	12.6	37.8
Kaplan et al,[29] 1989	25	24	41.7	24.1	61.7
Schmidt et al,[45] 1997	100	49	24.5	14.5	38.3
Williams et al,[49] 1978	33	24	19.2	8.2	38.7
Pooled effect		135	26.4	20.0	34.1

Note: Change criterion reflects change in symptom scores identified as necessary by investigator to say child benefitted from intervention. 100% symptom change means "normal range" behavior after intervention. All except Schmidt used Conners rating scale as the outcome measure. LL, UL, 95% confidence interval upper and lower limits.

the clinical question of response likelihood and to illustrate the methods and range of findings.

Kaplan and colleagues[29] examined 24 hyperactive preschool boys. They controlled all food given to the entire family during the weeks of the trial, with a diet that restricted not only food colors, but also chocolate, MSG, preservatives, caffeine, and any substance that families reported might affect their specific child. The diet was also low in simple sugars, and it was dairy-free if the family reported a history of possible problems with cow's milk. They defined a responder as 25% symptom improvement, and by this criterion, the response rate was nearly 50%.

Harley and colleagues[44] studied 36 school-aged children and 10 preschool children. Here only the school-aged children were considered because they were unable to obtain teacher ratings on the preschoolers (although there was some suggestion of a higher response rate in the preschoolers). They likewise removed all food from the house, delivered all food to the entire family, disguised the foods, and left the families unaware of what diet they were eating or which weeks they were eating the experimental diet. Thus, blinding of parents and teachers was carefully done. They defined a meaningful change as just a 10% change in the rating scale on the experimental diet. By this criterion, 30% of the mothers or fathers saw improvement. However, these effects tended to occur only when the experimental diet was the second diet tried, raising suspicion of rater artifact. In teacher rating (perhaps the best single rater), there was no such order effect and only 6 of 36 or 17% showed a minimal 10% improvement. Only 4 of 36 (11%) showed a 10% improvement agreed on by both teacher and at least one parent.

Williams and colleagues[49] gave a full elimination diet in an open-label fashion, but then conducted a double-blind trial using cookies with additives in them, thus providing a lower bound estimate on response. They required a 33% change in symptoms to define a responder. By that criteria, 5 of 26 (19%) were responders in teacher ratings; none of these were echoed in parent ratings.

Schmidt and colleagues[45] created a reasonable attempt at a double-blind, placebo-controlled oligoantigenic diet for 49 children. The outcome was judged based on ratings in a standardized setting by trained raters blinded to intervention condition. Twelve (24%) children responded, but notably, the response magnitude in those 12 children was judged to be similar to the response magnitude of children who received medication in the medication arm of the same trial. This small study thus suggests that the diet may work very well for some children.

Overall, studies that fully control the diet and conduct a double-blind trial to evaluate response rate are exceedingly rare, small, and outdated (none have been reported in nearly 2 decades if the studies by Pelsser and colleagues are excluded for inadequate blinding). More common are double-blind trials of food color additives. Taken together, the literature suggests that some children respond, but are almost certainly a minority of children with ADHD.

SUMMARY OF LITERATURE ON EFFECTIVENESS OF RESTRICTION DIET FOR ADHD

A small, but extensively discussed literature yields an emerging consensus that dietary intervention to remove food additives (color and perhaps preservatives) likely yields a small aggregate benefit, which is in the range of a standardized mean difference of about 0.3. Because this finding is based on a randomized, placebo-controlled trial, it verges on the strongest level of evidence rating (level 1) based on the guidelines from the Oxford Center for Evidenced Based Medicine. However, the small samples and now-dated methods of most studies, in conjunction with relatively small effect, suggest that the evidence rating might be conservatively graded at level 2. That said, and while the effect size of 0.3 is much smaller than a medication effect, it could be clinically significant in some cases. For example, a change of this magnitude across a group average is equivalent to a change from the 62nd to the 50th percentile.

Overall, for children presenting for ADHD treatment with no obvious gastrointestinal symptoms or strong prior evidence of a dietary effect, a strict elimination diet may have a 10% to 30% chance of providing a true effect detectable on a double-blind measurement, but this estimate is limited by very small samples and widely varying methods. The best estimate on the small literature is about a 25% rate of at least some symptom improvement. For some children, perhaps a minority of 10% of children with ADHD, response can include a full remission of symptoms equivalent to a successful medication trial. In short, the literature suggests that an elimination diet should be considered a possible treatment for ADHD, but one that will work partially or fully, and only in a potentially small subset of children.

LIMITATIONS AND RESEARCH DIRECTIONS

Two major limitations plague this literature and are noted by all reviewers. First, the data base is very small. In part, this is because doing these studies well is extremely difficult. Even if all elimination diet and food color challenge studies are taken as a whole, studies that used properly controlled procedures have examined only a few hundred children, and even fewer with ADHD. Much of this literature is in fact outdated, going back 3 decades. In the interim, understanding and assessment of ADHD have evolved; children's diets and average intake have changed, and the number of food additives used in the United States has increased. Thus, effects for today's children may look rather different than they did 30 years ago.

Furthermore, cultural and national differences in food content are notable, such that results in one nation may not generalize to another. For example, the number of food additives approved for use varies considerably between countries. Canada[50] and the European Union[51] both have less than 500 food additives approved for use. Contrast this with the United States, which has over 3000 food additives allowed to be used in food.[52] This much more liberal food policy results in a much larger exposure to chemicals in the United States. The issue of historical relevance is also notable, in that food content has changed. Stevens and colleagues[53] reported that the amount of artificial food colors and sweeteners allowed into foods has risen 5-fold in the past 60 years. This fact may suggest that prior studies have underestimated potential benefits for today's children, although there is as yet no evidence that the prevalence of ADHD differs among these nations.

The second major limitation is that the literature consistently shows that some children appear to respond to dietary intervention and some do not. Who are the responders, and how big is their response? This question has not yet received sufficient investigation to enable much beyond speculation given the very small, almost pilot nature of studies of individual differences to date. Although some studies suggested that response rate was predicted by parent suspicion of a dietary sensitivity, these effects were generally not formally defined, measured, or replicated. Thus, it is difficult to derive much clinical guidance from this research. Further comment is made in the "Future Directions" section.

CLINICAL ISSUES RELATED TO ATTEMPTING A RESTRICTION DIET

With the preceding in mind, dietary intervention for ADHD has less than a 50–50 chance of success and a notably lower chance of success than treatments such as pharmacotherapy. Clinical advice to parents interested in a restriction/elimination diet for children with ADHD might take a form along these lines: "An elimination diet has a chance of success between 0% and 50%, with our best guess being a 10% to 30% chance of successful completion and positive response." However, patients would need to be advised of the risks and difficulties of such interventions, including the risks of continued behavioral or learning problems, while other treatments which may have a 60% to 90% chance of benefit are delayed.

With that said, (1) many parents remain interested in dietary intervention, (2) the literature suggests that some children may benefit (a trial is not senseless), and (3), clinicians need some idea what the family would be getting into if they attempt a restriction diet. Therefore, a brief presentation of clinical considerations if such an intervention is going to be pursued follows.

First, a key issue for the mental health professional is often the lack of detailed nutrition education to adequately support a family embarking on an elimination diet. Each type of diet has different considerations based on potential difficulties with adherence and varying levels of safety. In general, elimination diets require discipline to sustain the diet over the testing period, major changes to food intake, and removal of highly palatable foods that are pleasurable due to their ability to release dopamine (high sugar-processed food)[54,55]; there is potential for conflict between parent and child if the child is unhappy with the dietary change. Thus, implementing these diets can be very challenging for the family and the clinician.

A "few foods" diet is by far the most challenging, because it is highly restrictive (initially allowing only a few foods with low allergenic potential) and then requiring testing of each food as it is reintroduced. Furthermore, the few foods diet must be overseen by a dietitian to ensure that the nutritional adequacy of the diet is maintained during the testing period. This dietary intervention is the most restrictive and the least nutritionally complete; therefore, it may be best viewed as a last resort option unless clear food allergy symptoms are present in addition to ADHD symptoms. At the same time, this diet can be very beneficial for identifying multiple food allergies in an individual. If a parent reports multiple known food allergies in their child and/or food allergy symptoms (described earlier) are present in addition to ADHD symptoms, then the few foods diet may be an appropriate place to start. Referral to an immunologist who can conduct skin prick allergy testing may also be beneficial, but dietary response may occur even with a negative skin prick test, if the response is due to a food intolerance rather than to an allergy. It remains unclear whether the presence of food allergy symptoms or allergy skin prick findings increase the likelihood that ADHD symptoms will respond to an elimination diet.

Second, if food allergy symptoms are *not* present, then a diet only restricting food additives may be a better choice. This diet is much less restrictive and hence is easier to implement and not as likely to cause an iatrogenic nutrient deficiency. Nonetheless, nutritional counseling is again advisable to ensure a nutritionally adequate diet is maintained during the trial and to counsel parents in learning how to read ingredient lists on food labels and how best to avoid food additives. In general, there is no risk to the exclusion of food additives per se, because most food additives, with the exception of vitamins and minerals, do not add nutritional value to the diet. Each food item in the diet can be replaced by a similar food item that excludes these additives. This concept helps prevent families from simply "excluding" foods. For example, a children's brand of breakfast cereal high in artificial colors can be replaced by oatmeal with added brown sugar and raisins. This approach can potentially steer the family toward a more whole-food, nutrient-dense diet that can increase their nutrient intake in addition to helping them avoid additives.

In short, a mental health professional can start this process, but generally should collaborate with a dietitian or other qualified professional with nutritional expertise. Patients can be given a list of food additives to avoid (for examples, see Appendix A) and can be instructed to look for ingredient labels that are short and easy to read and that have ingredients that they themselves could easily add to a food. For example, sodium benzoate would not be added by someone cooking at home, so that is an ingredient they would avoid.

It can be helpful to remind patients that nutrient-dense foods that have few to no additives are more often found on the outer aisles of a grocery store (fruits, vegetables, meat, dairy, and bread) and that bakery bread has the fewest additives. Other staple foods lower in additives can be found in the middle aisles (many times very low or very high on the shelves). These staples lower in additives include items like simple brown rice, oats, pasta, canned tomatoes, beans, nuts, and applesauce. Label reading will take more time initially, while safe foods are first being identified, and less time later.

With regard to duration, the diet can be tested over a 2- to 4-week period. It is important to emphasize that, to evaluate whether there is benefit of the diet, the diet must be followed strictly for a few weeks. Furthermore, during this period there is substantial possibility of placebo or expectancy effect, as would be seen with initiation of drug treatment. Regular standardized ratings (eg, using the 10-item Conners ADHD Index or Conners Global Index,[56] depending on target symptoms) could be obtained weekly, preferably from a teacher, in addition to the parent. A baseline rating should be obtained for a week or 2 before the trial. The mental health professional should review these ratings, score them, and examine them for reliable improvement, which means considering the 90% confidence interval around the scores (provided in the manual) to determine if the effect is likely to exceed chance variation in behavior. If after 4 weeks of strict adherence, no benefit is noted, then the patient could be switched to other treatments instead.

Note that there is one exception to the prior guideline. The few foods diet used for allergy testing does not follow this same time period. Allergy symptoms often remit within days of removing an allergen from the diet. Then, foods must be re-introduced individually over the next few weeks to test for a reaction. Therefore, if benefit is not noted after 1 week on the few foods diet, it can be discontinued.

RECOMMENDATIONS

A major recommendation coming out of this review, echoing prior reviews (see **Table 1**), is that dietary intervention for ADHD was abandoned too quickly in North America. Although it is likely that only a minority of children with ADHD will respond to dietary intervention, the evidence persistently suggests that for some children such intervention can be quite effective. Thus, where should the field go to develop and realize this possibility? Several additional future study and design considerations and suggestions were offered by Stevenson and colleagues.[46] The present authors highlight selected recommendations of their own here.

The first key future direction is clearly the need to improve personalized selection or treatment matching. Here, there are several levels of analysis that need to be pursued. It has already been noted that prior, albeit small studies, attempted to select children on the basis of either (1) allergy symptoms, or (2) ADHD status. These types of clinical predictors need to be more carefully re-evaluated in the contemporary context. In addition, advances in biological measurements suggest the potential to examine biomarkers of treatment response that may be of value. As one illustration, Stevenson and colleagues[57] found that histamine degradation genes moderated the effects of food additives in the data set reported by McCann and colleagues.[37] Further efforts in research to evaluate other biomarkers (eg, inflammatory biomarkers) may be valuable as understanding of these mechanisms increases.

Thus, the effect of diet on ADHD, and the identification of who benefits, would be greatly aided by better understanding of mechanisms in the ADHD population. To date, attempts in this vein have not yielded convincing results. Pelsser and colleagues[39] failed to find reliable prediction of diet response and IgE levels in blood, and use of IgG levels to identify challenge effects was similarly inconclusive, leading those authors to conclude that such tests did not add clinical value. This finding also suggests that food intolerance may be more likely than food allergy in this population.

Nonetheless, it is increasingly recognized that dietary additives, unhealthy food, emotional stress, and chemical toxicants in the environment may act synergistically and via common mechanisms, including in some instances inflammatory pathways. Studies of mechanisms and efforts to preidentify future responders to a dietary intervention can readily measure or at least obtain relevant sampling of stress (self-reports as well as cortisol measures), toxicant burden (urine or blood samples), along with food studies. Although assaying all of these measures at once is costly, such data and tissue banks will ultimately be needed to ensure maximal benefit of tailored lifestyle-related treatment and prevention approaches for ADHD.

Second, what is striking is the small scale of this literature relative to popular interest. Needed are fresh contemporary trials of elimination diets with well-controlled double-blind procedures as were pioneered decades ago. Contemporary trials of elimination diets are particularly needed, for the current readership, in North America, where trials of elimination diets essentially have been at a standstill for a generation. The same holds true for any nation that wants to evaluate pertinence of elimination diets in children with ADHD in their nation's specific context.

Third, the interplay of food reactivity with basic nutrition is increasingly in need of scrutiny. A modified diet may also be more nutritious. Thus, examining nutrient intake and maximizing nutrition while eliminating potential food intolerances or allergies may yield the most powerful effects. At the same time, the fact that supplementing with nutrients may be less burdensome than a few foods diet trial may open alternative avenues for treatment-tailoring.

Finally, which symptoms respond? Twenty years ago, Rowe and Rowe[48] suggested that it might be emotional symptoms, such as irritability, rather than inattention or hyperactivity that responds best to dietary intervention. This hypothesis has been often overlooked since then, yet may warrant renewed scrutiny in light of renewed and strong interest in the role of emotion regulation and irritability in ADHD.[58]

SUMMARY

Two generations ago, ADHD was seen by many as a neurotic reaction to a difficult upbringing. A decade ago, it was seen as primarily a genetic condition by many. Now it is seen, more appropriately, as likely to be an epigenetic condition triggered, in susceptible individuals, by varying environmental amplifiers. For a subgroup of children, these appear to include food intolerance, food allergy, or both. The literature clearly demonstrates that a minority of children with ADHD will benefit from an elimination diet. Research funders, scientists, and clinicians would do well to re-invigorate investigation of this intervention, while avoiding both excessive skepticism (clearly, it may work for some), and excess optimism (it probably only works for a minority). If it can be determined who benefits and why, important insights into the pathophysiology of ADHD could result. Because of likely heterogeneity of response, studies should focus on identifying the rate of responders by an a priori definition of clinically significant response and then examining predictors of response.

REFERENCES

1. Hurt EA, Arnold LE, Lofthouse N. Dietary and nutritional treatments for attention-deficit/hyperactivity disorder: current research support and recommendations for practitioners. Curr Psychiatry Rep 2011;13:323–32.
2. Rucklidge JJ, Johnstone J, Kaplan BJ. Nutrient supplementation approaches in the treatment of ADHD. Expert Rev Neurother 2009;9:461–76.
3. Rucklidge JJ, Frampton CM, Gorman B, et al. Vitamin-mineral treatment of attention-deficit hyperactivity disorder in adults: double-blind randomised placebo-controlled trial. Br J Psychiatry 2014;204:306–15.
4. Bloch MH, Qawasmi A. Omega-3 fatty acid supplementation for the treatment of children with attention-deficit/hyperactivity disorder symptomatology: systematic review and meta-analysis. J Am Acad Child Adolesc Psychiatry 2011;50: 991–1000.
5. Gillies D, Sinn J, Lad SS, et al. Polyunsaturated fatty acids (PUFA) for attention deficit hyperactivity disorder (ADHD) in children and adolescents. Cochrane Database Syst Rev 2012;(7):CD007986.
6. Sonuga-Barke EJ, Brandeis D, Cortese S, et al. Nonpharmacological interventions for ADHD: systematic review and meta-analyses of randomized controlled trials of dietary and psychological treatments. Am J Psychiatry 2013;170: 275–89.
7. Hawkey E, Nigg JT. Omega-3 fatty acid and ADHD: blood level analysis and meta-analytic extension of supplementation trials. Clin Psychol Rev, in press.
8. Rowe AH, editor. Elimination diets and the patient's allergies; a handbook of allergy. Philadelphia: Lea & Febiger; 1944.
9. Lapage CP. Allergy, metabolism, and the autonomic nervous system. Br Med J 1934;2:985–7.
10. Hall K. Allergy of the nervous system: a review. Ann Allergy 1976;36:49–64.
11. Grimshaw KE. Dietary management of food allergy in children. Proc Nutr Soc 2006;65:412–7.

12. Luyt D, Ball H, Makwana N, et al. BSACI guideline for the diagnosis and management of cow's milk allergy. Clin Exp Allergy 2014;44:642–72.
13. Kagalwalla AF. Dietary treatment of eosinophilic esophagitis in children. Dig Dis 2014;32:114–9.
14. Spergel JM. Eosinophilic esophagitis in adults and children: evidence for a food allergy component in many patients. Curr Opin Allergy Clin Immunol 2007;7: 274–8.
15. Mooney PD, Hadjivassiliou M, Sanders DS. Coeliac disease. BMJ 2014;348: g1561.
16. Mansueto P, Seidita A, D'Alcamo A, et al. Non-celiac gluten sensitivity: literature review. J Am Coll Nutr 2014;33:39–54.
17. Mari-Bauset S, Zazpe I, Mari-Sanchis A, et al. Evidence of the gluten-free and casein-free diet in autism spectrum disorders: a systematic review. J Child Neurol 2014;30:30.
18. Kanarek RB. Artificial food dyes and attention deficit hyperactivity disorder. Nutr Rev 2011;69:385–91.
19. Zukiewicz-Sobczak WA, Wroblewska P, Adamczuk P, et al. Causes, symptoms and prevention of food allergy. Postepy Dermatol Alergol 2013;30:113–6.
20. Allen DH, Van Nunen S, Loblay R, et al. Adverse reactions to foods. Med J Aust 1984;141:S37–42.
21. Pelsser LM, Buitelaar JK, Savelkoul HF. ADHD as a (non) allergic hypersensitivity disorder: a hypothesis. Pediatr Allergy Immunol 2009;20:107–12.
22. Kuriaki K, Wada I. Effect of tetrodotoxin on the mammalian neuro-muscular system. Jpn J Pharmacol 1957;7:35–7.
23. Lopez-Perez SJ, Urena-Guerrero ME, Morales-Villagran A. Monosodium glutamate neonatal treatment as a seizure and excitotoxic model. Brain Res 2010;4: 246–56.
24. Holton KF, Taren DL, Thomson CA, et al. The effect of dietary glutamate on fibromyalgia and irritable bowel symptoms. Clin Exp Rheumatol 2012;30:10–7.
25. Katz RS, Heard AR, Mills M, et al. The prevalence and clinical impact of reported cognitive difficulties (fibrofog) in patients with rheumatic disease with and without fibromyalgia. J Clin Rheumatol 2004;10:53–8.
26. Miller EM, Pomerleau F, Huettl P, et al. Aberrant glutamate signaling in the prefrontal cortex and striatum of the spontaneously hypertensive rat model of attention-deficit/hyperactivity disorder. Psychopharmacology 2014;28:28.
27. Maltezos S, Horder J, Coghlan S, et al. Glutamate/glutamine and neuronal integrity in adults with ADHD: a proton MRS study. Transl Psychiatry 2014;4: e373.
28. Chang JP, Lane HY, Tsai GE. Attention deficit hyperactivity disorder and N-methyl-D-aspartate (NMDA) dysregulation. Curr Pharm Des 2014;9:9.
29. Kaplan BJ, McNicol J, Conte RA, et al. Dietary replacement in preschool-aged hyperactive boys. Pediatrics 1989;83:7–17.
30. Lau K, McLean WG, Williams DP, et al. Synergistic interactions between commonly used food additives in a developmental neurotoxicity test. Toxicol Sci 2006;90:178–87.
31. Feingold BF. Hyperkinesis and learning disabilities linked to artificial food flavors and colors. Am J Nurs 1975;75:797–803.
32. Feingold BF. Why your child is hyperactive. New York: Random House; 1975.
33. Feingold BF. Food additives and child development. Hosp Pract 1973;8:10–21.
34. The National Advisory Committee on Hyperkinesis and Food Additives. Final report to the nutrition foundation. New York: The Nutrition Foundation, Inc; 1980.

35. Kavale KA, Forness SR. Hyperactivity and diet treatment: a meta-analysis of the Feingold hypothesis. J Learn Disabil 1983;16:324–30.

36. Schab DW, Trinh NH. Do artificial food colors promote hyperactivity in children with hyperactive syndromes? A meta-analysis of double-blind placebo-controlled trials. J Dev Behav Pediatr 2004;25:423–34.

37. McCann D, Barrett A, Cooper A, et al. Food additives and hyperactive behaviour in 3-year-old and 8/9-year-old children in the community: a randomised, double-blinded, placebo-controlled trial. Lancet 2007;370:1560–7. http://dx.doi.org/10.1016/S0140-6736(07)61306-3. pii:S0140-6736(07)61306-3.

38. UFDA, U. F. a. D. A. Summary of color additives for use in United States in foods, drugs, cosmetics and medical devices. 2011. Available at: http://www.fda.gov/forindustry/coloradditives/coloradditiveinventories/ucm115641.htm. Accessed June 1, 2014.

39. Pelsser LM, Frankena K, Toorman J, et al. Effects of a restricted elimination diet on the behaviour of children with attention-deficit hyperactivity disorder (INCA study): a randomised controlled trial. Lancet 2011;377:494–503.

40. Jacobson MF. Petition to Ban the Use of Yellow 5 and Other Food Dyes, in the Interim to Require a Warning on Foods Containing these Dyes, to Correct the Information the Food and Drug Administration Gives to Consumers On the Impact of These Dyes on the Behavior of Some Children, and to Require Neurotoxicity Testing of New Food Additives and Food Colors. Washington, DC: Center for Science in the Public Interest; 2008. Available at: http://tinyurl.com/yk9ghx8. Accessed June 1, 2014.

41. Stevens LJ, Kuczek T, Burgess JR, et al. Dietary sensitivities and ADHD symptoms: thirty-five years of research. Clin Pediatr (Phila) 2011;50:279–93. http://dx.doi.org/10.1177/0009922810384728. pii:0009922810384728.

42. Nigg JT, Lewis K, Edinger T, et al. Meta-analysis of attention-deficit/hyperactivity disorder or attention-deficit/hyperactivity disorder symptoms, restriction diet, and synthetic food color additives. J Am Acad Child Adolesc Psychiatry 2012;51:86–97.e88.

43. Egger J, Carter CM, Graham PJ, et al. Controlled trial of oligoantigenic treatment in the hyperkinetic syndrome. Lancet 1985;1:540–5. pii:S0140-6736(85)91206-1.

44. Harley JP, Ray RS, Tomasi L, et al. Hyperkinesis and food additives: testing the Feingold hypothesis. Pediatrics 1978;61:818–28.

45. Schmidt MH, Möcks P, Lay B, et al. Does oligoantigenic diet influence hyperactive/conduct-disordered children–a controlled trial. Eur Child Adolesc Psychiatry 1997;6:88–95.

46. Stevenson J, Buitelaar J, Cortese S, et al. Research review: the role of diet in the treatment of attention-deficit/hyperactivity disorder—an appraisal of the evidence on efficacy and recommendations on the design of future studies. J Child Psychol Psychiatry 2014;55:416–27.

47. Carter CM, Urbanowicz M, Hemsley R, et al. Effects of a few food diet in attention deficit disorder. Arch Dis Child 1993;69:564–8.

48. Rowe KS, Rowe KJ. Synthetic food coloring and behavior: a dose response effect in a double-blind, placebo-controlled, repeated-measures study. J Pediatr 1994;125:691–8.

49. Williams JI, Cram DM, Tausig FT, et al. Relative effects of drugs and diet on hyperactive behaviors: an experimental study. Pediatrics 1978;61:811–7.

50. Health Canada. Available at: http://www.hc-sc.gc.ca/fn-an/securit/addit/list/index-eng.php#a1. Accessed June 1, 2014.

51. European Commission. Available at: https://webgate.ec.europa.eu/sanco_foods/main/?sector=FAD&auth=SANCAS. Accessed June 1, 2014.
52. Federal Drug Administration. Available at: http://www.fda.gov/Food/Ingredients PackagingLabeling/FoodAdditivesIngredients/ucm115326.htm. Accessed June 1, 2014.
53. Stevens LJ, Burgess JR, Stochelski MA, et al. Amounts of artificial food dyes and added sugars in foods and sweets commonly consumed by children. Clin Pediatr 2014;24:24.
54. Hoebel BG, Avena NM, Bocarsly ME, et al. Natural addiction: a behavioral and circuit model based on sugar addiction in rats. J Addict Med 2009;3: 33–41.
55. Rada P, Avena NM, Hoebel BG. Daily bingeing on sugar repeatedly releases dopamine in the accumbens shell. Neuroscience 2005;134:737–44.
56. Conners CK. Conners-III rating scales. 3rd edition. Ontario (Canada): Mental Health Systems Inc; 2008.
57. Stevenson J, Sonuga-Barke E, McCann D, et al. The role of histamine degradation gene polymorphisms in moderating the effects of food additives on children's ADHD symptoms. Am J Psychiatry 2010;167:1108–15.
58. Shaw P, Stringaris A, Nigg J, et al. Emotion dysregulation in attention deficit hyperactivity disorder. Am J Psychiatry 2014;171:276–93.
59. Breakey J. The role of diet and behaviour in childhood. J Paediatr Child Health 1997;33:190–4.
60. Arnold LE, Hurt E, Lofthouse N. Attention-deficit/hyperactivity disorder: dietary and nutritional treatments. Child Adolesc Psychiatr Clin N Am 2013;22(3): 381–402, v.
61. Cook PS, Woodhill JM. The Feingold dietary treatment of the hyperkinetic syndrome. Med J Aust 1976;2:85–8, 90.
62. Rapp DJ. Double-blind confirmation and treatment of milk sensitivity. Med J Aust 1978;1:571–2.
63. Conners CK. Foods, food dyes, and allergies. In: Food additives and hyperactive children. New York: Plenum Press; 1980.
64. Holborow P, Elkins J, Berry P. The effect of the Feingold diet on "normal" school children. J Learn Disabil 1981;14:143–7.
65. Loblay R. Adverse reactions to tartrazine. Food Technol Aust 1985;37:508–14.
66. Rowe KS. Synthetic food colourings and 'hyperactivity': a double-blind crossover study. Aust Paediatr J 1988;24:143–7.
67. Sarantinos J, Rowe KS, Briggs DR. Synthetic food colouring and behavioural change in children with attention deficit disorder: a double-blind, placebo-controlled, repeated measures study. Proc Nutr Soc Australia 1990; 15:233.
68. Breakey J, Hill M, Reilly C, et al. A report on a trial of the low additive, low salicylate diet in the treatment of behavior and learning problems in children. Aust J Nutr Diet 1991;48:89–94.
69. Boris M, Mandel FS. Foods and additives are common causes of the attention deficit hyperactive disorder in children. Ann Allergy 1994;72:462–8.
70. Conners CK. A second challenge study. In: Food additives and hyperactive children. New York: Plenum Press; 1980.
71. Conners CK. Food, food dyes and allergies. In: Food additives and hyperactive children. New York: Plenum Press; 1980.
72. Conners CK. The Challenge Model. In: Food additives and hyperactive children. New York: Plenum Press; 1980.

APPENDIX A: EXAMPLE FOOD ADDITIVE LIST THAT COULD BE GIVEN TO A PATIENT

Food additives to avoid:

- All artificial colors
- All artificial flavors
- All artificial sweeteners, including aspartame, acesulfame K, neotame, saccharin, sucralose
- Sodium benzoate
- Butylated hydroxyanisole and Butylated hydroxytoluene
- Carrageenan
- Monosodium or monopotassium glutamate
- Any hydrolyzed, textured, or modified protein

An Integrated Dietary/ Nutritional Approach to ADHD

Elizabeth A. Hurt, PhD[a],*, L. Eugene Arnold, MD, M.Ed[b]

KEYWORDS

- Attention-deficit/hyperactivity disorder • Dietary treatments • Nutritional treatments
- Complementary treatment

KEY POINTS

- Children whose families are considering dietary/nutritional interventions should first be screened for nutritional deficiencies/insufficiencies through a detailed dietary history and physical examination, and laboratory tests as indicated by the findings.
- Diurnal appetite suppression from stimulants may unbalance a diet.
- Rarely will a patient be deficient/insufficient in only one nutrient; therefore it may be necessary to supplement with several and/or provide a "background" balanced vitamin/mineral supplement in recommended daily amounts.
- For children who have not responded optimally to stimulant medication, essential fatty acid (eg, fish oil) augmentation may be considered.
- Herbs should be obtained only from a reputable source because impurities such as lead have been found in some.
- When deciding on an individual patient trial, available evidence of effectiveness should be weighed against safety, difficulty, and expense.
- For children whose families are using traditional Chinese medicine, a trial of Yizhi capsule or Jingling oral liquid may be added to stimulant medication with careful monitoring.
- For a small number of children, a restricted elimination diet (RED) may be effective; however, family organizational skills and parents' level of control over the child's diet should be considered before attempting a RED.
- One risk of dietary intervention is the delay of evidence-based treatments; an appropriate timeline for a reasonable trial of dietary intervention should be discussed before beginning treatment.

[a] Wright State University, School of Professional Psychology, Ellis Human Development Institute, 9 North Edwin C. Moses Boulevard, Dayton, OH 45402, USA; [b] Nisonger Center, The Ohio State University, 1581 Dodd Drive, Columbus OH 43210, USA
* Corresponding author.
E-mail address: beth.hurt7478@gmail.com

Child Adolesc Psychiatric Clin N Am 23 (2014) 955–964
http://dx.doi.org/10.1016/j.chc.2014.06.002
1056-4993/14/$ – see front matter © 2014 Elsevier Inc. All rights reserved.

childpsych.theclinics.com

Abbreviations	
ADHD	Attention-deficit/hyperactivity disorder
EFA	Essential fatty acid
RCT	Randomized clinical trial
RDA/RDI	Recommended daily amount/recommended daily intake
RED	Restricted elimination diet
RUDE	Risky, unrealistic, difficult, or expensive
SECS	Safe, easy, cheap, and sensible
TCM	Traditional Chinese medicine

Three aspects of nutrition and diet in management of attention-deficit/hyperactivity disorder (ADHD) have been detailed in companion articles elsewhere in this issue. Nigg and Holton discuss elimination diets in "Restriction and Elimination Diets in ADHD Treatment," Bloch and Mulqueen discuss essential fatty acids in "Nutritional Supplements for the Treatment of Attention-Deficit Hyperactivity Disorder," and Ni and colleagues discuss traditional Chinese medicine in "Traditional Chinese Medicine in the Treatment of ADHD: A Review." This article integrates those contributions into a practical clinical approach, keeping in mind that health and disease result from the interaction of the genome with the environment, including the nutritional environment.

As described by Ni and colleagues elsewhere in this issue, traditional Chinese medicine (TCM), which includes attention to nutrition, has treated symptoms similar to those of ADHD for more than 2000 years. After the first Chinese workshop on ADHD in 1986, a system for treatment of ADHD using the TCM theoretic approach was developed. Western use of dietary intervention for ADHD accelerated in the 1970s after the proposal by Feingold[1] that ADHD could be treated by removing synthetic colors and flavors from the diet (see article by Nigg and Holton elsewhere in this issue). Based on the current available literature, including research cited in the 3 relevant articles in this issue, the following questions should be considered when designing a nutritional/dietary treatment for children with ADHD, either as an alternative treatment (used instead of conventional treatments) or as a complementary treatment (used as an adjunct to conventional treatment).

DOES THE CHILD HAVE ANY SUSPECTED/DOCUMENTED NUTRITIONAL DEFICIENCIES OR INSUFFICIENCIES?

Some,[2] but not all,[3] studies have documented deficiencies in minerals, such as iron, zinc, and magnesium, in children with ADHD relative to healthy controls. Various vitamins, most recently vitamin D, have also been suspected to be deficient in ADHD and other disorders (some of them often comorbid with ADHD). More common than frank deficiency is insufficiency, a borderline nutrient status slightly below the recommended level but not severe enough to cause classical deficiency signs, such as anemia, pellagra, or scurvy. A deficiency or insufficiency state could result from either insufficient intake or genetic requirement for greater-than-average intake. On average, Americans consume less than the recommended daily intake (RDI) of a half-dozen vitamins and minerals (**Fig. 1**).

Especially for families who are interested in nutritional treatment, the first step is an assessment of the child's baseline nutritional status to determine whether the child has any subthreshold or clinically significant nutritional deficiencies. A careful diet history can be illuminating. For example, a child whose only vegetable is potatoes in the

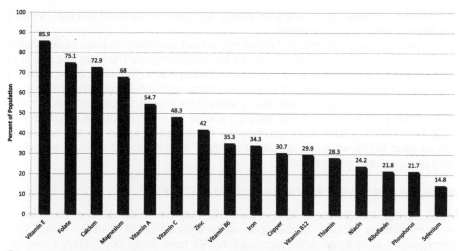

Fig. 1. Percentage of Americans who do not ingest the recommended daily allowance or recommended dietary intake of various essential minerals and vitamins. Note that, on average, each person has inadequate intake of 6 or 7 essential nutrients. The percentages of individuals not meeting the Dietary Reference Intakes (DRI) are based on day-1 nutrient intakes from the Continuing Survey of Food Intakes by Individuals and DRI values established from the mid-1990s to 2002. (*Data from* United States Department of Agriculture (USDA). Continuing Survey of Food Intakes by Individuals (CSFII) 1994–96. 1998. Available at: http://www.ars.usda.gov/Services/docs.htm?docid=11200. Accessed June 12, 2014.)

form of chips or fries and who rarely eats fruit can be assumed to be insufficient in several vitamins and minerals. A child who eats no or few dairy products in a northern climate may be assumed to have vitamin D deficiency in the winter and early spring. Equivocal cases may need tests of nutrient levels. Preschoolers and adolescents should be suspected of iron deficiency because those periods of rapid growth may outpace the body iron reserves. Vitamin D is worth testing in a child first presenting in winter or spring.

If any nutritional deficiencies are identified, well-monitored supplementation is standard treatment. The child's response to supplementation should be closely monitored, because some essential nutrients can be toxic in excess, and produce side effects (eg, constipation with iron supplement, diarrhea with magnesium, stomach discomfort with vitamins). Standardized rating scales of ADHD symptoms can check efficacy. Documentation that the nutrient has reached a normal level would indicate that the therapeutic dose can be tapered down to a recommended daily amount (RDA)/RDI level. It is also desirable, although not strictly necessary, to check nutrient blood levels to determine whether a change in a nutrient level is related to a change in ADHD symptoms. If the child has documented deficiencies, efficacy of supplementation should be evaluated before initiation of other dietary or conventional interventions.

DOES THE CHILD HAVE ANY SUSPECTED OR DOCUMENTED FOOD ALLERGIES?

As discussed in detail by Nigg and Holton elsewhere in this issue, children who have a documented food allergy may benefit from an exclusion diet of the one or more foods to which the child is allergic. Similar to supplementation for nutritional deficiencies, if the child has a documented food allergy, the elimination of the specific foods would be considered a standard conventional treatment rather than an alternative treatment.

For children who have a specific food allergy, symptoms may remit quickly—within a few days of removing the allergen.

A more common problem than food allergy is food sensitivity. In most cases of food sensitivity, an immune mechanism cannot be demonstrated. The child just reacts to the food (or food component) as if it were a noxious agent. In these cases, standard allergy testing is not useful, and the offending agent can only be identified by an elimination trial with challenge. Severe dietary restrictions should not be continued for long periods without demonstration of benefit because they can introduce dietary imbalance with nutritional deficiency/insufficiency. An exception to this caution is elimination of food additives, such as artificial colors, flavors, and preservatives, which have no inherent nutritional value.[4]

IS THE CHILD RECEIVING ADEQUATE GENERAL NUTRITION?

Some reports indicate the children with ADHD may have mild deficiencies in blood levels of vitamins, although neither open nor controlled trials of RDI/RDA vitamin supplementation in children with diagnosed ADHD have been conducted. However, adults with ADHD in a placebo-controlled randomized clinical trial (RCT) benefitted significantly from a 36-ingredient supplement with all known vitamins and essential minerals.[5] Results from 2 placebo-controlled trials[6,7] of RDA/RDI supplementation in nondiagnosed children documented improvement in nonverbal cognitive skills, attention, and hyperactivity, although effectiveness may be limited to children with poor diets.[8] Given that RDA/RDI supplementation carries little risk, with the exception of rare genetic disorders, it can be recommended as a complementary treatment, particularly for children who do not eat balanced diets and/or have stimulant-related appetite suppression.

IS THE CHILD TAKING STIMULANT MEDICATION? IF SO, WHAT IS APPROPRIATE NUTRITIONAL SUPPORT?

Many families choose to try nutritional treatments because their child has not responded to conventional treatments. Most dietary/nutritional treatments have evaluated the efficacy of dietary treatments as alternative treatments (used instead of conventional treatments) rather than as complementary treatments (used as an adjunct to conventional treatments). However, for families whose children are currently being treated with conventional treatments, particularly medication, a few studies have evaluated the adjunctive benefit of nutritional treatments.

Omega-3

The nutritional treatment with the most research as an adjunctive treatment is essential fatty acid (EFA) supplementation. Although EFAs have considerable RCT evidence for a small but significant effect as monotherapy, the evidence for adjunctive treatment is equivocal, possibly because of a ceiling effect from the large benefit of stimulant medication in good responders. In one double-blind, placebo-controlled trial,[9] EFA supplementation did not add significant benefit to methylphenidate for children who were considered to be medication responders. In 2 additional studies of children not selected for previous methylphenidate response,[10,11] EFA supplementation also did not produce additional benefit when added to methylphenidate, although in the unblinded study,[11] children who received EFA supplementation as an adjunct to stimulant could be maintained on a significantly lower dose of methylphenidate and were less likely to experience appetite suppression (70.0% for methylphenidate and 33.3% for methylphenidate with EFA). Whether the lower rate of appetite suppression was specifically related to the lower stimulant dose or whether EFA supplementation itself directly decreased appetite suppression is unclear. This finding (lower methylphenidate dose and decreased side effects with EFA supplementation) requires replication before a standard-of-care recommendation can be made for providing EFA supplementation solely for reducing dosage and side effects (in the absence of additional benefit to ADHD symptoms) for children who respond well to stimulant medication.

On the other hand, in a recent study,[12] children judged to have had an unsatisfactory response to a combination of conventional treatments (methylphenidate and behavior therapy) were randomized to placebo or adjunctive EFA supplementation for 6 months. Children randomized to EFA supplementation were rated by parents as significantly more improved than those randomized to placebo. Thus, adjunctive EFA supplementation may be beneficial for children who do not have satisfactory response to conventional treatment.

Zinc

Three double-blind, placebo-controlled trials[13–15] have evaluated the benefit of zinc supplementation as an adjunct to stimulant medication. In 44 children treated with methylphenidate,[13] the authors found significantly greater benefit compared with placebo based on parent and teacher ratings. However, adjunctive zinc supplementation had no benefit on ADHD symptoms in the later 2 trials,[14,15] and children's zinc levels were not significantly affected by supplementation. However, in one trial,[14] children randomized to zinc supplementation at 30 mg/d, near the tolerable upper limit, required lower doses of D-amphetamine to optimize clinical benefit relative to those randomized to placebo. This finding requires replication before a recommendation can be made to consider zinc supplementation near the tolerable upper limit solely for reduction in stimulant dosage. Thus, zinc supplementation currently can not be recommended as an adjunctive treatment to conventional treatments for ADHD unless the child has documented zinc deficiency, for which zinc supplementation would be a standard treatment.

Traditional Chinese Herbs

As detailed by Ni and colleagues elsewhere in this issue, 2 Chinese medicine herbal treatments have been evaluated as adjunctive treatments to methylphenidate. In a 12-week trial,[16] children were randomized to receive Yizhi mixture (a combination of 10 herbs designed to affect Yin/Yang liver functions), methylphenidate, or combination treatment. ADHD symptoms improved significantly more in children randomized to combination treatment than in those randomized to either individual treatment. Fewer side effects were reported by children randomized to either the Yizhi mixture alone or combination treatment than by those randomized to methylphenidate alone. Similarly, children randomized to combination treatment with Jingling oral liquid and methylphenidate experienced greater improvement in ADHD and tic symptoms than children who were treated with methylphenidate alone.[17] The safety profile for Jingling liquid was not clear.

Given these results, supplementation with essential fatty acids or zinc does not seem warranted in children who respond well to conventional treatments. For families using a TCM approach, a carefully monitored individual trial of Yizhi or Jingling oral liquid may be considered as an adjunct to stimulant medication. Dietary supplementation has not been studied empirically as an adjunct to other medications for ADHD (atomoxetine, guanfacine extended release, clonidine extended release); therefore, children whose ADHD has responded only partially to these medications and whose families are considering adding an individual trial of a dietary intervention will require careful monitoring by their physician for efficacy and side effects.

CAN HERBS BE USED AS THE PRIMARY TREATMENT?

A few herbal preparations have been shown to be effective as monotherapy for ADHD. As described by Bloch and Mulqueen elsewhere in this issue, clinical trials evaluating herbal preparations by Western practitioners are limited. Pycnogenol (French maritime pine bark) showed significant benefit according to teacher, but not parent, ratings of ADHD symptoms in a double-blind, placebo-controlled trial.[18] St John's Wort, however, did not show improvement relative to placebo.[19] When compared with methylphenidate in a double-blind randomized trial,[20] children treated with gingko biloba experienced significantly less improvement of symptoms, although a controlled trial comparing gingko biloba and placebo has not been completed.

In addition to Chinese herbal medicine being evaluated as an adjunctive treatment to stimulant medication (see article by Ni and colleagues elsewhere in this issue), 2 Chinese medicinal herbs have been evaluated as alternative treatments. Improvement seen with duodongning[21] and Ningdong[22] granules was similar to that seen with methylphenidate in each trial, and fewer side effects were reported with Chinese herbal medication than with methylphenidate. These positive findings require replication. Herbs usually contain more than one psychoactive substance and may have additive or interactive effects. Families who try herbal preparations to treat ADHD symptoms should work with their practitioners to closely monitor efficacy and side effects.

WHAT IS THE CURRENT FAMILY ENVIRONMENT AND LEVEL OF CHILD COMPLIANCE?

Some dietary interventions may require limited time and effort (eg, giving the child a tablet or liquid formulation 1 or even 3 times per day), similar to the time and effort required by conventional medications. However, some treatments, such as the use of an elimination diet, require significant time, effort, and family organizational skills. As detailed by Nigg and Holton elsewhere in this issue, an elimination diet involves removing foods that are suspected to cause a behavioral reaction, and systematically adding them back to the diet to assess the child's reaction. Approximately 25% of children may show improvement on an elimination diet, and a minority (perhaps 8%–10%) may experience a full remission of symptoms. Recent research suggests[23] that families for whom a restricted elimination diet (RED) may be the most effective are those who are highly motivated and have a positive family environment. Because a RED requires a significant level of organizational skill, if the family has difficulty with organization and structure, these skills may require remediation before the RED can be implemented. Furthermore, if child compliance during mealtimes is already poor and/or the child is resistant to change, the family may benefit from parent training and/or family therapy to improve child compliance and parent-child communication before the RED is implemented, although this has not been evaluated in the literature.

Families who choose to implement a RED should first consider the level of control they will have over the child's dietary intake. Parents may need to plan to begin the RED when they will have the most control (eg, during a school holiday). Some children, especially those who are more astute, may notice the difference in how they feel and commit voluntarily to dietary adherence. Clinicians should attempt to cultivate this commitment in the child.

HOW MUCH SAFER THAN CONVENTIONAL MEDICATION ARE DIETARY AND NUTRITIONAL TREATMENTS? WHAT ABOUT HERBS?

Many people think that because dietary, nutritional, and herbal treatments are "natural," they are automatically safer than conventional medication. However, rattlesnake venom, tobacco, poison ivy, and deadly nightshade are also natural. Although many dietary/nutritional treatments are considerably safer than conventional medication (at least in moderation), and some may even promote general health (eg, omega-3 EFAs for heart health), others may confer risks as great as the FDA-approved medications. For example, megadoses of some vitamins or minerals (greater than the official upper tolerable limit) can cause liver damage, neuropathy, or deficiency of other vitamins or minerals through interfering with their absorption or metabolism. The dictum of Paracelsus, "The dose alone makes the poison," is especially apt for nutrients.

Herbs do not always have the same quality control as drugs and may have impurities that can be more dangerous than drugs. It is important to check that the source of the herbs is reputable. Even when of standard quality, herbs are essentially crude drugs and should be treated with the same respect, with careful monitoring of side effects and the requirement of evidence of efficacy to justify the risk. Fish oil also has the potential for mercury contamination; none should be used that is not labeled as United States Pharmacopeia (USP) or "refined to eliminate mercury."

Even eliminating dietary components can be risky through unbalancing the diet. When undertaking a rigorous elimination regimen, it is important to have dietary consultation regarding balance and sufficiency of each nutrient. A precautionary multivitamin/mineral in the RDA/RDI amounts is probably advisable in these cases.

WITH THE EVIDENCE BASE SO MIXED AND UNCERTAIN, HOW CAN A CLINICIAN DECIDE WHETHER TO RECOMMEND A GIVEN INTERVENTION?

A basic common sense guideline is that an intervention that is safe, easy, cheap, and sensible in light of other knowledge (SECS) does not require as much evidence of efficacy to justify an individual patient trial as one that is risky, unrealistic, difficult, or expensive (RUDE).[24] For example, daily omega-3 EFA in moderate doses is reasonably safe (if refined to eliminate heavy metals); involves only swallowing 1 or 2 capsules a day with meals; costs less than most prescription copays; and is good for cardiovascular and other general health even if it does not help ADHD, thus fulfilling the SECS criteria. On the other hand, a RED is difficult, has the potential to unbalance nutritional intake and/or cause parent-child friction, and may require extra food expense; therefore, it requires more evidence of its efficacy and closer monitoring of the risk-benefit ratio. The dose may factor into the SECS-RUDE equation. A vitamin or mineral in RDA/RDI amounts, especially a balanced multi-ingredient formulation, seems to fulfill the SECS criteria, but megavitamin therapy in huge doses considerably greater than published upper tolerable limits, especially with a single vitamin or mineral, carries enough risk to require convincing evidence of efficacy.

OVERALL CLINICAL RECOMMENDATIONS

When considering nutritional/dietary treatments for treatment of ADHD, the following general clinical recommendations seem appropriate:

- Families should meet with a physician or certified nurse practitioner, and preferably also a dietician, to discuss options for nutritional treatment.
  - Before starting treatment, a comprehensive physical evaluation should be performed and a history of the child's current diet should be documented.
  - Based on the results of the dietary history, children may benefit from RDI/RDA dietary supplementation if they are not currently eating a varied diet and/or if they are experiencing appetite suppression from stimulant medication.

- Documented specific nutritional deficiencies or insufficiencies (eg, zinc, iron, magnesium, vitamin D) should be treated with specific therapeutic supplementation as standard treatment before other interventions are considered.
- Similarly, if the child has documented food allergies or sensitivities, those foods or food components should be eliminated from the diet, and the child's symptoms then reevaluated before other interventions are considered.
- Regardless of the type of intervention, the dietary/nutritional intervention should be monitored closely by a practitioner with experience working with children with ADHD. Treatment efficacy should be monitored with standardized rating scales. Adverse events should also be monitored closely, particularly because of the lack of safety data regarding the use of many complementary and alternative treatments. Common side effects of supplements (eg, constipation with iron) should be explained, as with a drug. Herbs, when used, require special attention to safety.
- The SECS versus RUDE guideline should be applied,[24] considering safety, ease/difficulty, expense, and how sensible the intervention is for the patient's situation in light of available efficacy evidence.
- One risk of dietary intervention that is often overlooked is the risk of delaying other treatment with a better evidence base. Determining whether a dietary treatment is effective may take up to a few months; therefore, parents should consider, with professional consultation, whether their child first needs a trial of a standard treatment (eg, if the child is having significant problems at school), which may produce a faster response.
  - The lack of an immediate response to a dietary treatment does not necessarily mean the treatment will not be effective with a reasonable trial. Reasonable trial lengths will vary per individual treatment (eg, a few weeks for dietary elimination, 3 months for essential fatty acid supplementation). Parents are encouraged to keep in mind that no dietary intervention works as quickly as stimulant medication, and therefore patience is needed.
- Another factor to consider when using dietary/nutritional interventions is the time, effort, and other resources (eg, money) they may require. Parents should consider whether they have the time to administer the treatment as prescribed; this is particularly important when planning elimination diets, which require considerable time, effort, and organization.
- Parents (and practitioners) may be tempted to initiate more than one treatment at a time to increase the likelihood that something will be effective; however, the use of multiple treatments simultaneously may actually be less effective than the well-monitored use of one treatment. One treatment may interfere with the potential benefits of another treatment, and parents may not be able to carefully administer more than one treatment, which may result in a less-than-adequate trial of each. Therefore, except for RDA/RDI multivitamins/minerals, which are compatible with all the others, the authors recommend that one treatment be initiated at a time, and the child's response systematically monitored before adding an additional treatment.

REFERENCES

1. Feingold BF. Hyperkinesis and learning disabilities linked to artificial food flavors and colors. Am J Nurs 1975;75:797–803.
2. Toren P, Elder S, Sela B, et al. Zinc deficiency in attention-deficit hyperactivity disorder. Biol Psychiatry 1996;40(12):1308–10.

3. McGee R, Williams S, Anderson J, et al. Hyperactivity and serum and hair zinc levels in 11-year-old children from the general population. Biol Psychiatry 1990; 28(2):165–8.
4. Arnold LE, Lofhouse NL, Hurt EA. Artificial food colors and attention-deficit/ hyperactivity symptoms: conclusions to dye for. Neurotherapeutics 2012;9:599–609.
5. Rucklidge JL, Frampton CM, Gorman B, et al. Vitamin-mineral treatment of attention-deficit hyperactivity disorder in adults: double-blind randomized placebo-controlled trial. Br J Psychiatry 2014. http://dx.doi.org/10.1192/bjp.bp.113.132126.
6. Benton D, Roberts G. Effects of vitamin and mineral supplementation on intelligence of a sample of schoolchildren. Lancet 1998;1(8578):140–3.
7. Benton D, Cook R. Vitamin and mineral supplements to improve the intelligence scores and concentration of six-year-old children. Pers Individ Dif 1991;12(11): 1151–8.
8. Benton D, Buts JP. Vitamin/mineral supplementation and intelligence. Lancet 1990;335(8698):1158–60.
9. Voight RG, Liarente AM, Jenden CL, et al. A randomized double-blind placebo-controlled trial of docosahexaenoic acid supplementation in children with attention-deficit/hyperactivity disorder. J Pediatr 2001;139(2):189–96.
10. Behdani F, Hebrani P, Naseraee A, et al. Does omega-3 supplement enhance the therapeutic results of methylphenidate in attention deficit hyperactivity disorder patients? J Res Med Sci 2013;18(8):653–8.
11. Barragan E, Breuer D, Dopfner M. Efficacy and safety of omega-3/6 fatty acids, methylphenidate, and a combined treatment in children with ADHD. J Atten Disord 2014. http://dx.doi.org/10.1177/1087054713518239.
12. Perera H, Jeewandara KC, Seneviratne S, et al. Combined omega-3 and omega-6 supplementation in children with attention-deficit hyperactivity disorder (ADHD) refractory to methylphenidate treatment: a double-blind, placebo controlled study. J Child Neurol 2012;27(6):747–53.
13. Akhondzadeh S, Mohammadi MR, Khademi M. Zinc sulfate as an adjunct to methylphenidate for the treatment of attention deficit hyperactivity disorder in children: a double blind and randomized trial. BMC Psychiatry 2004;4:9.
14. Arnold LE, DiSilvestro RA, Bozzolo D, et al. Zinc for attention-deficit/hyperactivity disorder: placebo-controlled double-blind pilot trial along and combined with amphetamine. J Child Adolesc Psychopharmacol 2011;21(1):1–19.
15. Zamora J, Valasquez A, Trancoso L, et al. Zinc in the therapy of the attention-deficit/hyperactivity disorder in children: a preliminary randomized controlled trial. Arch Latinoam Nutr 2011;61(3):242–6.
16. Ding GA, Yo GH, Chen SF. Assessment of effect of treatment for childhood hyperkinetic syndrome by combined therapy of yizhi mixture and Ritalin. Zhongguo Zhong Xi Yi Jie He Za Zhi 2002;22(4):255–7 [in Chinese].
17. Wang MJ, Wei H, Zhang Y, et al. Clinical observation of Jingling oral liquid combined with methylphenidate in the treatment of ADHD with transient Tic disorder. Chinese Traditional Patent Medicine 2011;33(9):1638–9 [in Chinese].
18. Trebaticka J, Kopasova S, Hiradecna Z, et al. Treatment of ADHD with French maritime pine bark extract, Pycnogenol. Eur Child Adolesc Psychiatry 2006;15(6):329–35.
19. Weber W, Vander Stoep A, McCarty RL, et al. Hypericum perforatum (St. John's wort) for attention-deficit/hyperactivity disorder in children and adolescents: a randomized controlled trial. JAMA 2008;299(2):2633–41.
20. Salehi B, Imani R, Mohammadi MR, et al. Gingko biloba for attention-deficit/ hyperactivity disorder in children and adolescents: a double-blind, randomized controlled trial. Prog Neuropsychopharmacol Biol Psychiatry 2010;34(1):76080.

21. Li X, Chen Z. Clinical comparative observation on duodongning and Ritalin in treating child hyperkinetic syndrome. Zhongguo Zhong Xi Yi Jie He Za Zhi 1999;19(7): 410–1 [in Chinese].

22. Li JJ, Li ZW, Wang SZ, et al. Ningdong granule: a complementary and alternative therapy in the treatment of attention-deficit/hyperactivity disorder. Psychopharmacology 2011;216(4):501–9.

23. Pelsser LM, van Steijn DJ, Frankena K, et al. A randomized controlled pilot study into the effects of a restricted elimination diet on family structure in families with ADHD and ODD. Child Adol Mental Hlth 2013;18(1):39–45.

24. Arnold LE, Hurt EA, Mayes T, et al. Ingestible alternative and complementary treatments for attention-deficit/hyperactivity disorder. In: Hoza B, Evans SW, editors. Treating attention deficit hyperactivity disorder: assessment and intervention in developmental context. Kingston (NJ): Civic Research Institute; 2011. p. 15-1–15-24.

Towards an Evidence-based Taxonomy of Nonpharmacologic Treatments for ADHD

(R) CrossMark

Stephen V. Faraone, PhD[a,b],*, Kevin M. Antshel, PhD[c]

KEYWORDS

- ADHD • Children • Treatment • Medications • Psychosocial • Therapy
- Alternative treatments

KEY POINTS

- Some parents seek nonpharmacologic treatments for their children with attention-deficit/hyperactivity disorder (ADHD).
- Research about nonpharmacologic treatments has grown rapidly in recent years.
- An evidence-based approach can help clinicians explain to parents the relative utility of ADHD treatments.

Attention-deficit/hyperactivity disorder (ADHD) is perhaps the most well-known of all psychiatric disorders. In part, this is because of its high prevalence[1] and the multiple impairments[2] that affect children and adolescents, concern parents, and in most

All authors of this article have seen and approved the submission of this version of the article and take full responsibility for the article.

In the past year, Dr S.V. Faraone received consulting income, travel expenses, and/or research support from Ironshore, Shire, Akili Interactive Labs, Alcobra, VAYA, and Neurovance; and research support from the National Institutes of Health (NIH). His institution is seeking a patent for the use of sodium-hydrogen exchange inhibitors in the treatment of ADHD. In previous years, he received consulting fees or was on advisory boards or participated in continuing medical education programs sponsored by: Shire, Alcobra, Otsuka, McNeil, Janssen, Novartis, Pfizer, and Eli Lilly. Dr S.V. Faraone receives royalties from books published by Guilford Press (*Straight Talk about Your Child's Mental Health*) and Oxford University Press (*Schizophrenia: The Facts*). Dr K.M. Antshel has no conflicts of interests or financial relationships to disclose.

[a] Department of Psychiatry, SUNY Upstate Medical University, 750 East Adams Street, Syracuse, NY 13210, USA; [b] Department of Neuroscience and Physiology, SUNY Upstate Medical University, 750 East Adams Street, Syracuse, NY 13210, USA; [c] Department of Psychology, 802 University Avenue, Syracuse, NY 13244, USA

* Corresponding author. SUNY Upstate Medical University, 750 East Adams Street, Syracuse, NY 13210.

E-mail address: sfaraone@childpsychresearch.org

Child Adolesc Psychiatric Clin N Am 23 (2014) 965–972
http://dx.doi.org/10.1016/j.chc.2014.06.003
1056-4993/14/$ – see front matter © 2014 Elsevier Inc. All rights reserved.

childpsych.theclinics.com

Abbreviations	
ADHD	Attention-deficit/hyperactivity disorder
OCEBM	Oxford Center for Evidence-Based Medicine

cases lead to a difficult transition into adulthood.[3] ADHD has gained the attention of the public and is a popular topic in print, on television, and on the Internet. A search for ADHD on YouTube (4/7/2014) found 480,000 videos. ADHD is very much in the public eye. We are in favor of increased access to information about ADHD, especially when provided by reputable organizations such as family support groups (www. chadd.org), the National Institutes of Mental Health (www.nimh.nih.gov), or the American Professional Society of ADHD and Related Disorders (www.apsard.org; www. adhdinadults.com). However, an unfortunate side effect of media and Internet attention to ADHD is that much of the available information is wrong or misleading. Our search for alternative ADHD treatment on www.google.com produces 83,100 results (4/7/14). How can clinicians and parents decide which of these links provides valid information?

To help answer that question, we have created an evidence-based guide for the clinicians who must explain to parents the pros and cons of treatment choices. Many parents have been convinced by the media, the Internet, or friends that medications for ADHD are dangerous and that nonmedication alternatives exist that are as good or better. The clamor for nonmedical treatments has likely increased in the wake of media reports that doctors overprescribe ADHD medications or that ADHD medications have serious side effects. Such reports typically simplify and/or exaggerate results from the scientific literature. The result is that many parents bring children to treatment in search of nonmedical treatments or favoring a specific nonmedical treatment that they heard about through the Internet. This situation increases the burden on clinicians to know which nonmedical treatments work and which do not. To restate this from an evidence-based perspective, they need to know the level of evidence that supports the use of a nonmedical treatment of ADHD. This article uses the term evidence-based in the strict sense applied by the Oxford Center for Evidence-Based Medicine (OCEBM; http://www.cebm.net/). The OCEBM guidelines are applied here and in the companion articles to help readers understand the degree to which nonpharmacologic treatments are supported by the scientific literature. This overview and the companion articles provide clinicians with the tools they need to advise parents and to implement nonmedical treatments that will help their patients.

LEVEL OF EVIDENCE AND MAGNITUDE OF TREATMENT EFFICACY

Figs. 1 and 2 summarize the relative efficacy of treatments based on meta-analyses in the literature[4,5] and information provided in this issue. Fig. 1 provides the OCEBM level of evidence for each treatment. The levels have been scaled so that larger numbers indicate a higher level of evidence. The levels are defined as follows:

1. Mechanism-based reasoning
2. Case series, case-control studies, or historically controlled studies
3. Non–randomized controlled studies
4. Single randomized trial or observational study with clear effect
5. Systematic review of randomized trials

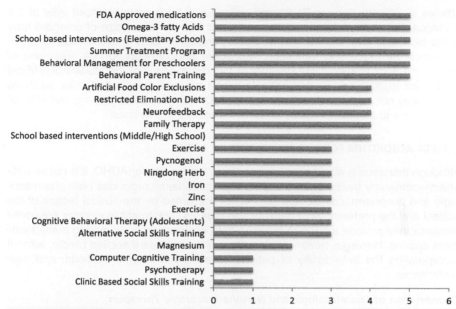

Fig. 1. OCEBM evidence strength for ADHD treatments.

Fig. 1 summarizes the quality of the evidence, and **Fig. 2** gives the magnitude of the treatment effect expressed as the standardized mean difference effect size (also known as the Cohen D). **Fig. 2** uses the results from blinded studies and relies on Faraone and colleagues[6,7] (updated with newer data) for medication effects, and the companion articles in this issue and Sonuga-Barke and colleagues[4] for nonpharmacologic treatments. **Fig. 2** shows that stimulant medications are more effective than nonstimulant medications and that both types of medication are more effective than nonpharmacologic treatments. These figures are presented as a broad overview that must be considered in light of several limitations. Of most importance, they refer to the evidence for the ability of treatments to change ADHD symptoms. They do not refer to the ability of treatments to create clinically significant changes in functioning. For example, much evidence supports the ability of behavioral parent training to change child behaviors for the better, even though the effect on ADHD symptoms is small. These figures present mean values across many studies and thus provide only a rough guide to the literature. We encourage readers to consult the companion

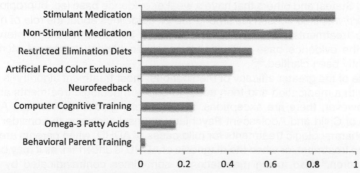

Fig. 2. ADHD treatment effect sizes.

articles along with Sonuga-Barke and colleagues[4] for a more nuanced view of the evidence. For example, the evidence suggests that the effect size of omega-3 fatty acids increases with the fraction of eicosapentaenoic acid in the formulation. See the article by Bloch and Mulqueen: Nutritional Supplements for the Treatment of Attention-Deficit Hyperactivity Disorder in this issue. Many of the studies of artificial food color exclusions selected patients based on food color sensitivities, so these results may not apply to all patients with ADHD. See the article by Nigg and Holton: Restriction and Elimination Diets in ADHD Treatment in this issue.

A META-ALGORITHM FOR THE TREATMENT OF ADHD

Although this issue is about nonpharmacologic treatments for ADHD, it is not an anti-pharmacotherapy treatise. Any competent practitioner incorporates both pharmacologic and nonpharmacologic approaches as warranted by the clinical picture of the patient and the preferences of patients and parents. Treatment algorithms are useful because they provide a concise guide to help clinicians choose among many treatment options. However, treatment algorithms are worthless if applied blindly, without incorporating the individuality of patients, their environmental contexts, and their preferences.

Coordination of Pharmacologic and Nonpharmacologic Therapies

How should pharmacologic and nonpharmacologic therapies be coordinated when treating children and adolescents with ADHD? The answer to this question usually depends on the training of the practitioner. A child with ADHD referred to a physician is likely to be prescribed an ADHD medication. The same child referred to a psychologist is likely to be seen as a candidate for behavior therapy. The same child seen by a nutritionist may only get nutritional therapy. However, it is a mistake for physicians to only consider medications and for nonphysician mental health practitioners to only consider nonpharmacologic treatments. Both treatments play key roles in treating youth with ADHD. Our view is consistent with Seixas and colleagues[8] summary of treatment guidelines: start with the most efficacious treatment acceptable to the family and add additional treatments as needed to attain an optimal level of outcome.

Medication Selection

Regarding which medications to use, Seixas and colleagues[8] reviewed 26 treatment guidelines for ADHD from around the world. All guidelines recommended stimulants as the first-line treatment, followed by nonstimulants approved by regulatory authorities (eg, atomoxetine and extended-release versions of guanfacine and clonidine in the United States) and others that have a weaker evidence base (eg, bupropion, modafinil). There was little consensus among the 26 guidelines about the role of nonpharmacologic treatments, although most recognized the need for these interventions because the evidence base for nonpharmacologic blinded treatment studies has only recently been clarified.[4,5]

Because of the greater efficacy of medications, most treatment algorithms suggest starting with a medication and then adding nonpharmacologic treatments as appropriate. However, there are exceptions. For example, guidelines from the American Academy of Child and Adolescent Psychiatry counsel clinicians to consider starting with nonpharmacologic treatments for mild cases of ADHD, when parents are against medication treatment, or when the diagnosis of ADHD is uncertain, as it may be in very young children.[9] Also, using medication is sometimes contraindicated by medical issues such as preexisting cardiac problems. Although a history of adverse reactions to medications also contraindicates their use, treatment guidelines for ADHD have otherwise used efficacy, not adverse reactions, to choose among available treatments. The reason for this choice is that, for all treatments, all but the very rare adverse reactions are typically not serious and can be alleviated by changing the dose or type of treatment. Nonpharmacologic treatments can also have adverse reactions, especially herbs or poorly formulated supplements. This topic is discussed by Hurt and Arnold elsewhere in this issue, along with a warning that delaying the use of an efficacious treatment (eg, medication) for a less efficacious treatment exposes many patients to the adverse effects of their ADHD symptoms, which are considerable.[10–12]

Broad-band Versus Narrow-band Treatments

Given these considerations, if there are no contraindications to medication, treatment of the typical school-aged child or adolescent with ADHD ought to start with a medication regimen and then incorporate nonpharmacologic treatments for specific purposes, which can be roughly classified into broad-band and narrow-band categories. When medications cannot achieve full remission of ADHD symptoms, nonpharmacologic treatments could be used in the broad-band sense as an adjunct treatment with the goal of reducing as many ADHD symptoms and functional impairments as possible. Examples of broad-band treatments for ADHD are traditional Chinese medicine (TCM; see the article Traditional Chinese Medicine in the Treatment of ADHD by Ni and colleagues in this issue), omega-3 fatty acids (see the article Omega-3 and other Supplements by Bloch in this issue), and diet (see the article Restriction and Food Color Exclusion Diets for ADHD by Nigg in this issue). These treatments do not focus on a set of specific symptoms, behaviors, or impairments. Instead, like pharmacologic treatments, they seek overall reductions in ADHD symptoms and, by doing so, also aim to reduce ADHD-associated impairments. In contrast, narrow-band nonpharmacologic treatments focus on a subset of symptoms, behaviors, or impairments. By strengthening skills, increasing adaptive behaviors, and/or decreasing maladaptive behaviors, these narrow-band treatments directly target the behavioral effects of ADHD. Examples include social skills training (see the article Social Skills Training by Mikami in this issue), cognitive behavioral therapy (see the article CBT in Adolescents by Antshel in this issue), and school-based interventions (see the article School-based Interventions for Elementary School by DuPaul in this issue). Even if these treatments have low effect sizes for the treatment of ADHD symptoms (see **Fig. 2**), they may improve specific behaviors or life skills required for the child to improve family, school, or social functioning.

A Schematic for the Treatment of ADHD

This article provides a schematic of this treatment approach in **Fig. 3**. For a similar schematic giving more details about medication management, see Warikoo and Faraone.[13] For details about how to coordinate dietary and nutritional treatments with other treatments see Hurt and Arnold elsewhere in this issue. The treatment of ADHD starts with education as recommended by the American Academy of Child and Adolescent Psychiatry.[9] The logic is clear: patients and parents cannot make treatment decisions without information about the comparative effectiveness, costs, and side effects of the treatment options. If medications are contraindicated because of medical issues or family preferences, then it makes sense to start with one or more broad-band nonpharmacologic trials. Otherwise, one or more medication trials are indicated following standard guidelines.[9,13] This article uses the word trials to emphasize that more than one treatment may need to be tried before achieving an optimal response.

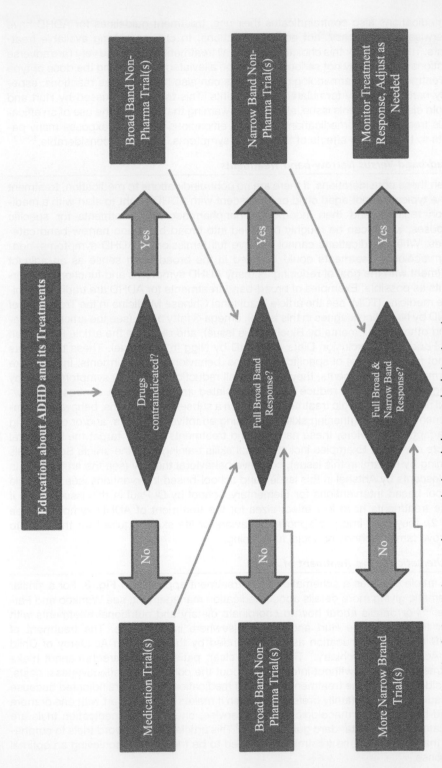

Fig. 3. Meta-algorithm for integrating nonpharmacologic and pharmacologic treatments.

Whether the first broad-band treatment is pharmacologic or not, one or more trials of different methods may be needed to obtain a full broad-band response. This article defines the broad-band response as the degree of overall reduction in ADHD symptoms and ADHD-associated impairments. To be considered successful, this treatment should reduce ADHD symptoms to a subdiagnostic level. All impairing symptoms should ideally be eliminated.[14] After the fullest broad-band response has been achieved, the clinician should consider narrow-band nonpharmacologic treatments. At this stage, one or more narrow-band nonpharmacologic treatments could be used to address any residual problems not adequately addressed by the broad-band treatment(s).

Our algorithm provides a framework for thinking about how to integrate pharmacologic and nonpharmacologic treatments. It cannot replace clinical training, clinical experience, or factors deriving from the unique situation of patients and their families. It is also not possible to address all permutations of treatment. For example, a natural question is whether and how a pharmacologic treatment could be combined with broad-band treatments such as omega-3 supplementation or TCM. In some cases (eg, omega-3) little is known about combined therapies; in others (eg, TCM) an evidence base is available. The companion articles provide some guidance on these issues, but algorithmic statements require a larger evidence base.

SUMMARY

In summary, the past decade has seen many advances in nonpharmacologic treatments for ADHD. There are new approaches such as working memory and neurofeedback training and more research on older treatments (eg, diet, TCM, behavior therapy) that allows a more systematic evaluation of their efficacy. Perhaps, more importantly, nonpharmacologic interventions have embraced an evidence-based approach that motivates quality research and makes it easier for clinicians to make recommendations to their patients. With this in mind, clinicians can help patients achieve the optimal outcomes that Rostain and colleagues[14] and others target as the ultimate goal of a comprehensive ADHD treatment regimen.

REFERENCES

1. Faraone SV, Sergeant J, Gillberg C, et al. The worldwide prevalence of ADHD: is it an American condition? World Psychiatry 2003;2(2):104–13.
2. Gordon M, Antshel K, Faraone S, et al. Symptoms versus impairment: the case for respecting DSM-IV's criterion D. J Atten Disord 2006;9(3):465–75.
3. Biederman J, Petty CR, Woodworth KY, et al. Adult outcome of attention-deficit/ hyperactivity disorder: a controlled 16-year follow-up study. J Clin Psychiatry 2012;73(7):941–50.
4. Sonuga-Barke EJ, Brandeis D, Cortese S, et al. Nonpharmacological interventions for ADHD: systematic review and meta-analyses of randomized controlled trials of dietary and psychological treatments. Am J Psychiatry 2013;170(3): 275–89.
5. Bloch MH, Qawasmi A. Omega-3 fatty acid supplementation for the treatment of children with attention-deficit/hyperactivity disorder symptomatology: systematic review and meta-analysis. J Am Acad Child Adolesc Psychiatry 2011;50(10): 991–1000.
6. Faraone SV, Glatt SJ. A comparison of the efficacy of medications for adult attention-deficit/hyperactivity disorder using meta-analysis of effect sizes. J Clin Psychiatry 2010;71(6):754–63.

7. Faraone SV, Buitelaar J. Comparing the efficacy of stimulants for ADHD in children and adolescents using meta-analysis. Eur Child Adolesc Psychiatry 2010; 19(4):353–64.

8. Seixas M, Weiss M, Muller U. Systematic review of national and international guidelines on attention-deficit hyperactivity disorder. J Psychopharmacol 2012; 26(6):753–65.

9. Pliszka S. Practice parameter for the assessment and treatment of children and adolescents with attention-deficit/hyperactivity disorder. J Am Acad Child Adolesc Psychiatry 2007;46(7):894–921.

10. Biederman J, Monuteaux MC, Spencer T, et al. Do stimulants protect against psychiatric disorders in youth with ADHD? A 10-year follow-up study. Pediatrics 2009;124(1):71–8.

11. Hammerness P, Joshi G, Doyle R, et al. Do stimulants reduce the risk for cigarette smoking in youth with attention-deficit hyperactivity disorder? A prospective, long-term, open-label study of extended-release methylphenidate. J pediatr 2013;162(1):22–27, e2.

12. Spencer TJ, Brown A, Seidman LJ, et al. Effect of psychostimulants on brain structure and function in ADHD: a qualitative literature review of magnetic resonance imaging-based neuroimaging studies. J Clin Psychiatry 2013;74(9): 902–17.

13. Warikoo N, Faraone SV. Background, clinical features and treatment of attention deficit hyperactivity disorder in children. Expert opin pharmacother 2013;14(14): 1885–906.

14. Rostain A, Jensen PS, Connor DF, et al. Toward quality care in ADHD: defining the goals of treatment. J Atten Disord 2013. [Epub ahead of print].

Index

Note: Page numbers of article titles are in **boldface** type.

Child Adolesc Psychiatric Clin N Am 23 (2014) 973–981
http://dx.doi.org/10.1016/S1056-4993(14)00070-4
1056-4993/14/$ – see front matter © 2014 Elsevier Inc. All rights reserved.
childpsych.theclinics.com

United States Postal Service

Statement of Ownership, Management, and Circulation
(All Periodicals Publications Except Requestor Publications)

1. Publication Title	2. Publication Number	3. Filing Date
Child and Adolescent Psychiatric Clinics of North America	0 1 1 - 3 6 8	9/14/14

4. Issue Frequency	5. Number of Issues Published Annually	6. Annual Subscription Price
Jan, Apr, Jul, Oct	4	$310.00

7. Complete Mailing Address of Known Office of Publication (Not printer) (Street, city, county, state, and ZIP+4®)

Elsevier Inc.
360 Park Avenue South
New York, NY 10010-1710

Contact Person
Stephen R. Bushing
Telephone (Include area code)
215-239-3688

8. Complete Mailing Address of Headquarters or General Business Office of Publisher (Not printer)

Elsevier Inc., 360 Park Avenue South, New York, NY 12010-1710

9. Full Names and Complete Mailing Addresses of Publisher, Editor, and Managing Editor (Do not leave blank)

Linda Belfus, Elsevier Inc., 1600 John F. Kennedy Blvd., Su te 1800, Philadelphia, PA 19103-2899
Publisher (Name and complete mailing address)

Joanne Husovski, Elsevier Inc., 1600 John F. Kennedy Blvd. Suite 1800, Philadelphia, PA 19103-2839
Editor (Name and complete mailing address)

Adrianne Brigido, Elsevier Inc., 1600 John F. Kennedy Blvd., Suite 1800, Philadelphia, PA 19103-2899
Managing Editor (Name and complete mailing address)

10. Owner (Do not leave blank. If the publication is owned by a corporation, give the name and address of the corporation immediately followed by the names and addresses of all stockholders owning or holding 1 percent or more of the total amount of stock. If not owned by a corporation, give the names and addresses of the individual owners. If owned by a partnership or other unincorporated firm, give its name and address as well as those of each individual owner. If the publication is published by a nonprofit organization, give its name and address.)

Full Name	Complete Mailing Address
Wholly owned subsidiary of	1600 John F. Kennedy Blvd, Ste. 1800
Reed/Elsevier, US holdings	Philadelphia, PA 19103-2899

11. Known Bondholders, Mortgagees, and Other Security Holders Owning or Holding 1 Percent or More of Total Amount of Bonds, Mortgages, or Other Securities. If none, check box. ☐ None

Full Name	Complete Mailing Address
N/A	

12. Tax Status (For completion by nonprofit organizations authorized to mail at nonprofit rates) (Check one)
The purpose, function, and nonprofit status of this organization and the exempt status for federal income tax purposes:
☐ Has Not Changed During Preceding 12 Months
☐ Has Changed During Preceding 12 Months (Publisher must submit explanation of change with this statement)

PS Form 3526, August 2012 (Page 1 of 3 (Instructions Page 3)) PSN 7530-01-000-9931 PRIVACY NOTICE: See our Privacy policy in www.usps.com

---

13. Publication Title	14. Issue Date for Circulation Data Below
Child and Adolescent Psychiatric Clinics of North America	July 2014

15. Extent and Nature of Circulation		Average No. Copies Each Issue During Preceding 12 Months	No. Copies of Single Issue Published Nearest to Filing Date
a. Total Number of Copies (Net press run)		519	514
b. Paid Circulation (By Mail and Outside the Mail)	(1) Mailed Outside-County Paid Subscriptions Stated on PS Form 3541. (Include paid distribution above nominal rate, advertiser's proof copies, and exchange copies)	305	290
	(2) Mailed In-County Paid Subscriptions Stated on PS Form 3541 (Include paid distribution above nominal rate, advertiser's proof copies, and exchange copies)		
	(3) Paid Distribution Outside the Mails Including Sales Through Dealers and Carriers, Street Vendors, Counter Sales, and Other Paid Distribution Outside USPS®	55	61
	(4) Paid Distribution by Other Classes Mailed Through the USPS (e.g. First-Class Mail®)		
c. Total Paid Distribution (Sum of 15b (1), (2), (3), and (4))		360	351
d. Free or Nominal Rate Distribution (By Mail and Outside the Mail)	(1) Free or Nominal Rate Outside-County Copies Included on PS Form 3541	69	78
	(2) Free or Nominal Rate In-County Copies Included on PS Form 3541		
	(3) Free or Nominal Rate Copies Mailed at Other Classes Through the USPS (e.g. First-Class Mail)		
	(4) Free or Nominal Rate Distribution Outside the Mail (Carriers or other means)		
e. Total Free or Nominal Rate Distribution (Sum of 15d (1), (2), (3) and (4))		69	78
f. Total Distribution (Sum of 15c and 15e		429	429
g. Copies not Distributed (See instructions to publishers #4 (page #3))		90	85
h. Total (Sum of 15f and g)		519	514
i. Percent Paid (15c divided by 15f times 100)		83.92%	81.82%

16. Total circulation includes electronic copies. Report circulation on PS Form 3526-X worksheet.

17. Publication of Statement of Ownership
If the publication is a general publication, publication of this statement is required. Will be printed in the October 2014 issue of this publication.

18. Signature and Title of Editor, Publisher, Business Manager, or Owner

Stephen R. Bushing

Stephen R. Bushing – Inventory Distribution Coordinator

Date
September 14, 2014

I certify that all information furnished on this form is true and complete. I understand that anyone who furnishes false or misleading information on this form or who omits material or information requested on the form may be subject to criminal sanctions (including fines and imprisonment) and/or civil sanctions (including civil penalties).

PS Form 3526, August 2012 (Page 2 of 3)

Printed and bound by CPI Group (UK) Ltd, Croydon, CR0 4YY

03/10/2024

01040495-0009